Best of Five MCQs for the Gastroenterology SCE

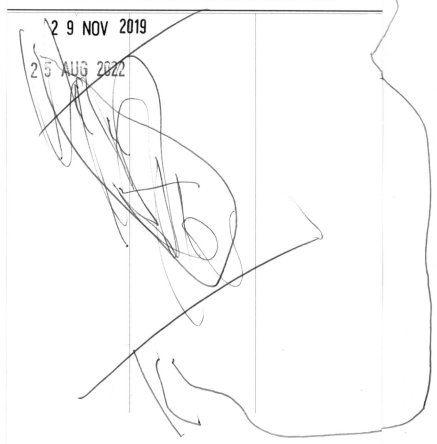

Best of Five MCQs for the Gastroenterology SCE

Edited by

Dr Charlotte Rutter
Gastroenterology Specialty Registrar, Gloucester Royal Hospital, Gloucester, UK

Dr Leonard Griffiths
Gastroenterology Specialty Registrar and Clinical Research Fellow, Department of Biology and Biochemistry, University of Bath, Bath, UK

Dr Tina Mehta
Consultant Gastroenterologist, Royal United Hospital, Bath, UK

Professor Chris Probert
Professor of Gastroenterology, Institute of Translational Medicine, University of Liverpool, Liverpool, UK

OXFORD
UNIVERSITY PRESS

Great Clarendon Street, Oxford OX2 6DP
United Kingdom

Oxford University Press is a department of the University of Oxford.
It furthers the University's objective of excellence in research, scholarship,
and education by publishing worldwide. Oxford is a registered trade mark of
Oxford University Press in the UK and in certain other countries

© Oxford University Press, 2013

The moral rights of the author have been asserted

First Edition published in 2013
Reprinted 2014

Published in the United States of America by Oxford University Press
198 Madison Avenue, New York, NY 10016, United States of America

British Library Cataloguing in Publication Data
Data available

Library of Congress Cataloging in Publication Data
Data available

ISBN 978-0-19-965302-7

FOREWORD

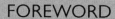

The Specialist Certificate Exam is a relatively new (and final) hurdle for the aspiring Gastroenterologist to jump. The 'best of five' format is particularly challenging and requires a synthesis of knowledge, experience, data analysis, and clinical problem solving. Practice at this is essential to avoid disappointment and the expense of retakes. Nothing concentrates the mind more than the prospect of sitting an exam in the morning and thus who better to ask to write the questions than Specialty Registrars, hopefully at the top of their form and brim full of knowledge in preparation for their own attempts. This book I believe is a unique achievement.

It also represents a long project full of experience in communication, cooperation, cajoling and time-management for the editors and contributors who are all Trainees in the Severn and South West Peninsula Deaneries. As the Head of School (Medicine) for Severn I am proud to have been asked to write this foreword and grateful to my consultant colleagues who supported this venture. Reading this book and answering the practice questions will provide invaluable experience for the entrant. The supplementary information provided with the answers will be very instructional, but needs to be supported by up to date information in the form of Specialist Guidelines, NICE etc. Simply ploughing through these is often unrewarding because it is unfocussed. Attempting some of these questions first helps identify what you don't know and provides the impetus to go to the guidelines and books in earnest. Then do some more questions to reinforce what you have learnt and hopefully enjoy the reward of an improved performance!

Enjoy this book, tell your friends (but make them buy their own copy).

Stirling Pugh
PhD MSc (Med Ed) FRCP FHEA
Head of School (Medicine) Severn Deanery
Associate Postgraduate Dean

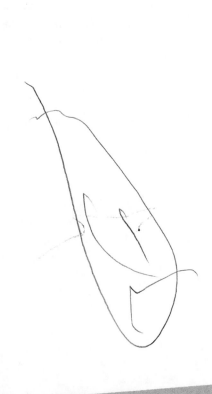

PREFACE

Introduced in 2008, the Gastroenterology SCE (Speciality Certificate Examination) is compulsory for trainees to gain a CCT (Certificate of Completion of Training) in this specialty. Candidates who have sat their written MRCP are familiar with the 'best of 5' format, where they select the best of five plausible comparable answers. This requires both knowledge and exam technique, which is often best achieved through practice questions.

Currently exam preparation is hampered by the lack of available reliable practice questions. This textbook seeks to fill that void, consisting of 'best of 5 questions' that resemble the exam format, alongside explanatory answers. The question material was written with the 2010 syllabus in mind, and based on contemporary guidelines from the relevant bodies. These are cited for the reader along the way.

Our goal was to create a valuable tool for all trainees revising for the SCE exam, as well as reference material for other professionals working in the specialty of gastroenterology.

The questions were contributed by 13 Severn and South West Peninsula Deanery gastroenterology specialty trainees and the three of us; many of the authors have sat the SCE. Our authors were supported by consultants in the region and we offer our thanks to them all.

We would also like to extend a 'thank you' to our friends and families, who might otherwise have seen more of us during the writing and editing process, but despite this offered support and encouragement.

Finally a big thank you to Professor Chris Probert, without whose dedication and experience in editing, this book would not have been possible.

Charlotte Rutter,
Tina Mehta, *and*
Leonard Griffiths

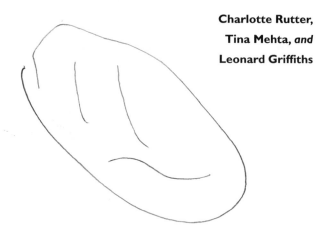

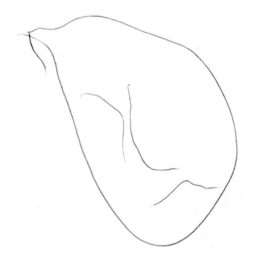

CONTENTS

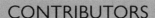

CONTRIBUTORS

Dr Iftikhar Ahmed   Gastroenterology Specialty Registrar, Musgrove Park Hospital, Taunton, UK
Chapter 3, Inflammatory Bowel Disease

Dr Elizabeth Arthurs   Clinical Research Fellow in Gastroenterology, Bristol Royal Infirmary, Bristol, UK
Chapter 4, Nutrition; Chapter 7, Endoscopy

Dr Sandip Bhatt   Gastroenterology Specialty Registrar, Yeovil District Hospital, Yeovil, UK
Chapter 1, Upper Gastrointestinal Tract Disorders

Dr Uthayanan Chelvaratnam   Gastroenterology Specialty Registrar, Bristol Royal Infirmary, Bristol, UK
Chapter 5, Hepatology

Dr Michael Fung   Gastroenterology Specialty Registrar, Royal Devon & Exeter Hospital, Exeter, UK
Chapter 2, Intestinal Disorders

Dr Leonard Griffiths   Gastroenterology Specialty Registrar and Clinical Research Fellow, Department of Biology and Biochemistry, University of Bath, Bath, UK
Chapter 3, Inflammatory Bowel Disease

Dr Simon Hazeldine   Gastroenterology Specialty Registrar, Bristol Royal Infirmary, Bristol, UK
Chapter 5, Hepatology; Chapter 7, Endoscopy

Dr Hiruni Jayasena   Gastroenterology Clinical Research Fellow, Clinical Research Unit – Gastroenterology, Bristol Royal Infirmary, Bristol, UK
Chapter 1, Upper Gastrointestinal Tract Disorders

Dr Tina Mehta   Consultant Gastroenterologist, Royal United Hospital Bath, Bath, UK
Chapter 3, Inflammatory Bowel Disease; Chapter 7, Endoscopy

Dr Joanna Rimmer   Gastroenterology Specialty Registrar, Derriford Hospital, Plymouth, UK
Chapter 2, Intestinal Disorders

Dr Charlotte Rutter   Gastroenterology Specialty Registrar, Gloucester Royal Hospital, Gloucester, UK
Chapter 3, Inflammatory Bowel Disease; Chapter 4, Nutrition

Dr Aye Aye Thi   LAS Gastroenterology Registrar, Diana, Princess of Wales Hospital, Grimsby, UK
Chapter 5, Hepatology

Dr Talal Valliani   Gastroenterology Specialty Registrar, Frenchay Hospital, Bristol, UK
Chapter 5, Hepatology

Dr Louisa Vine   Gastroenterology Specialty Registrar, Derriford Hospital, Plymouth, UK
Chapter 3, Inflammatory Bowel Disease; Chapter 4, Nutrition

Dr Gareth Walker LAT Gastroenterology Registrar, Cheltenham General Hospital, Cheltenham, UK
Chapter 5, Hepatology

Dr Kathy Woolson Gastroenterology Specialty Registrar, Royal Cornwall Hospital, Truro, UK
Chapter 6, Pancreatic and Biliary Disorders

CONSULTANT EDITORS

Dr John Anderson Consultant Gastroenterologist, Cheltenham General Hospital, Cheltenham, UK
Chapter 7, Endoscopy

Dr Peter Collins Consultant Hepatologist, Bristol Royal Infirmary, Bristol, UK
Chapter 5, Hepatology

Dr Paul Dunckley Consultant Gastroenterologist, Gloucester Royal Hospital, Gloucester, UK
Chapter 3, Inflammatory Bowel Disease

Dr Melanie Lockett Consultant Gastroenterologist, Frenchay Hospital, Bristol, UK
Chapter 4, Nutrition

Dr Richard Makins Consultant Gastroenterologist, Cheltenham General Hospital, Cheltenham, UK
Chapter 1, Upper Gastrointestinal Tract Disorders

Dr Julia Maltby Consultant Gastroenterologist, Royal United Hospital Bath, Bath, UK
Chapter 2, Intestinal Disorders

Dr Jim Portal Consultant Hepatologist, Bristol Royal Infirmary, Bristol, UK
Chapter 5, Hepatology

Dr Robert Przemioslo Consultant Gastroenterologist, Frenchay Hospital, Bristol, UK
Chapter 6, Pancreatic and Biliary Disorders

Dr Ian Shaw Consultant Gastroenterologist, Gloucester Royal Hospital, Gloucester, UK
Chapter 3, Inflammatory Bowel Disease

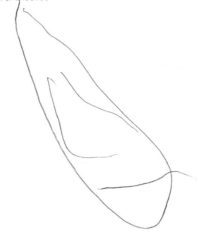

ABBREVIATIONS

5-ASA	5-aminosalicylic acid
AASLD	American Association for the Study of Liver Disease
ACE	angiotensin-converting enzyme
AH	alcoholic hepatitis
AICD	automated implantable cardioverter–defibrillator
AIP	autoimmune pancreatitis
AJCC	American Joint Committee on Cancer
ALD	alcohol related liver disease
ALF	acute liver failure
ALT	alanine aminotransferase
AN	anorexia nervosa
ANCA	anti-neutrophil cytoplasmic antibody
anti-HBs	antibody to hepatitis B surface antigen
anti-HBc IgG	IgG antibody to hepatitis B core antigen
anti-HBc IgM	IgM antibody to hepatitis B core antigen
anti-Hbe	antibody to hepatitis B extracellular antigen
anti-TNF	anti-tumour necrosis factor
anti-TTG	anti-tissue transglutaminase antibodies
APC	adenomatous polyposis coli
AST	aspartate aminotransferase
ATN	acute tubular necrosis
AZA	azathioprine
BAM	bile acid malabsorption
BAPEN	British Association for Parenteral and Enteral Nutrition
BCLC	Barcelona Clinic Liver Cancer
BD	'bis die'; twice daily
BER	base excision repair
BMI	body mass index
BRCA	breast cancer susceptibility gene
BSG	British Society of Gastroenterology
CAM	complementary and alternative medicines

CBD	common bile duct
CCK	cholecystokinin
CD	Crohn's disease
CDAI	Crohn's Disease Activity Index
CDI	*Clostridium difficile* infection
CEA	carcinoembryonic antigen
CHRPE	congenital hypertrophy of the retinal pigment epithelium
CJD	Creutzfeldt–Jakob disease
CLD	chronic liver disease
CMV	cytomegalovirus
COPD	chronic obstructive pulmonary disease
COX2	COX-2 selective inhibitor
CRC	colorectal cancer
CRP	C-reactive protein
CSF	cerebrospinal fluid
CT	computed tomography
CTP	Child–Turcotte–Pugh (score)
CTZ	chemoreceptor trigger zone
DEXA	dual-emission X-ray absorptiometry
D-IBS	diarrhoea-predominant irritable bowel syndrome
DILI	drug induced liver injury
DM	diabetes mellitus
DNA	deoxyribonucleic acid
DU	duodenal ulcer
EASL	European Association for the Study of the Liver
EBL	endoscopic band ligation
EBV	Epstein–Barr virus
ECAD	extracorporeal albumin dialysis
ECCO	European Crohn's and Colitis Organisation
EIA	enzyme immunoassay
EIM	extra intestinal manifestation
EMA	endomysial antibodies
EMR	endoscopic mucosal resection
EN	erythema nodosum
ERCP	endoscopic retrograde cholangiopancreatography
ESD	endoscopic submucosal dissection
ESPEN	European Society for Parenteral and Enteral Nutrition
ESR	erythrocyte sedimentation rate
EUA	examination under anaesthetic
EUS	endoscopic ultrasound

EVR	early virological response
FAP	familial adenomatous polyposis
FBC	full blood count
FFP	fresh frozen plasma
FNA	fine needle aspiration
FOB	faecal occult blood
g	gram
GAVE	gastric antral vascular ectasia
GCS	Glasgow Coma Scale
GDH	glutamate dehydrogenase antigen
GFR	glomerular filtration rate
gGT	gamma glutamyl transferase
GI	gastrointestinal
GIP	glucose-dependent insulinotropic polypeptide or gastric inhibitory polypeptide
GORD	gastro-oesophageal reflux disease
GOV	gastro-oesophageal varices
GP	general practitioner
GRS	Global Rating Scale
GU	gastric ulcer
HAS	human albumin solution
Hb	haemoglobin
HBsAg	hepatitis B surface antigen
HBcAg	hepatitis B core antigen
HBeAg	hepatitis B extracellular antigen
HBV	hepatitis B virus
HCC	hepatocellular carcinoma
HCV	hepatitis C virus
HE	hepatic encephalopathy
HELLP	haemolysis, elevated liver enzymes, and low platelets (syndrome)
HIV	human immunodeficiency virus
HNPCC	hereditary non-polyposis colorectal cancer
HPV	human papillomavirus
HRS	hepatorenal syndrome
HSV	herpes simplex virus
HVPG	hepatic venous pressure gradient
IBD	inflammatory bowel disease
IBS	irritable bowel syndrome
IBS-C	constipation-predominant irritable bowel syndrome
IBS-D	diarrhoea-predominant irritable bowel syndrome
ICP	intrahepatic cholestasis of pregnancy

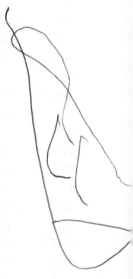

IDA	iron deficiency anaemia
IF	intrinsic factor
IGV	isolated gastric varices
IMA	inferior mesenteric artery
IMCA	Independent Mental Capacity Advocate
IPMN	intraductal papillary mucinous neoplasm
ISMN	isosorbide mononitrate
IV	intravenous
JAG	Joint Advisory Group on GI Endoscopy
JCV	John Cunningham virus; JC polyomavirus
JPS	juvenile polyposis syndrome
KUB	kidneys, ureter, and bladder (X-ray or CT scan)
LDH	lactate dehydrogenase
LFT	liver function test
LGV	Chlamydia lymphogranuloma venereum
LKB1	liver kinase B1
MAP	MUTYH-associated polyposis
μg	micrograms
MCN	mucinous cystic neoplasm
MCP	mercaptopurine
MCV	mean corpuscular volume
MDF	Maddrey's discriminant function
MDT	multidisciplinary team
MELD	Model for End-Stage Liver Disease
mg	milligrams
MMR gene	mismatch repair gene
MRCP	magnetic resonance cholangiopancreatography
MRI	magnetic resonance imaging
MSH	DNA MMR gene for HNPCC
MSI	microsatellite instability
MYH	MutY human homologue gene
NAAT	nucleic acid amplification tests
NACC	National Association for Colitis and Crohn's disease
NAFLD	non-alcoholic fatty liver disease
NAPQI	para amino benzoquinoneimine
NASH	non-alcoholic steatohepatitis
Nd-YAG	neodymium-doped yttrium aluminium garnet; Nd:Y3Al5O12
NG	nasogastric
NHS	National Health Service
NICE	National Institute for Health and Clinical Excellence

NJ	nasojejunal
NNH	number needed to harm
NNT	number needed to treat
NPV	negative predictive value
NSAID	non-steroidal anti-inflammatory drug
NSBB	non-selective beta blocker
OGD	oesophagogastroduodenoscopy
OGTT	oral glucose tolerance test
PBC	primary biliary cirrhosis
PCR	polymerase chain reaction
PDT	photodynamic therapy
PEG	percutaneous endoscopic gastrostomy
PG	pyoderma gangrenosum
PHG	portal hypertensive gastropathy
PJS	Peutz–Jegher's syndrome
PML	progressive multifocal leukoencephalopathy
PMN	polymorphonuclear leucocytes
PN	parenteral nutrition
PO	'per os'; by mouth
PONV	post-operative nausea and vomiting
PP	pancreatic polypeptide family
PPI	proton pump inhibitor
PPV	positive predictive value
PSC	primary sclerosing cholangitis
QDS	'quater die sumendus'; four times a day
RAA	renin–angiotensin–aldosterone (system)
RBC	red blood cell
RCT	randomized controlled trial
RFA	radiofrequency ablation
RIG	radiologically inserted gastrostomy
RUQ	right upper quadrant
SAAG	serum-ascites albumin gradient
SBBO	small bowel bacterial overgrowth
SBP	spontaneous bacterial peritonitis
SCFA	short chain fatty acid
SeHCAT	selenium 75-labelled homotaurocholic acid test
SIGN	Scottish Intercollegiate Guidelines Network
SMA	superior mesenteric artery
SOD	sphincter of Oddi dysfunction
SSRI	selective serotonin reuptake inhibitor

STK11	serine/threonine kinase 11
SVR	sustained virological response
TACE	transarterial chemoembolization
TB	tuberculosis
TDS	'ter die sumendum'; three times a day
TI	terminal ileum
TIPSS	transjugular intrahepatic portosystemic shunt
TPMT	thiopurine methyltransferase
U&E	urea and electrolytes
UC	ulcerative colitis
UKELD	United Kingdom End-Stage Liver Disease
ULN	upper limit of normal
USS	ultrasound scan
VH/CD	villous height/crypt depth (ratio)
VIP	vasoactive intestinal peptide
VTE	venous thromboembolism
VZV	Varicella zoster virus
WCC	white cell count
WDHA	watery diarrhoea, hypokalaemia, and achlorhydria (syndrome)
WHO	World Health Organization
ZES	Zollinger–Ellison syndrome

NORMAL RANGES

Haematology

haemoglobin
    males   g/L (130–180)
    females   g/L (115–165)
red cell count
    males $\times 10^{12}$/L (4.3–5.9)
    females $\times 10^{12}$/L (3.5–5.0)
haematocrit
    males   (0.40–0.52)
    females   (0.36–0.47)
mean corpuscular volume   fL (80–96)
mean corpuscular haemoglobin   pg (28–32)
mean corpuscular haemoglobin concentration   g/dL (32–35)
white cell count $\times 10^{9}$/L (4.0–11.0)
neutrophil count $\times 10^{9}$/L (1.5–7.0)
lymphocyte count $\times 10^{9}$/L (1.5–4.0)
monocyte count $\times 10^{9}$/L (< 0.8)
eosinophil count $\times 10^{9}$/L (0.04–0.40)
basophil count $\times 10^{9}$/L (< 0.1)
platelet count $\times 10^{9}$/L (150–400)
reticulocyte count $\times 10^{9}$/L (25–85)
reticulocyte count   % (0.5–2.4)
CD4 count $\times 10^{6}$/L (430–1690)

erythrocyte sedimentation rate
  under 50 years of age:
    males   mm/1st hour (< 15)
    females   mm/1st hour (< 20)
  over 50 years of age:
    males   mm/1st hour (< 20)
    females   mm/1st hour (< 30)

plasma viscosity (25°C)   mPa/second (1.50–1.72)

Coagulation screen

prothrombin time   seconds (11.5–15.5)
international normalized ratio   (< 1.4)
activated partial thromboplastin time   seconds (30–40)
thrombin time   seconds (15–19)

fibrinogen   g/L (1.8–5.4)
bleeding time   minutes (3.0–8.0)

Coagulation factors

factors II, V, VII, VIII, IX, X, XI, XII   IU/dL (50–150)
von Willebrand factor antigen   IU/dL (45–150)
von Willebrand factor activity   IU/dL (50–150)
protein C   IU/dL (80–135)
protein S   IU/dL (80–120)
antithrombin   IU/dL (80–120)
activated protein C resistance   (2.12–4.00)
fibrin degradation products   mg/L (< 100)
D-dimer   mg/L (< 0.5)

Haematinics

serum iron μmol/L (12–30)
serum iron-binding capacity μmol/L (45–75)
serum ferritin μg/L (15–300)
serum transferrin   g/L (2.0–4.0)
serum vitamin B_{12} ng/L (160–760)
serum folate μg/L (2.0–11.0)
red cell folate μg/L (160–640)
serum haptoglobin   g/L (0.13–1.63)
zinc protoporphyrin:haemoglobin ratio μmol/mol haemoglobin (< 70)

haemoglobinopathy screen:
    haemoglobin A   % (> 95)
    haemoglobin A_2 % (2–3)
    haemoglobin F   % (< 2)
    haemoglobin S   % (0)
transferrin saturations   % (20–50)
methaemoglobin   % (< 1)

Chemistry

Blood

serum sodium   mmol/L (137–144)
serum potassium   mmol/L (3.5–4.9)
serum chloride   mmol/L (95–107)
serum bicarbonate   mmol/L (20–28)
anion gap   mmol/L (12–16)
serum urea   mmol/L (2.5–7.0)
serum creatinine μmol/L (60–110)
estimated glomerular filtration rate (MDRD)   mL/minute (> 60)
serum corrected calcium   mmol/L (2.20–2.60)
serum ionized calcium   mmol/L (1.13–1.32)
serum phosphate   mmol/L (0.8–1.4)
serum total protein   g/L (61–76)
serum albumin   g/L (37–49)

serum globulin	g/L (24–27)
serum total bilirubin	µmol/L (1–22)
serum conjugated bilirubin	µmol/L (< 3.4)
serum alanine aminotransferase	U/L (5–35)
serum aspartate aminotransferase	U/L (1–31)
serum alkaline phosphatase	U/L (45–105)
serum gamma glutamyl transferase	
males	U/L (< 50)
females	U/L (4–35)
serum lactate dehydrogenase	U/L (10–250)
serum acid phosphatase	U/L (2.6–6.2)
serum creatine kinase	
males	U/L (24–195)
females	U/L (24–170)
serum creatine kinase MB fraction	% (< 5)
serum troponin I	µg/L (< 0.1)
serum troponin T	µg/L (< 0.01)
fasting plasma glucose	mmol/L (3.0–6.0)
haemoglobin A_{1c}	% (4.0–6.0); mmol/mol (20–42)
serum α_1-antitrypsin	g/L (1.1–2.1)
serum copper	µmol/L (12–26)
serum caeruloplasmin	mg/L (200–350)
serum aluminium	µg/L (< 10)
blood lead	µmol/L (< 0.5)
serum magnesium	mmol/L (0.75–1.05)
serum zinc	µmol/L (6–25)
serum urate	
males	mmol/L (0.23–0.46)
females	mmol/L (0.19–0.36)
plasma lactate	mmol/L (0.6–1.8)
plasma ammonia	µmol/L (12–55)
serum angiotensin-converting enzyme	U/L (25–82)
plasma fructosamine	µmol/L (< 285)
serum amylase	U/L (60–180)
plasma osmolality	mosmol/kg (278–300)
plasma osmolar gap	mosmol (< 10)
thiopurine methyltransferase	U/L (> 25)

Urine

glomerular filtration rate	mL/minute (70–140)
24-hour urinary total protein	g (< 0.2)
24-hour urinary albumin	mg (< 30)
24-hour urinary creatinine	mmol (9–18)
24-hour urinary calcium	mmol (2.5–7.5)
24-hour urinary copper	µmol (0.2–0.6)
24-hour urinary urate	mmol (< 3.6)
24-hour urinary oxalate	mmol (0.14–0.46)
24-hour urinary urobilinogen	µmol (1.7–5.9)
24-hour urinary coproporphyrin	nmol (< 300)

24-hour urinary uroporphyrin	nmol (6–24)
24-hour urinary δ-aminolevulinate	μmol (8–53)
24-hour urinary 5-hydroxyindoleacetic acid	μmol (10–47)
urinary osmolality	mosmol/kg (350–1000)
urinary osmolality after dehydration	mosmol/kg (> 750)

urinary albumin:creatinine ratio

males	mg/mmol (< 2.5)
females	mg/mmol (< 3.5)
urinary protein:creatinine ratio	mg/mmol (< 30)

urine microscopy:

| white cells | /μL (< 10) |

Faeces

stool weight (non-fasting)	g (< 200)
24-hour faecal nitrogen	mmol (70–140)
24-hour faecal urobilinogen	μmol (50–500)
24-hour faecal coproporphyrin	μmol (0.018–1.200)
faecal coproporphyrin	mmol/g dry weight (0.46)
24-hour faecal protoporphyrin	μmol (< 4)
faecal protoporphyrin	nmol/g dry weight (< 220)

faecal total porphyrin

ether soluble	nmol/g dry weight (10–200)
ether insoluble	nmol/g dry weight (< 24)
24-hour faecal fat (on normal diet)	mmol (< 20)
osmolality	mosmol/kg (300)
osmolar gap [300 − 2 × (faecal Na + K)]	mosmol/kg (< 100)
faecal calprotectin	μg/g (< 50)
faecal elastase	μg/g (> 200)
faecal α_1-antitrypsin	μg/g (< 300)

Body mass index

| body mass index | kg/m^2 (18–25) |

Lipids and lipoproteins

serum cholesterol	mmol/L (< 5.2)
serum LDL cholesterol	mmol/L (< 3.36)
serum HDL cholesterol	mmol/L (> 1.55)
fasting serum triglycerides	mmol/L (0.45–1.69)

Arterial blood gases, breathing air

PO_2	kPa (11.3–12.6)
PCO_2	kPa (4.7–6.0)
pH	(7.35–7.45)
H^+	nmol/L (35–45)
bicarbonate	mmol/L (21–29)
base excess	mmol/L (±2)
lactate	mmol/L (0.5–1.6)

carboxyhaemoglobin:

| non-smoker | % (< 2) |
| smoker | % (3–10) |

oxygen saturations   % (94–99)
methaemoglobin   % (< 1)

Endocrinology

Adrenal steroids (blood)

plasma renin activity
    (after 30 minutes supine)   pmol/mL/hour (1.1–2.7)
    (after 30 minutes upright)   pmol/mL/hour (3.0–4.3)

plasma aldosterone (normal diet)
    (after 30 minutes supine)   pmol/L (135–400)
    (after 4 hours upright)   pmol/L (330–830)
plasma aldosterone:renin ratio   (< 25)
plasma angiotensin II   pmol/L (5–35)

serum cortisol (09.00 hours)   nmol/L (200–700)
serum cortisol (22.00 hours)   nmol/L (50–250)

overnight dexamethasone suppression test (after 1 mg dexamethasone):
    serum cortisol   nmol/L (< 50)

low-dose dexamethasone suppression test (2 mg/day for 48 hours):
    serum cortisol   nmol/L (< 50)

high-dose dexamethasone suppression test (8 mg/day for 48 hours):
    serum cortisol   nmol/L (should suppress to < 50%
                                     of day 0 value)

short tetracosactide (Synacthen®) test (250 micrograms):
    serum cortisol (30 minutes after tetracosactide)   nmol/L (> 550)

plasma 11-deoxycortisol   nmol/L (24–46)
serum dehydroepiandrosterone (09.00 hours)   nmol/L (7–31)
serum dehydroepiandrosterone sulphate
    males   μmol/L (2–10)
    females   μmol/L (3–12)
serum androstenedione
    males   nmol/L (1.6–8.4)
    females   nmol/L (0.6–8.8)
    post-menopausal   nmol/L (0.9–6.8)
serum 17-hydroxyprogesterone
    males   nmol/L (1–10)
    females
      follicular   nmol/L (1–10)
      luteal   nmol/L (10–20)
serum oestradiol
    males   pmol/L (< 180)
    females
      post-menopausal   pmol/L (< 100)
      follicular   pmol/L (200–400)
      mid-cycle   pmol/L (400–1200)
      luteal   pmol/L (400–1000)

serum progesterone
    males   nmol/L (< 6)
    females
        follicular   nmol/L (< 10)
        luteal   nmol/L (> 30)

serum testosterone
    males   nmol/L (9–35)
    females   nmol/L (0.5–3.0)

serum dihydrotestosterone
    males   nmol/L (1.0–2.6)
    females   nmol/L (0.3–9.3)

serum sex hormone binding protein
    males   nmol/L (10–62)
    females   nmol/L (40–137)

Adrenal steroids (urine)

24-hour urinary aldosterone   nmol (14–53)
24-hour urinary free cortisol   nmol (55–250)

Pancreatic and gut hormones

oral glucose tolerance test (75 g)
    2-hour plasma glucose   mmol/L (< 7.8)
plasma gastrin   pmol/L (< 55)
plasma or serum insulin
    overnight fasting   pmol/L (< 186)
    after hypoglycaemia
    (plasma glucose < 2.2 mmol/L)   pmol/L (< 21)
serum C-peptide   pmol/L (180–360)
plasma glucagon   pmol/L (< 50)
plasma pancreatic polypeptide   pmol/L (< 300)
plasma vasoactive intestinal polypeptide   pmol/L (< 30)

Anterior pituitary hormones

plasma adrenocorticotropic hormone (09.00 hours)   pmol/L (< 18)
plasma follicle-stimulating hormone
    males   U/L (1.0–7.0)
    females
        follicular   U/L (2.5–10.0)
        mid-cycle   U/L (25–70)
        luteal   U/L (0.32–2.10)
        post-menopausal   U/L (> 30)

plasma growth hormone
    basal, fasting and between pulses   µg/L (< 0.4)
    2 hours after glucose tolerance test (75 g)   µg/L (< 1)

insulin-induced hypoglycaemia (blood glucose < 2.2 mmol/L):
    plasma growth hormone   µg/L (> 3)
    serum cortisol   nmol/L (> 580)

plasma luteinizing hormone
    males   U/L (1.0–10.0)
    females
        follicular   U/L (2.5–10.0)
        mid-cycle   U/L (25–70)
        luteal   U/L (1.0–13.0)
        post-menopausal   U/L (> 30)
plasma prolactin   mU/L (< 360)
plasma thyroid-stimulating hormone   mU/L (0.4–5.0)

Posterior pituitary hormones

plasma antidiuretic hormone   pmol/L (0.9–4.6)

Thyroid hormones

plasma thyroid-binding globulin   mg/L (13–28)
plasma T_4 nmol/L (58–174)
plasma free T_4 pmol/L (10.0–22.0)
plasma T_3 nmol/L (1.07–3.18)
plasma free T_3 pmol/L (3.0–7.0)

serum thyroid-stimulating hormone receptor
   antibodies   U/L (< 7)
serum anti-thyroid peroxidase antibodies   IU/mL (< 50)
serum thyroid-receptor antibodies   U/L (< 10)
technetium-99m scan of thyroid (20-minute uptake)   % (0.4–3.0)

Catecholamines (blood)

(Plasma recumbent with venous catheter in place for 30 minutes before collection of sample)
plasma adrenaline   nmol/L (0.03–1.31)
plasma noradrenaline   nmol/L (0.47–4.14)

Catecholamines (urine)

24-hour urinary vanillylmandelic acid   µmol (5–35)
24-hour urinary dopamine   nmol (< 3100)
24-hour urinary adrenaline   nmol (< 144)
24-hour urinary noradrenaline   nmol (< 570)

Others

plasma parathyroid hormone   pmol/L (0.9–5.4)
plasma calcitonin   pmol/L (< 27)
serum cholecalciferol (vitamin D_3)   nmol/L (60–105)
serum 25-OH-cholecalciferol   nmol/L (45–90)
serum 1,25-$(OH)_2$-cholecalciferol   pmol/L (43–149)

serum insulin-like growth factor 1
    13–20 years   nmol/L (9.3–56.0)
    21–40 years   nmol/L (7.5–37.3)
    41–60 years   nmol/L (5.6–23.3)
    > 60 years   nmol/L (3.3–23.3)
serum IGF1:IGF2 ratio   (< 10)

Immunology/Rheumatology

serum complement C3	mg/dL (65–190)
serum complement C4	mg/dL (15–50)
total serum haemolytic complement activity CH50	U/L (150–250)
serum C-reactive protein	mg/L (< 10)
serum immunoglobulin G	g/L (6.0–13.0)
serum immunoglobulin A	g/L (0.8–3.0)
serum immunoglobulin M	g/L (0.4–2.5)
serum immunoglobulin E	kU/L (< 120)
serum immunoglobulin D	mg/L (20–120)
serum immunoglobulin G4	g/L (0.08–1.30)
serum β_2-microglobulin	mg/L (< 3)
serum mast cell tryptase (1 hour post-reaction)	µg/L (2–14)

Autoantibodies

anti-acetylcholine-receptor antibodies	
anti-adrenal antibodies	(negative at 1:10 dilution)
anticentromere antibodies	(negative at 1:40 dilution)
anticardiolipin antibodies:	
immunoglobulin G	U/mL (< 23)
immunoglobulin M	U/mL (< 11)
anti-cyclic citrullinated peptide antibodies	
anti-double-stranded DNA antibodies (ELISA)	U/mL (< 73)
anti-glomerular basement membrane antibodies	
anti-lactoferrin antibodies	
anti-neutrophil cytoplasmic antibodies:	
c-ANCA	
p-ANCA	
PR3-ANCA	U/mL (< 10)
MPO-ANCA	U/mL (< 10)
antinuclear antibodies	(negative at 1:20 dilution)
extractable nuclear antigen	
gastric parietal cell antibodies	(negative at 1:20 dilution)
intrinsic factor antibodies	
interstitial cells of testis antibodies	(negative at 1:10 dilution)
anti-Jo-1 antibodies	
anti-La antibodies	
antimitochondrial antibodies	(negative at 1:20 dilution)
anti-RNP antibodies	
anti-Scl-70 antibodies	
anti-Ro antibodies	
anti-skeletal muscle antibodies	(negative at 1:60 dilution)
anti-Sm antibodies	
anti-smooth muscle antibodies	(negative at 1:20 dilution)
anti-thyroid colloid and microsomal antibodies	(negative at 1:10 dilution)
anti-gliadin antibodies	IU/L (< 10)
anti-endomysial antibodies	

anti-tissue transglutaminase antibodies	U/mL (< 15)
rheumatoid factor	kIU/L (< 30)
antistreptolysin titre	IU/mL (< 200)

Hepatitis virus serology

HBs Ag	IU/mL (lower detection limit 50)
HBV DNA	IU/mL (lower detection limit 250)
Hepatitis B genotype	A–H
HCV RNA	IU/mL (lower detection limit 15)
Hepatitis C genotype	1–6

Tumour markers

serum α-fetoprotein	kU/L (< 10)
serum carcinoembryonic antigen	µg/L (< 10)
serum neuron-specific enolase	µg/L (< 12)
serum prostate-specific antigen	
males < 40 years of age	µg/L (< 2)
males > 40 years of age	µg/L (< 4)
serum β-human chorionic gonadotropin	U/L (< 5)
serum CA 125	U/mL (< 35)
serum CA 19–9	U/mL (< 33)

Viral loads

cytomegalovirus viral load	copies/mL (lower detection limit 400)
Epstein–Barr viral load	copies/mL (lower detection limit 250)
hepatitis B viral load	IU/mL (lower detection limit 250)
hepatitis C viral load	IU/mL (lower detection limit 15)
HIV viral load	copies/mL (lower detection limit 40)
human herpesvirus-6 viral load	copies/mL (lower detection limit 50)
human herpesvirus-8 viral load	copies/mL (lower detection limit 50)

Therapeutic drug concentrations

plasma carbamazepine	µmol/L (34–51)
blood ciclosporin	nmol/L (100–150)
blood tacrolimus	
≤ 12 months following transplant	nmol/L (8–12)
> 12 months following transplant	nmol/L (5–10)
plasma digoxin (taken at least 6 hours post-dose)	nmol/L (1.0–2.0)
serum gentamicin (peak)	mg/L (5–7)
pre-dose	mg/L (< 1)
1 hour post-dose	mg/L (3–5)
serum vancomycin (trough)	mg/L (10–15)
serum lithium	mmol/L (0.5–1.2)
serum phenobarbital	µmol/L (65–172)
serum phenytoin	µmol/L (40–80)
serum primidone	µmol/L (23–55)
plasma theophylline	µmol/L (55–110)

Cerebrospinal fluid

opening pressure	mmH$_2$O (50–180)
total protein	g/L (0.15–0.45)
albumin	g/L (0.066–0.442)
chloride	mmol/L (116–122)
glucose	mmol/L (3.3–4.4)
lactate	mmol/L (1.0–2.0)
cell count	/μL (≤ 5)
white cell count	/μL (≤ 5)
red cell count	/μL (0)
lymphocyte count	/μL (≤ 3.5)
neutrophil count	/μL (0)
immunoglobulin G:albumin ratio	(≤ 0.26)
immunoglobulin index	(≤ 0.88)

Synovial fluid

white cell count	/mL (< 200)

Pulmonary function

transfer factor for CO (TL$_{CO}$)	% (80–120) mmol/minute/kPa
transfer coefficient (K$_{CO}$)	% (100) mmol/minute/kPa

Cardiac pressures

mean arterial pressure	mmHg (96)
mean right atrial pressure	mmHg (3)
mean pulmonary arterial pressure	mmHg (15)
mean pulmonary arterial wedge pressure	mmHg (9)
mean cardiac output	L/min (5)

Hepatic venous pressures

portal venous pressure	mmHg (4–8)
hepatic venous pressure	mmHg (2–4)
hepatic venous pressure gradient	mmHg (< 5)

ECG measurements

PR interval	ms (120–200)
QRS complex	ms (40–120)

Ascites

white cell count	< 250 cells/mm^3

UPPER GASTROINTESTINAL TRACT DISORDERS

1. **A 46-year-old teacher presented with a 5-month history of profuse diarrhoea despite fasting, and associated abdominal bloating. She complained of increasing fatigue and appeared dehydrated.**

   Investigations:

haemoglobin	125 g/L (130–180)
serum sodium	138 mmol/L (137–144)
serum potassium	1.9 mmol/L (3.5–4.9)
serum urea	7.3 mmol/L (2.5–7.0)
serum creatinine	105 µmol/L (60–110)
plasma viscosity	1.76 mPa/s (1.50–1.72)

   Which of the following is the most likely diagnosis?

   A. Bile salt malabsorption
   B. Coeliac disease
   C. Irritable bowel syndrome
   D. Ulcerative colitis
   E. VIPoma

2. **A 43-year-old housewife with a history of ischaemic heart disease and a body mass index of 37 was referred for gastric bypass surgery. She was included in a research study investigating the effects of satiety hormones before Roux-en-Y gastric bypass.**

   Which of the following statements best describes the behaviour of ghrelin before and after meal ingestion?

   A. Ghrelin level falls before meal ingestion but gradually rises in the next 2 hours
   B. Ghrelin level remains unchanged
   C. Ghrelin level rises sharply before and remains high after meal ingestion
   D. Ghrelin level sharply rises before and falls shortly after meal ingestion
   E. Ghrelin level unchanged before meal ingestion and fall rapidly afterwards

3. **A 46-year-old man was reviewed in clinic with troublesome symptoms of reflux occurring at any time of day, for the last 2 years. He had a gastroscopy six months ago which was normal. He had taken omeprazole 40 mg BD and metoclopramide 10 mg TDS for eight months. He had previously tried an H2-receptor antagonist in addition to this, with no benefit. He had no lifestyle risk factors for reflux.**

    What is the next most appropriate management step?

    A. Ambulatory oesophageal pH and manometry studies
    B. Barium swallow
    C. Fasting gastrin level
    D. Peripheral blood eosinophil count
    E. Repeat endoscopy

4. **A 58-year-old man underwent an OGD for investigation of reflux symptoms. Macroscopically he was found to have an area suggestive of Barrett's oesophagus. This was biopsied and his histology report was returned to you.**

    Which of the following histological features best supports the endoscopic diagnosis of Barrett's oesophagus with no dysplasia?

    A. Cardiac-type columnar cells bordering squamous mucosa
    B. Columnar mucosa with nuclear pleomorphism in all cells seen
    C. Gastric-type mucosa with a similarity in nuclear/cytological appearances in the crypt base cells to those at the surface epithelium
    D. Increased foci of mitotic activity seen at the gastro-oesophageal junction
    E. Intestinal metaplastic glandular mucosa with adjacent oesophageal ducts

5. **A 58-year-old woman under surveillance for Barrett's oesophagus was found to have high-grade dysplasia in four biopsies at gastroscopy. Repeat gastroscopy and further biopsies confirmed this. The Barrett's segment appeared uncomplicated macroscopically, and was circumferential and 5 cm in length (Prague C5M5). She was taking a high-dose proton pump inhibitor. She declined surgical intervention.**

    Which of the following is the most appropriate management step?

    A. Argon plasma coagulation
    B. Endoscopic mucosal resection
    C. Laser ablation
    D. Multipolar electrocoagulation
    E. Radio-frequency ablation

6. **A 72-year-old man presented with a 3-week history of dysphagia and was found to have a large oesophageal adenocarcinoma at 37 cm.**

Which of the following is the most significant predisposing factor in the pathogenesis of oesophageal adenocarcinoma?

A. Alcohol excess

B. *Helicobacter pylori* infection

C. Obesity

D. Smoking

E. Social deprivation

7. **A 37-year-old Brazilian man who complained of chest pain was referred to the gastroenterology clinic by cardiology. He had a history of episodic dysphagia and occasional regurgitation; his GP had adequately trialled PPI and prokinetics.**

Investigations:

gastroscopy	normal
oesophageal pH studies	DeMeester score 11
oesophageal motility studies	simultaneous high-amplitude contractions with 40% of swallows, but intermittently normal peristaltic waves and a high resting pressure at the lower oesophageal sphincter (LOS). There is normal relaxation during swallowing

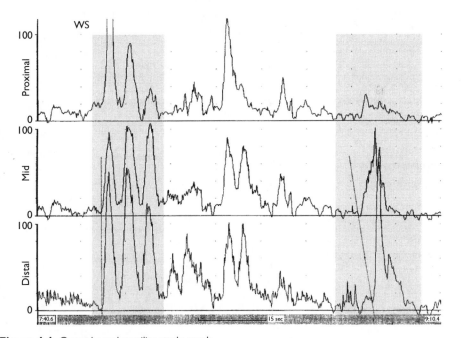

Figure 1.1 Oesophageal motility study result

Reproduced from *Gut*, Spechler SJ, Castell DO, 'Classification of oesophageal motility abnormalities', 49, 1, pp. 145–151. Copyright 2001, with permission from BMJ Publishing Group Ltd and British Society of Gastroenterology.

What is the most likely diagnosis?

A. Achalasia

B. Chagas disease

C. Diffuse oesophageal spasm

D. Gastro-oesophageal reflux disease

E. Nutcracker oesophagus

8. **A 28-year-old Brazilian man who complained of chest pain was referred to the gastroenterology clinic by cardiology. He had a 1-year history of episodic dysphagia and occasional regurgitation; his GP had adequately trialled PPI and prokinetics. You organized gastroscopy, oesophageal manometry, and pH studies, the results of which have been reported as being consistent with achalasia. Protozoal serology is negative.**

   In this scenario, which of the following is the most appropriate first-line management step?

   A. Benznidazole

   B. Botulinum toxin injection of the lower oesophageal sphincter

   C. Surgery

   D. Trial of calcium-channel blockers

   E. Weight loss

9. **A 70-year-old woman with a WHO performance status of 3 and COPD was found to have a 2 x 6 cm flat adenocarcinoma of the oesophagus at 35 cm on OGD, not bordering the gastro-oesophageal junction.**

   Investigations:

endoscopic ultrasound	no evidence of lymphadenopathy
CT abdomen and pelvis	no evidence of lymphadenopathy, no distant metastases

   Which is the next best option in her management?

   A. Chemoradiotherapy

   B. Endoscopic mucosal resection

   C. Endoscopic submucosal dissection

   D. Radiofrequency ablation

   E. Surgery with pre-operative chemotherapy

10. **A 56-year-old man presented with a 3-month history of intermittent vomiting. He had no past medical history, drank 10 units of alcohol a week, and was a non-smoker.**

Investigations:
gastroscopy   4 cm antral tumour
histopathology   adenocarcinoma

With regard to the initial staging of gastric cancer, which is the most useful modality as an adjunct to CT scanning?

A. Barium meal
B. Endoscopic mucosal resection
C. Endoscopic ultrasound
D. Laparoscopy
E. Magnetic resonance imaging

11. **A 76-year-old man was referred by his GP for endoscopy complaining of a 6-month history of dyspepsia, despite adequate trials of a PPI. His *Helicobacter pylori* breath test was negative. His stepmother died from gastric carcinoma.**

Among patients who are referred for gastroscopy for alarm features, the prevalence of gastric cancer is most appropriately described as:

A. 0.8%
B. 4%
C. 16%
D. 28%
E. 32%

12. **A 33-year-old woman of Indian origin was referred for endoscopy with dyspepsia. This had been resistant to omeprazole 20 mg orally daily and metoclopramide 10 mg three times daily, which she was taking at the time of gastroscopy. She was on no other medications.**

Investigations:
gastroscopy   antral erosions and three large duodenal
                           ulcers in D1 (Forrest class III)
antral rapid urease test   negative
haemoglobin   138 g/L (130–180)
plasma viscosity   1.70 mPa/s (1.50–1.72)
serum C-reactive protein   8 mg/L (< 10)
plasma gastrin   90 pmol/L (<55)

Which of the following is the most likely diagnosis?

A. Crohn's disease
B. *Helicobacter pylori* infection
C. Human immunodeficiency virus
D. Tuberculosis
E. Zollinger–Ellison syndrome

13. A 75-year-old man with a coffee ground vomit was referred for an OGD on your list. His notes state that he had a Billroth II procedure 20 years ago.

Which of the following most accurately describes his surgery?

A. Division of the vagus nerve and a gastrojejunostomy

B. Division of the vagus nerve and lateral division of the pylorus, followed by longitudinal resuturing

C. Formation of gastric pouch; small bowel divided at the duodenal-jejunal junction; anastomosis of the jejunum to the gastric pouch; anastamosis of the duodenum to the small bowel distal to the jejunal anastamosis

D. Longitudinal division of the pylorus

E. Resection of gastric antrum, gastrojejunostomy and closure of the first part of the duodenum and gastric outflow

14. A 76-year-old man presenting with dysphagia was found to have inoperable oesophageal adenocarcinoma. He has an endoscopically placed oesophageal stent for palliation of his symptoms, but unfortunately found it very painful, and it was removed a few days later. There is no perforation. He asks whether there are any other treatment options to help with his symptoms.

Which of the following modalities is an appropriate first-line treatment option to discuss?

A. Band ligation

B. Botulinum toxin injection

C. Brachytherapy

D. Local ethanol injection

E. Photodynamic therapy

15. A 72-year-old man was admitted with a 1-day history of melaena. He had no relevant past medical history and took no regular medications.

What percentage of patients who are admitted with apparent acute upper gastrointestinal bleeding do not reveal a cause at initial gastroscopy?

A. 10%

B. 20%

C. 30%

D. 40%

E. 50%

16. **A previously fit and well 35-year-old woman, who was on an SSRI for depression, took high doses of ibuprofen for rheumatoid arthritis. She was subsequently diagnosed with an upper GI bleed. At endoscopy she had a bleeding gastric ulcer with an adherent clot which was treated with adrenaline and heater probe. The endoscopist was satisfied that haemostasis was optimally achieved. A *Helicobacter pylori* test was not performed. She was stable following her endoscopy, and returned to the ward.**

    Regarding her post-endoscopic care, which of the following most accurately represents current guidelines?

    A. Change her ibuprofen to naproxen
    B. Consider switching from an SSRI to an alternative antidepressant
    C. Empirical *Helicobacter pylori* eradication therapy for 1 week
    D. High-dose IV PPI infusion for 48 hours
    E. Oral PPI indefinitely after discharge

17. **A 37-year-old woman with stigmata of chronic liver disease was admitted on the acute medical take with fresh red haematemesis. She was adequately fluid resuscitated and received terlipressin and IV antiobiotics prior to an urgent OGD. She had three bleeding oesophageal varices at endoscopy, and six bands were applied at multiple sites. There were no gastric varices. Post procedure she continued to have fresh haematemesis.**

    What is the definitive treatment of choice?

    A. Balloon tamponade
    B. H-graft portocaval shunting
    C. Laparotomy
    D. Repeat endoscopy and radiofrequency ablation
    E. Transjugular intrahepatic portosytemic shunt (TIPSS)

18. **A 40-year-old man with known gastric varices was admitted with melaena. He was resuscitated with blood and fluids and started on terlipressin and broad-spectrum antibiotics. His gastric varices were injected with cyanoacrylate glue.**

    Why is glue considered to be the first-line treatment for bleeding gastric varices?

    A. It has a lower risk of mortality than TIPSS
    B. It has a lower risk of re-bleeding than TIPSS
    C. It is better at achieving haemostasis than TIPSS
    D. It is more cost-effective than TIPSS
    E. It leads to a lower requirement for blood transfusions than TIPSS

19. **A 68-year-old man with a background history of Parkinson's disease on levodopa was admitted with vomiting and abdominal pain.**

    Which of the following anti-emetics is the first-line treatment for nausea and vomiting in patients with Parkinson's disease?

    A. Domperidone
    B. Haloperidol
    C. Metoclopromide
    D. Ondansetron
    E. Prochlorperazine

20. **A 45-year-old woman attended her general practitioner with recurrent nausea and vomiting associated with travel. She had tried cyclizine to no effect.**

    What is the next choice of medication for her motion sickness?

    A. Betahistine
    B. Hyoscine
    C. Metoclopromide
    D. Ondansetron
    E. Prochlorperazine

21. **A 32-year-old woman with type 1 diabetes mellitus attended the nutrition outpatient clinic with persistent bloating, nausea, and vomiting. She was diagnosed with gastroparesis on the basis of gastric emptying studies, and had tried prokinetics for the last 3 months, but with only marginal effect. She is struggling to maintain her weight. Her most recent HbA1C was 5.8% (range 4.0–6.0%).**

    What would be the most appropriate next step to consider in management?

    A. Botulinum injection to pylorus
    B. Gastric pacemaker device
    C. Nasojejunal feeding
    D. Pancreatic islet cell transplantation
    E. Surgical jejunostomy

22. **A 34-year-old man presented with symptoms suggestive of delayed gastric emptying.**

    With regard to the physiology of gastric emptying, which of the following cells are responsible for controlling the slow-wave phase in the distal stomach?

    A. Chief cells
    B. Enterochromaffin cells
    C. Interstitial cells of Cajal
    D. Mucous neck cells
    E. Parietal cells

1. E. This patient exhibits the symptoms of watery profuse diarrhoea, abdominal pain, fatigue, and bloating that are found in VIPoma, or Verner–Morrison syndrome. Patients complain of high-volume diarrhoea despite fasting and are found to have achlorhydria, hypokalaemia (serum potassium < 3 mmol/L), hyperglycaemia, and hypercalcaemia with signs of dehydration. VIPoma results in high levels of vasoactive intestinal peptide (VIP). VIP usually stimulates fluid and electrolyte secretion from intestinal epithelium and bile duct cholangiocytes, and thus overactivity leads to symptoms of VIPoma.

VIPoma is a rare form of cancer that affects an estimated 1 in 10 million people per year, and consists of typically solitary lesions which are found in the tail of the pancreas (up to 75%). They are usually diagnosed in adults, most commonly in the age range 30–50 years, and are more common in women than in men.

Diagnosis is made by measuring fasting plasma VIP levels. Treatment is mostly surgical, but up to 50% of cases can be metastatic at the time of diagnosis. VIPomas are extremely responsive to octreotide, which results in tumour necrosis and inhibition of growth.

Gut peptide	Actions
Gastrin Two forms of gastrin: G34 and G17 Production: gastric antrum Release: • High pH stimulates secretion, low pH inhibits it • Stimulated by protein, peptides, and amino acids	(1) Stimulates gastric acid secretion (2) Growth-promoting effects on gastric mucosa Note: Hypergastrinaemia occurs in: • Decreased acid production (e.g. atrophic gastritis) • Overuse of acid-suppressive medication • Zollinger–Ellison syndrome
Cholecystokinin (CCK) Production: I cells of small intestine Acts on CCK_1 receptors on gallbladder, pancreas, stomach, smooth muscle, and peripheral nerves Release: • Stimulated by ingested fat and protein	(1) Regulates gastric emptying and bowel motility to induce satiety (2) Main hormonal regulator of gallbladder contraction (3) Regulates meal-stimulated pancreatic secretion Note: • Low CCK is implicated in coeliac disease and bulimia • High CCK is reported in chronic pancreatitis
Secretin Production: small intestine S cells Release: influenced by acid in duodenum G-protein-coupled receptor	(1) Pancreatic and bicarbonate secretion causing neutralization of acidic chyme in intestine (2) Inhibits gastric acid, gastric secretion, and intestinal motility (3) Aids in osmoregulation in hypothalamus, pituitary and kidney

Gut peptide	Actions
Vasoactive intestinal polypeptide (VIP)	
Production and release: neurons within gut, pancreas, suprachiasmatic nuclei of hypothalamus	(1) Potent vasodilator causing smooth muscle relaxation
G-protein-coupled receptor	(2) Stimulates fluid and electrolyte secretion from intestinal epithelium and bile duct cholangiocytes
	(3) Neuromodulator of sphincters of GI tract
	Note:
	• Lack of VIP innervation leads to Hirschsprung's disease and/or achalasia
	• Very high levels occur in watery-diarrhoea–hypokalaemia–achlorhydria (WDHA)/Verner–Morrison syndrome
Glucagon	
Production: alpha cells of pancreas	(1) Regulates glucose homeostasis via:
Release: ileum, colon, and alpha cells	• Gluconeogenesis
G-protein-coupled receptor	• Glycogenolysis
	• Lipolysis
Glucose-dependent insulinotropic polypeptide (GIP) (also called gastric inhibitory polypeptide)	(1) Inhibits gastric acid secretion
Production: K cells on duodenum, jejunum mucosa	(2) Stimulates release of insulin only in hyperglycaemic status
	(3) Augments triglyceride storage contributing to fat accumulation
	Note: it is proposed that GIP may have a role in obesity and insulin resistance associated with type 2 DM
Pancreatic polypeptide family (PP)	
Production: secreted from and stored by pancreatic endocrine cells	(1) Self-regulation of pancreatic secretory activity
	(2) Affects hepatic glycogen levels and gastrointestinal secretions
Somatostatin	
Production: D cells in gastric and intestinal mucosa, islets of pancreas	(1) Regulation of gastric acid secretion in stomach
Release:	(2) Reduction of pepsinogen secretion
• Influenced by pH	(3) Inhibits pancreatic enzyme, fluid bicarbonate secretion
• Mechanical stimulation	(4) Reduces bile flow
• Dietary components (fats/protein/glucose)	(5) Reduces splanchnic blood flow
	(6) Inhibits tissue growth and proliferation within the gut
	(7) Reduces gut motility
Leptin	
Blood levels reflect total body fat store	(1) Regulation of food ingestion by lowering neuropeptide Y, a potent stimulant of food intake within the brain
Secreted from adipocytes and gastric chief cells of stomach	
Ghrelin	
Production: by P/D1 cells gastric fundus, intestine, pancreas, pituitary, and kidneys	(1) Stimulation of gastric contraction
Acts on vagus nerve	(2) Enhances stomach emptying
	(3) Initiation of ingestion
	Note:
	• In gastric bypass patients there is *no* pre-meal rise in ghrelin levels
	• In Prader–Willi patients, ghrelin levels remain high after meals, which leads to hyperphagia

Gut peptide	Actions
Motilin	
Production: endocrine cells in duodenum	(1) Increase the migrating myoelectric complex of GI motility
Secretion:	(2) Stimulation of pepsin production
• Is periodic	(3) Peristalsis in the small intestine in preparation of gut for the next meal
• Is *not* stimulated by ingestion	
Substance P	
Primary mediator of neurogenic inflammation	(1) Activation of vomiting reflex
	(2) Involvement in nociception
	Note: high levels of substance P receptors are found in UC and CD

Feldman M, Friedman LS and Brandt LJ (eds). Gastrointestinal hormones and neurotransmitters. In: *Sleisenger and Fordtran's Gastrointestinal and Liver Disease: pathophysiology, diagnosis, management,* 8th edition. Philadelphia, PA: Saunders Elsevier; 2006. pp. 3–24.

American Association of Endocrine Surgeons. *Patient Education Site.* http://endocrinediseases.org/neuroendocrine/vipoma.shtml (accessed 20 October 2011).

2. D. Satiety signals share several functions.

• Cholecystokinin	• Delays rate of gastric emptying
	• Signals termination of food ingestion
• Ghrelin	• Initiates meal ingestion
	• Levels rise rapidly before the onset of meal and fall rapidly afterwards
• Glucagon-like peptide-1	• Delays gastric emptying
	• Increases satiety
• Leptin	• There is contradictory evidence
	• Reduces food intake
	• Produces greater reduction in body weight
• Neuropeptide Y	• Increases food intake
	• Increases proportion of food stored as fat
	• Stimulates intermittent pattern of licking and delayed satiation
• Peptide YY	• Reduce calorie intake
	• Inhibits gastric motility
	• Increases water and electrolyte absorption in colon

Recent research show that the levels of circulating ghrelin over a 24-hour period increased after diet-induced weight loss. However, the same study showed that ghrelin levels in patients with gastric bypass surgery did not change in relation to meals, and were in fact abnormally low.

Beglinger C and Degena L. Gastrointestinal satiety signals in humans: physiologic roles for GLP-1 and PYY? *Physiology & Behavior* 2006; 89: 460–464.

Feldman M, Friedman LS and Brandt LJ (eds). Gastrointestinal hormones and neurotransmitters. In: *Sleisenger and Fordtran's Gastrointestinal and Liver Disease: pathophysiology, diagnosis, management,* 8th edition. Philadelphia, PA: Saunders Elsevier; 2006. pp. 3–24.

Cummings DE, Wiegle DS, Frayo RS *et al.* Plasma ghrelin levels after diet-induced weight loss or gastric bypass surgery. *New England Journal of Medicine* 2002; 346: 1623–1630.

Borg CM, Le Roux CW and Ghatei MA. Progressive rise in gut hormone levels after Roux-en-Y gastric bypass suggests gut adaptation and explains altered satiety. *British Journal of Surgery* 2006; 93: 210–215.

3. A. This patient still has symptomatic gastro-oesophageal reflux disease (GORD) despite optimal medical therapy with acid suppression and a prokinetic. He may benefit from anti-reflux surgery with a fundoplication, but it would be sensible to try to determine whether his symptoms correlate with physiological reflux, and whether there is an element of dysmotility, prior to asking for a surgical opinion.

Surgery for GORD is an area with debatable efficacy, is associated with a morbidity and mortality risk, and can lead to problems with post-operative dysphagia. However, there is a role for surgery performed by an experienced operator in patients with resistant reflux with optimized medical therapy and lifestyle factors. Proven dysmotility makes symptoms less likely to respond to surgery, and this should be discussed with the patient before proceeding to surgical referral.

The BSG guidelines state that oesophageal pH studies have no role in the initial investigation of patients with established oesophagitis at endoscopy, but that there is a role in the work-up for anti-reflux surgery if patients are still symptomatic despite optimal medical treatment. Correlation of symptoms with acidic reflux helps to select those more likely to benefit.

Indications for oesophageal pH manometry:

- Assessment of suitability for anti-reflux surgery
- Diagnosis of motility disorders
- Investigation of patient with persistent symptoms despite surgery or dilatation/botulinum toxin treatment.

Use is restricted to those patients whose symptoms are resistant to first-line PPI and prokinetic. Barium testing can be useful if there are symptoms suggestive of dysmotility, but are unlikely to add anything above manometry. Serum gastrin testing is not indicated in this scenario.

H_2-receptor antagonists can be used in patients with nocturnal breakthrough symptoms, although this tends to be of only short-term benefit and demonstrates tachyphylaxis.

If found by rapid urease test or breath test, *Helicobacter pylori* eradication in endoscopy negative reflux disease with resistant symptoms is often undertaken as a measure to try to improve symptoms when all else has failed. This is a consensus approach in this circumstance, although evidence is conflicting. The role of *Helicobacter pylori* in endoscopically visible oesophagitis is also controversial, but at present eradication is not advised. There is some evidence that infection is negatively associated with GORD (i.e. is potentially protective). In contrast with this, but evidence based, *Helicobacter pylori* testing and eradication 'test and treat' is recommended in uninvestigated dyspepsia and non-ulcer dyspepsia which has not responded to a trial of PPI without alarm symptoms.

Endoscopic radiofrequency ablation, endoluminal gastroplication, lower oesophageal sphincter bulking agents, and hydrogel implantation have all been considered for GORD, but have not received NICE approval at review.

With regard to GORD that is resistant to medical treatment, optimal management includes:

1. Addressing lifestyle issues such as diet, timing of meals, alcohol, smoking, and weight
2. Reviewing compliance with medications to ensure an adequate trial of at least 2 months of therapy
3. Working through a logical differential diagnosis for the patient's symptoms if there are suggestive features for an alternative explanation (e.g. biliary or cardiac disease)
4. Considering whether patients are likely to benefit from anti-reflux surgery by assessing the correlation of symptoms to reflux using ambulatory oesophageal pH studies and manometry
5. Excluding complications

Unusual presentations of GORD	Complications of GORD
Chest pain	Barrett's oesophagus
Chronic cough	Peptic stricture
Sore throat	Oesophageal adenocarcinoma
Globus	
Dysphonia	

Peripheral eosinophil count can be elevated in patients with eosinophilic oesophagitis, but can also be normal, so is not very discriminatory.

Eosinophilic oesophagitis

Clinical features	Often young and male
	History of atopy
	GORD
	Dysphagia or food bolus obstruction
	Chest pain
Investigations	May have eosinophilia
Endoscopic appearances	May be normal
	Trachealized oesophagus (concentric circular rings)
	Linear furrowing
	Strictures or Schatzki ring
	White exudates
Biopsy appearances	Eosinophils > 15 cells per high-powered field
	Eosinophilic microabscesses
Treatment	PPI
	Fluticasone inhaled preparation swallowed BD
	Systemic steroids in resistant cases

Bodger K and Trudgill N. *Guidelines for Oesophageal Manometry and pH Monitoring*. BSG Guidelines in Gastroenterology, 2006. www.bsg.org.uk/clinical-guidelines/general/guidelines-by-date.html (accessed 12 March 2011).

North of England Dyspepsia Guideline Development Group (UK). *Dyspepsia: managing dyspepsia in adults in primary care*. London: National Institute for Health and Clinical Excellence; 2004.

NICE Interventional Procedures Advisory Committee. *Endoscopic Radiofrequency Ablation for Gastro-Oesophageal Reflux Disease*. London: National Institute for Health and Clinical Excellence; 2009. http://guidance.nice.org.uk/IPG292 (accessed 12 March 2011).

NICE Interventional Procedures Advisory Committee. *Endoluminal Gastroplication for Gastro-Oesophageal Reflux Disease*. London: National Institute for Health and Clinical Excellence; 2011. http://guidance.nice.org.uk/IPG404 (accessed 3 July 2011).

NICE Interventional Procedures Advisory Committee. *Endoscopic Injection of Bulking Agents for Gastro-Oesophageal Reflux Disease*. London: National Institute for Health and Clinical Excellence; 2004. http://guidance.nice.org.uk/IPG55 (accessed 12 March 2011).

NICE Interventional Procedures Advisory Committee. *Endoscopic Augmentation of the Lower Oesophageal Sphincter Using Hydrogel Implants for the Treatment of Gastro-Oesophageal Reflux Disease*. London: National Institute for Health and Clinical Excellence; 2007. http://guidance.nice.org.uk/IPG222 (accessed 12 March 2011).

4. E. Current UK guidelines define Barrett's oesophagus as endoscopically visible columnar epithelium replacing the normal squamous lining of the oesophagus. Histology is used to confirm or corroborate the diagnosis. Changes of intestinal metaplasia (IM) juxtaposed with oesophageal structures such as oesophageal glands or submucous glands provide the strongest evidence. Biopsies showing gastric-type mucosa without evidence of IM can still be consistent with Barrett's oesophagus but are not diagnostic, because they could originate from the gastro-oesophageal junction, stomach, or hiatus hernia. Thus B is the best answer, although A could still be consistent with the diagnosis.

Recommendations for identifying dysplasia in Barrett's oesophagus suggest that greatest accuracy is obtained when two experienced GI pathologists review specimens where inflammatory change has been minimized with PPI therapy. All of the features described in C, D, and E might suggest dysplasia (whether in Barrett's oesophagus or not) to an examining pathologist. However, none of the features are as useful as those in B in the diagnosis of Barrett's oesophagus.

The early case series are widely held to have overstated the relationship between Barrett's oesophagus and development of oesophageal adenocarcinoma. Meta-analysis of the data suggests an incidence of oesophageal cancer in these patients of approximately 0.5–1% per annum. Progression to oesophageal carcinoma is more common in males. The widely practised 2-yearly surveillance strategy is not evidence based, although the BOSS study currently under way is hopeful of resolving this.

There is no robust evidence to suggest that anti-reflux surgery is better than medical acid suppression in the prevention of progression to cancer, and this is not a recommended indication for surgery.

The link between *H.pylori* and oesophageal adenocarcinoma is not firmly established, but it may offer some protective effect. One theory behind this is a reduction in acidic refluxate caused by *H.pylori* pangastritis.

Barr H and Shepherd NA. *Management of Dysplasia. Guidelines for the diagnosis and management of Barrett's columnar-lined oesophagus.* London: British Society of Gastroenterology; 2005. www.bsg.org.uk/clinical-guidelines/oesophageal/guidelines-for-the-diagnosis-and-management-of-barrett-s-columnar-lined-oesophagus.html (accessed 5 January 2011).

5. E. The Prague classification attempts to standardize reporting in Barrett's oesophagus by quantifying endoscopically visible segments. From the GOJ, **C** the maximal length in centimetres of circumferential Barrett's mucosa is measured, as well as **M** the maximal length (including tongues) of Barrett's. Thus in the question the segment described is a 5 cm circumferential area of Barrett's without any tongues of mucosa extending above.

Ablative therapy for Barrett's oesophagus with high-grade dysplasia or intramucosal cancer was considered by NICE in 2010. The guidelines suggested that that the modalities suitable for initial monotherapy were:

- Endoscopic mucosal resection (EMR)
- Radiofrequency ablation (RFA)
- Photodynamic therapy (PDT)

EMR can be followed by adjunctive ablative therapy including RFA, PDT, and argon plasma coagulation (APC). However, APC, laser ablation, and multipolar electrocoagulation have insufficient evidence for use at this time.

The choice of endoscopic therapy rather than surgery for definitive management depends on:

- The discussion and steering of treatment options occurring at a specialist centre with an oesophago-gastric multidisciplinary team
- Patient preference

- Suitability for surgery
- Stage of oesophageal cancer—the use of endoscopic therapy not recommended for lesions invading beyond the muscularis mucosa (AJCC stage T1b)

The choice between the different endoscopic therapies was less clear, due to heterogeneity of evidence. EMR is less suitable for circumferential lesions, as it is associated with a high rate of stricture formation post procedure. Therefore it is most useful for localized lesions. RFA and PDT were felt to be of equivalent effectiveness for flat high-grade dysplasia (not intramucosal cancer). For these reasons, radiofrequency ablation is considered the best answer. The nature of the evidence base in this field makes statements about the relative efficacy of each modality difficult and will require further study in randomized controlled trials.

National Institute for Health and Clinical Excellence. *Ablative Therapy for the Treatment of Barrett's Oesophagus*. London: National Institute for Health and Clinical Excellence; 2010. http://guidance.nice. org.uk/CG106 (accessed 31 March 2011).

Rice TW, Blackstone EH and Rusch VW. 7th edition of the AJCC Cancer Staging Manual: esophagus and esophagogastric junction. *Annals of Surgical Oncology* 2010; 17: 1721–1724.

6. C. Obesity is a recognized risk factor for oesophageal adenocarcinoma. Other risk factors include:

- Below average fruit and vegetable consumption
- GORD
- Barrett's oesophagus
- Family history
- Smoking (to a lesser extent than obesity).

H. pylori is a recognized risk factor for gastric adenocarcinoma, but its relationship with oesophageal adenocarcinoma is not clear; some data suggest that it may have a protective effect.

Alcohol excess, smoking, and social deprivation are recognized risk factors for squamous-cell carcinoma of the oesophagus and gastric cancer. Social deprivation and alcohol excess are not risk factors for oesophageal adenocarcinoma.

Scottish Intercollegiate Guidelines Network. *Management of Oesophageal and Gastric Cancer: a national clinical guideline*. Edinburgh: Scottish Intercollegiate Guidelines Network; 2006. www.sign.ac.uk/guidelines/published/index.html (accessed 3 March 2011).

Allum WH, Blazeby J, Griffin SM *et al.* Guidelines for the management of oesophageal and gastric cancer. *Gut* 2011; 60: 1449–e1472. doi: 10.1136/gut.2010.228254.

7. C. The condition described by the report is diffuse oesophageal spasm (DOS). Treatment can be challenging, and the options are summarized later in the chapter. Achalasia could also present like this, but the manometry is more suggestive of DOS. Important mimics of achalasia (sometimes referred to as *pseudoachalasia*) include Chagas disease and carcinoma of the GOJ. Chagas disease is caused by *Trypanosoma cruzi* infection and can be treated with antibiotic agents. The diagnosis is confirmed by using serology. As well as DOS, other hypercontractile oesophageal motility disorders have been described:

1. hypertensive LOS: normal peristalsis and LOS relaxation but elevated LOS pressure
2. nutcracker oesophagus: normal peristalsis but higher-amplitude contractions (mean > 180 mmHg)

There is an overlap between primary dysmotility syndromes and also a group of patients who have atypical features that do not fit any of the patterns described. This can further complicate diagnosis and treatment.

Secondary causes of oesophageal dysmotility include scleroderma/connective tissue diseases, amyloidosis, diabetes, and neurological disease (e.g. MS).

With regard to the differential diagnosis of dysphagia, the following should be considered:

- Oropharyngeal (high) vs. oesophageal (low) dysphagia
- Mechanical vs. functional
- Mechanical: extramural, mural, and luminal causes
- Mechanical: malignant vs. benign
- Functional: neuromuscular, systemic, and idiopathic

Spechler SJ and Castell DO. Classification of oesophageal motility abnormalities. *Gut* 2001; 49: 145–151.

	Diffuse oesophageal spasm	**Achalasia**
Presentation	Dysphagia Non-cardiac chest pain Regurgitation Reflux	Dysphagia Non-cardiac chest pain Regurgitation Weight loss
Pathology	Not well characterized	Myenteric plexus degeneration—trigger not known
Barium swallow appearances	Can be normal. May show corkscrew pattern	Dilated oesophagus, food or fluid level, and 'bird's beak' at the LOS
Manometric features	LOS relaxation usually normal LOS pressure can be high, low, or normal Loss of sequential oesophageal peristalsis with simultaneous high-amplitude contractions in > 10% of swallows	LOS relaxation incomplete Often LOS resting pressure is increased Loss of sequential oesophageal peristalsis with simultaneous low-amplitude contractions (although variant vigorous achalasia is recognized)

8. C.

Condition	Treatment options
Achalasia	Nifedipine/nitrates
	Botox injection of LOS (often requires repeating)
	Endoscopic dilatation
	Laparoscopic Heller's myotomy and fundoplication; well-described surgical option
Diffuse oesophageal spasm	Nifedipine/nitrates/tricyclic antidepressants/SSRIs, and phosphodiesterase inhibitors
Nutcracker oesophagus	Multiple-level botox has been used
Hypertensive LOS	Endoscopic dilatation can be used if overlap features of achalasia
	Surgery is not usually useful

In a young and otherwise fit patient with achalasia a skilful and experienced surgeon can offer long-term benefit with a laparoscopic myotomy to disrupt the LOS. Endoscopic treatment with balloon dilatation is also an effective treatment with similar efficacy and relapse rate to surgery at 2 years in a recent trial. Surgical myotomy may offer better outcomes in young (< 40 years) male patients and those with high resting LOS pressures. However, there is probably more risk of post-procedural reflux and also associated risks of a surgical procedure. The decision is therefore made on an individual basis following a risk–benefit discussion. It is possible that this patient has Chagas disease, but serology is negative and in chronic infection anti-protozoal treatment is not usually helpful for the achalasia-like syndrome, so surgery is still probably the most appropriate option.

Endoscopic LOS injection with botox is effective but will require regular re-treatment, often within a year of initial therapy, so in a young patient is probably not as helpful.

Medication can offer some benefit, but the results are variable, tolerability is a problem, and patients may continue to lose weight while they are trialled. Therefore it is usually used as a bridging method or as a last resort if all other treatments are unsuccessful or contraindicated.

The treatment of DOS and the other hypercontractile dysmotility syndromes is less well described, and represents a heterogenous group of patients whose symptoms can be difficult to manage. Optimization of anti-reflux treatments is essential. Standard medical therapy with nitrates or nifedipine can be poorly tolerated due to headache and other symptoms attributable to systemic vasodilation. There is some evidence for symptomatic benefit of treatment with tricyclic antidepressants. Phosphodiesterase inhibitors and SSRIs have also been used. Surgery and endoscopic therapy are not standard treatment, although they have been described and can be considered in resistant cases.

Boeckxstaens GE, Annese V, Bruely des Varannes B et al. Pneumatic dilation versus laparoscopic Heller's myotomy for idiopathic achalasia. New England Journal of Medicine 2011; 364: 1807–1816.

9. B. EMR is a useful modality in staging and treatment of oesophageal carcinoma. It allows histological assessment of tumour invasion, and can be used as a potentially curative technique if the lesion is confined to mucosa (T1a disease). Therefore it is a useful option in patients for whom major surgery carries a high risk, or who have refused surgery.

Tumour staging at diagnosis is an important determinant of survival, of which lymph node involvement is by far the most important factor to consider. The TNM staging for oesophageal cancer is as follows:

T1	Tumour in lamina propria or submucosa
T1a	No invasion of submucosa
T1b	Tumour in submucosa NOT in muscularis propria
T2	Tumour in muscularis propria
T3	Tumour invades adventitia
T4 [T4a, T4b]	Tumour invades adjacent structures
T4a	Tumour grown into pleura/pericardium/diaphragm
T4b	Tumour grown into trachea/vertebrae/major blood vessels
N0	Lymph nodes containing cancer cells
N1	One or two nearby lymph nodes involved
N2	Three to six nearby lymph nodes involved
N3	Seven or more nearby lymph nodes involved
M0	No tumour spread to other organs
M1	Distant tumour metastases

Patients without distant metastasis and with limited lymph node involvement are most likely to receive benefit from curative treatment. SIGN guidelines recommend radical surgery for patients with T1b, T2, and T3 tumours, provided that they have a relatively low lymph node burden and are fit for the procedure. EMR is recommended as a curative modality for T1a lesions, and is an important step in staging more extensive disease. Patients without distant metastasis and with limited lymph node involvement are most likely to benefit from curative treatment. The 2011 BSG guidelines agree that EMR should be considered for staging and/or treatment of early oesophageal cancer.

Patients with distant metastasis in any of the three compartments (neck, mediastinum, and abdomen), or T4 disease involving structures that cannot be easily resected, should not undergo surgery as their quality of life has been shown to be reduced by operating in this context.

There is limited evidence on the efficacy of endoscopic submucosal dissection (ESD) in patients with oesophageal adenocarcinoma or high-grade dysplasia in Barrett's oesophagus, and it is limited to use in clinical trials. There are also safety concerns about the risk of oesophageal perforation.

The BSG 2011 guidelines suggest that chemoradiation is a valid radical treatment option for patients with oesophageal cancer who are unfit for surgery. Indeed in localized squamous carcinoma of the proximal oesophagus this is the treatment of choice over surgery. It can also be used in mid to lower oesophageal lesions with or without surgery. The evidence for effectiveness in adenocarcinoma is less convincing. There is no credible evidence showing survival advantage at 5 years with chemoradiation therapy.

Scottish Intercollegiate Guidelines Network. *Management of Oesophageal and Gastric Cancer: a national clinical guideline.* Edinburgh: Scottish Intercollegiate Guidelines Network; 2006. www.sign.ac.uk/guidelines/published/index.html (accessed 3 March 2011).

Allum WH, Blazeby J, Griffin SM *et al.* Guidelines for the management of oesophageal and gastric cancer. *Gut* 2011; 60: 1449–e1472. doi: 10.1136/gut.2010.228254.

10. D. There is good evidence indicating that laparoscopy should be considered in patients with oesophageal tumours extending to the proximal stomach and in staging of gastric tumours. The BSG suggests all patients with gastric cancer should have a diagnostic laparoscopy in order to accurately stage for local spread and metastatic disease.

Barium studies are sensitive in diagnosing malignancy. However, they have been shown to be less sensitive than endoscopy for identifying cancer *in situ* or T1 cancers.

MRI has similar rates of accuracy to CT in TNM staging, and therefore will not add anything in this case.

EUS is often useful in detecting local spread or nodal disease. EMR can be used to accurately stage the depth of invasion in small, early disease. However, the presence or absence of metastatic disease will be critical in this patient's management. Therefore laparoscopy is likely to be more discriminatory.

PET-CT scanning can also be helpful in staging. The BSG suggests its utilization in oesophageal and oesophagogastric junctional tumours, as it provides additional functional and anatomical data to optimize M and N staging pre-treatment.

Allum WH, Blazeby J, Griffin SM et al. Guidelines for the management of oesophageal and gastric cancer. *Gut* 2011; 60: 1449–e1472. doi: 10.1136/gut.2010.228254.

11. B. Patients who are worried about cancer are common in clinical practice. However, not all patients who present with dyspepsia require endoscopy; alarm features (see list) are an indication for urgent endoscopy. However, among those who are referred the prevalence of gastric cancer is around 4%.

Alarm features:

- Weight loss
- Iron-deficiency anaemia
- GI bleeding
- Persistent vomiting
- Dysphagia
- Epigastric mass
- Abnormal barium imaging

Those patients who have truly resistant symptoms despite best medical therapy may require a specialist gastroenterology opinion and/or an endoscopy. NICE 2004 guidance attempted to identify a further specific subset of patients who should be offered endoscopy.

Patients over the age of 55 years who have persistent symptoms of dyspepsia despite adequate acid suppression and eradication of *H. pylori* should be considered for endoscopy if there is:

- Previous gastric ulcer
- Previous gastric surgery
- Continuing need for NSAID treatment
- Anxiety about cancer
- Increased risk of gastric cancer

Family history, gastric ulcers, polyps or polyposis syndromes, Lynch syndrome, previous gastric surgery, Ménétrier's disease, and pernicious anaemia are all associated with an increased risk of gastric carcinoma. Lifestyle factors associated with gastric cancer are alcohol excess, smoking, and social deprivation.

North of England Dyspepsia Guideline Development Group (UK). *Dyspepsia: managing dyspepsia in adults in primary care.* London: National Institute for Health and Clinical Excellence; 2004. www.nice. org.uk/nicemedia/live/10950/29459/29459.pdf (accessed 13 October 2011).

12. B. Rapid urease testing (e.g. CLO® test) sensitivity is well recognized as being compromised by acid-suppressing therapy, and patients should ideally withhold these medications for 2 weeks prior to testing. If patients are still taking their medication at the time of endoscopy, there is a risk of obtaining false-negative results.

PPI treatment is also associated with an elevated serum gastrin due to the interruption of the normal negative feedback loop.

The most likely diagnosis is of a false-negative rapid urease test in a patient with *H. pylori* infection, and she should be offered non-invasive *H. pylori* testing off PPI, with eradication if positive.

Zollinger–Ellison syndrome (ZES) is a cause of peptic ulceration in 0.1–1% of cases. Features suggestive of ZES include:

- Severe or resistant ulceration in the absence of NSAIDs or *H. pylori* infection
- Unusual sites of ulceration (e.g. D2 or more distally)
- Diarrhoea
- Large gastric folds
- Fasting serum gastrin levels > 1000 pg/ml off PPI treatment

Fasting serum gastrin levels can be intermediate in ZES, so if there is strong suspicion clinically, the next step would be a secretin provocation test. Other causes of intermediate elevated fasting serum gastrin levels include atrophic gastritis and/or pernicious anaemia, gastric outlet obstruction, renal failure, and small bowel resection.

All of the differential diagnoses listed in the question can lead to ulceration, and the raised gastrin levels may be due to the concomitant PPI usage. HIV infection predisposes to CMV and HSV which can cause ulcers resistant to standard treatment. Crohn's disease is characterized by trans-mural ulceration, although this is uncommon in the upper GI tract. Tuberculosis is a rare cause of ulceration. The normal blood tests make these diagnoses less likely.

Travis SPL, Ahmad T, Collier J et al. *Pocket Consultant Gastroenterology.* Malden, MA: Blackwell Publishing, Inc.; 2005.

13. E.
A is as described.
B is a vagotomy and pyloroplasty.
C is a Roux-en-Y gastric bypass.
D is pyloromyotomy.
Please refer to diagram in Chapter 4, Answer 12 (Fig. 4.1, p. 137).

14. C. The question of palliation of dysphagia in oesophageal cancer is reviewed in detail in the British Society of Gastroenterology guidance published in 2011. Chemotherapy and radiotherapy have evidence to support their use in palliation of those patients who are fit enough to tolerate treatment. In this situation radiotherapy is often used.

Brachytherapy (internalized radiotherapy treatment with a radioactive source) when compared with endoscopic stent insertion was felt to be superior in long-term symptom relief in dysphagic patients with a prognosis greater than 3 months. Onset of symptom relief was not as rapid with brachytherapy—hence the time consideration.

Laser therapy and argon plasma therapy have also been used successfully in this context and could be considered, depending on local expertise and resources.

Photodynamic therapy was felt to have insufficient evidence to recommend its use currently. Ethanol injection has been shown to exacerbate dysphagia and pain and was not recommended.

Band ligation and botulinum toxin injection are less likely to have a role in this situation.

Allum WH, Blazeby J, Griffin SM et al. Guidelines for the management of oesophageal and gastric cancer. Gut 2011; 60: 1449–e1472. doi: 10.1136/gut.2010.228254.

15. B. B is the correct answer. Peptic ulcer (44%) is the commonest cause of gastrointestinal (GI) bleeding. Other causes in order of relative frequency are:

- Oesophagitis: 28%
- Gastritis/erosions: 26%
- Erosive duodenitis: 15%
- Varices: 13%
- Portal hypertensive gastropathy: 7%
- Malignancy: 5%
- Mallory–Weiss tear: 5%
- Vascular malformation: 3%

Scottish Intercollegiate Guidelines Network. Management of Acute Upper and Lower Gastrointestinal Bleeding. Edinburgh: Scottish Intercollegiate Guidelines Network; 2008. www.sign.ac.uk/pdf/sign105.pdf (accessed 13 June 2011).

16. B. The correct answer here is B. D is partially correct, but the trials/guidelines use 72 hours of therapy.

SSRI treatment can increase the risk of upper GI bleeding, especially in those at high risk and taking concomitant NSAIDs or aspirin. Number needed to harm per year was calculated as 411 for SSRI alone and 106 with concomitant NSAIDs. The relative risk of upper GI bleeding with alternative antidepressants is much lower. Therefore it is appropriate to switch the patient to an alternative non-SSRI antidepressant prior to discharge. Swapping to a non-selective NSAID does not necessarily reduce the risk of ulcer-related complications in a patient with a complicated NSAID-related ulcer.

The optimum dose of PPI for prevention of NSAID-induced ulcer complications is unclear. Studies have demonstrated that esomeprazole 20 mg is just as effective as 40 mg daily for ulcer prevention. There are no studies comparing the combination of COX-2 inhibitor and PPI with non-selective NSAID and PPI in patients with a history of ulcer bleeding. As generic PPIs have become cheaper, their use has become highly cost-effective for users of COX-2 inhibitors and NSAIDs, which has led to the recommendation for their use by NICE. For high-risk patients (those who have already experienced a life-threatening gastric ulcer bleed), the subsequent use of a COX-2 inhibitor with a PPI was remarkably associated with no recurrent events at all.

The patient should be tested for H. pylori status before commencing eradication therapy, either with a rapid urease test (e.g. CLO® test) at endoscopy, or if endoscopic biopsy is not done, by urea breath testing. If the patient tests positive, it is recommended that they go on to receive eradication therapy for 1 week and a further 3 weeks of PPI therapy to promote ulcer healing. In the absence of evidence to support a shorter treatment course, three weeks of ulcer healing PPI therapy is recommended following H. pylori eradication. There is no evidence to suggest that H. pylori influences rates of re-bleeding in the acute phase of peptic ulcer bleeding.

Loke YK, Trivedi AN and Singh S. Meta-analysis: gastrointestinal bleeding due to interaction between selective serotonin uptake inhibitors and non-steroidal anti-inflammatory drugs. *Alimentary Pharmacology and Therapeutics* 2008; 27: 31–40.

Scheiman JM, Yeomans ND, Talley NJ et al. Prevention of ulcers by esomeprazole in at-risk patients using non-selective NSAIDs and COX-2 inhibitors. *American Journal of Gastroenterology* 2006; 101: 701–710.

Norman A and Hawkey CJ. What you need to know when you prescribe a proton pump inhibitor. *Frontline Gastroenterology* 2011; 2: 199–205.

Gisbert JP, Khorrami S, Carballo F et al. *H. pylori* eradication therapy vs. antisecretory non-eradication therapy (with or without long-term maintenance antisecretory therapy) for the prevention of recurrent bleeding from peptic ulcer (Cochrane Review). In: *The Cochrane Library*, Issue 4. London: John Wiley & Sons Ltd; 2005.

Scottish Intercollegiate Guidelines Network. *Management of Acute Upper and Lower Gastrointestinal Bleeding*. Edinburgh: Scottish Intercollegiate Guidelines Network; 2008. www.sign.ac.uk/pdf/sign105.pdf (accessed 13 June 2011).

17. E. TIPSS is the recommended treatment of choice for uncontrolled variceal bleeding. Even though there is evidence to suggest that H-graft portocaval shunting may be more effective than TIPSS in uncontrolled variceal haemorrhage, the proportion of patients treated with surgical shunting on an emergency basis is much lower than the proportion treated with TIPSS.

Balloon tamponade is only a temporary measure until definitive treatment can be arranged with either TIPSS, endoscopic, or surgical treatment. It has an 80–95% rate of haemostasis in patients with either gastric or oesophageal varices. However, bleeding tends to recur when the balloon is deflated. In addition, complications such as pneumonia, oesophageal tears, and discomfort are significantly more common when compared with sclerotherapy or drug treatment.

Options C and D are not routinely used as treatment options for uncontrolled variceal bleeding.

Scottish Intercollegiate Guidelines Network. *Management of Acute Upper and Lower Gastrointestinal Bleeding*. Edinburgh: Scottish Intercollegiate Guidelines Network; 2008. www.sign.ac.uk/pdf/sign105.pdf (accessed 13 June 2011).

18. D. Option D is the correct answer regarding cyanoacrylate. Although it has been the treatment of choice for gastric varices, according to the SIGN guidelines it does not offer a lower mortality rate than TIPSS. In fact studies have found that there is no significant difference in mortality between the two treatment modalities. Instead they have found that the use of cyanoacrylate is more cost-effective than TIPSS.

The superiority of cyanoacrylate therapy over band ligation in treatment of gastric varices is due to the following:

1. Higher initial haemostatic rate (ie. no bleeding for 72 hours after treatment)
2. Lower re-bleeding rates
3. Lower treatment-induced ulcer bleeding
4. Lower amount of blood transfusions

Mahadeva S, Bellamy MC, Kessel D et al. Cost-effectiveness of N-butyl-2-cyanoacrylate (histoacryl) glue injections versus transjugular intrahepatic portosystemic shunt in the management of acute gastric variceal bleeding. *American Journal of Gastroenterology* 2003; 98: 2688–2693.

Lo GH, Lai KH, Cheng JS et al. A prospective, randomized trial of butyl cyanoacrylate injection versus band ligation in the management of bleeding gastric varices. *Hepatology* 2001; 33: 1060–1064.

19. A. A is the correct answer. Domperidone, despite being an anti-dopaminergic agent, does not cross the blood–brain barrier, so is not able to induce the central effects that other dopamine antagonists could. It acts on dopaminergic receptors in the upper gastrointestinal tract as well as the chemoreceptor trigger zone (CTZ), which lacks a true blood–brain barrier. Given the fact that in Parkinson's disease there is already impaired gastric emptying, domperidone's prokinetic effect makes it the most useful anti-emetic in this situation.

There are two important areas within the medulla that initiate nausea and vomiting: the emetic centre and the CTZ within the area postrema. The CTZ has five different receptors that may activate it:

1. 5-HT$_3$ receptors
2. Histamine H1 receptors
3. Muscarinic receptors
4. Dopamine D2 receptors
5. Substance P (also called neurokinin-1 neuropeptide)

Chemicals such as hormones, ketoacids, uraemia, opioids, and ipecac are all carried in the blood or CSF and can directly stimulate the CTZ due to lack of a true blood–brain barrier. During pregnancy, oestrogen is thought to be the cause of morning sickness due to its direct action at the CTZ.

Gastric irritation and distension, especially at the duodenum (a particularly strong stimulus), causes massive uptake of 5HT by 5HT$_3$ receptors within the postrema. Anti-emetics that work at this site are 5HT$_3$ receptor antagonists such as ondansetron and granisetron. These are therefore safe for use in Parkinson's disease. However, they do not carry the prokinetic effect that metoclopramide or domperidone have. They could therefore be used as a second-line anti-emetic in this situation.

Dopamine antagonists such as metoclopramide and prochlorperazine are effective anti-emetics. These dopamine antagonists freely cross the blood–brain barrier and have no selectivity for dopamine receptors in the CTZ. Therefore they can act on dopaminergic systems in other parts of the brain, worsening the symptoms of Parkinson's disease.

Haloperidol also has a strong anti-dopaminergic action, thereby worsening the symptoms of Parkinson's disease when used in affected patients.

Gan TJ, Meyer T, Apfel CC et al. Consensus guidelines for managing postoperative nausea and vomiting. *Anesthesia and Analgesia* 2003; 97: 62–71.

Pleuvry B. Physiology and pharmacology of nausea and vomiting. *Anaesthesia and Intensive Care Medicine* 2003; 4: 349–352.

Vella-Brincat J and Macleod AD. Haloperidol in palliative care. *Palliative Medicine* 2004; 18: 195–201.

20. B. Dopamine antagonists are not useful in motion sickness. Vestibular nuclei contain muscarinic and histaminic receptors, not dopaminergic receptors. Anti-muscarinic (hyoscine) and anti-histaminic (cyclizine) drugs are used in motion sickness, as both receptors are present in vestibular nuclei.

Studies have shown that, in early pregnancy, pyridoxine is more effective than placebo and other newer drugs in reducing the severity of nausea but not of vomiting. There is no evidence that it is useful in hyperemesis gravidarum.

Serotonin-receptor antagonists such as ondansetron have been found to be effective in managing postoperative nausea and vomiting (PONV), due to their ability to reduce activity at the vagus nerve, thereby reducing stimulation at the vomiting centre. It has also been found to be effective in managing chemotherapy-induced nausea and vomiting.

Metoclopramide is a dopamine antagonist, but in motion sickness it is not effective by itself. It is used in combination with hyoscine for its added advantage of being a prokinetic. Therefore in practice a combination of the two is routinely used.

Opioids cross the blood–brain barrier and stimulate the CTZ directly to induce the vomiting response. Dopamine-receptor antagonists which also cross the blood–brain barrier are thus recommended as the first-line treatment for opioid-induced nausea and vomiting.

Pleuvry B. Physiology and pharmacology of nausea and vomiting. *Anaesthesia and Intensive Care Medicine* 2003; 4: 349–352.

Mazzotta P and Magee LA. A risk–benefit assessment of pharmacological and nonpharmacological treatments for nausea and vomiting of pregnancy. *Drugs* 2000; 59: 781–800.

Jewell D and Young G. Interventions for nausea and vomiting in early pregnancy. In: *The Cochrane Library*, Issue 2. London: John Wiley & Sons; 2008.

21. C. Impaired gastric emptying is present in over 50% of patients with long-standing diabetes mellitus type I or II. It takes at least 10 years with diabetes mellitus before symptoms of gastroparesis such as nausea, vomiting, early satiety, and bloating develop. Gastric emptying is delayed during acute hyperglycaemic states.

Treatment initially involves tightening of glycaemic control in patients with appropriate anti-diabetic medication and symptom relief with prokinetics such as metoclopramide, domperidone, or erythromycin. Diet and social habits are also addressed. Patients are advised to reduce alcohol and tobacco consumption and to cut down on high-fibre foods, animal fat, and vegetable oils, which can all contribute to delayed gastric emptying.

If simple dietary measures and medication fail, and the patient is struggling to maintain weight, clinical practice is to consider artificial enteral feeding. A trial of nasojejunal feeding is therefore recommended in this patient. If a trial of nasojejunal feeding is well tolerated, the patient should be carefully considered for PEJ/surgical jejunostomy for managing their long-term nutritional needs.

Botulinum toxin is only used in clinical trial stages. It is thought to be useful as there is observational evidence which suggests that botulinum toxins help to inhibit pylorospasms and thereby improve symptoms. However, this is still only at clinical trial stages, and its use is still under evaluation.

Studies have shown that symptoms of nausea and vomiting as well as quality of life and nutritional status all improve following implantation of a gastric pacing device. Electrical stimulation is delivered by two electrodes (implanted laparoscopically or at laparotomy) on to the greater curve of the stomach overlying the pacemaker site. However, the mechanism of action is still unclear. Implantation is an invasive procedure and thus carries with it risks associated with surgery and especially that of infection. The procedure is noted to carry substantial morbidity and mortality rates. There are only a few centres in the UK with much experience of this procedure, and therefore it is not widely available. Most case series suggest that it is most helpful in patients with intractable and refractory gastroparesis.

Horowitz M and Fraser R. Disordered gastric motor function in diabetes mellitus. *Diabetologia* 1994; 37: 543–551.

Enck P, Rathmann W, Spiekermann M et al. Prevalence of gastrointestinal symptoms in diabetic patients and non-diabetic subjects. *Zeitschrift für Gastroenterologie* 1994; 32: 637–641.

Kashyap P and Farrugia G. Diabetic gastroparesis: what we have learned and had to unlearn in the past 5 years. *Gut* 2010; 59: 1716–1726.

Friedenberg FK, Palit A, Parkman HP et al. Botulinum toxin A for the treatment of delayed gastric emptying. American Journal of Gastroenterology 2008; 103: 416–423.

Epstein O and Patrick A. Review article: gastroparesis. Alimentary Pharmacology and Therapeutics 2008; 27: 724–740.

22. C. Option C is the correct answer, as there are two types of waves in the distal stomach:

- the slow wave—controlled by the interstitial cells of Cajal
- phasic contractions—controlled by the migrating motor complex.

Chief cells—present in stomach	(1) Production of pepsinogen
Enterochromaffin cells—present in the lumen of GI and respiratory tracts	(1) Stores serotonin
	(2) Mediation of serotonin release
Mucous neck cells—present in gastric mucosa and pits	(1) Protects gastric mucosa from corrosive gastric acid
Parietal cells—stomach epithelial cells	(1) Secretion of gastric acid and intrinsic factor

The proximal stomach serves as a reservoir for food and at its maximum relaxation, gastric barostat studies have shown that it can allow over 1 L of nutrients to be ingested. In addition, the proximal stomach also helps to regulate the gastroduodenal flow rate and provides the space and time for pepsin and hydrochloric acid to initiate digestion.

The duration of post-prandial motor activity varies according to the volume ingested as well as the chemical characteristics of the ingested foods. The maximum duration of post-prandial motor activity is 120 minutes.

CCK and GIP are hormones involved in producing a negative feedback to slow gastric emptying. CCK regulates gastric emptying and bowel motility to induce satiety, thus delaying gastric emptying. GIP is thought to inhibit gastric acid secretion and reduce the rate at which food is transferred through the stomach, thereby delaying gastric emptying.

Varón AR and Zuleta J. From the physiology of gastric emptying to the understanding of gastroparesis. Revista Colombiana de Gastroenterologia 2010; 25: 207–213.

Haans JJ and Masclee AA. Review article: The diagnosis and management of gastroparesis. Alimentary Pharmacology and Therapeutics 2007; 26: 37–46.

Ahluwalia NK, Thompson DG and Barlow J. Effect of distension and feeding on phasic changes in human proximal gastric tone. Gut 1996; 39: 757–761.

Feldman M, Friedman LS and Brandt LJ. Sleisenger and Fordtran's Gastrointestinal and Liver Disease: pathophysiology, diagnosis, management, 8th edition. Philadelphia, PA: Saunders Elsevier; 2006.

1. **A 55-year-old housewife had suffered diarrhoea, bloating, and weight loss for many years. The patient had started a strict gluten-free diet after reading about coeliac disease on the Internet and her symptoms dramatically improved. She had made an appointment to see her GP to discuss this.**

   Investigations:

   haemoglobin   107 g/L (115–165)
   mean cell volume   77.2 fL (80–96)

   She was referred for a gastroscopy, and duodenal biopsies were taken.

   Which one of the following duodenal histological features is most suggestive of a Marsh I classification of coeliac disease?

   A. Crypt hyperplasia
   B. Flat atrophic mucosa
   C. Increased mitotic activity
   D. Lymphocytic infiltration on the lamina propria
   E. Villous height/crypt depth ratio reduced

2. **A 32-year-old man with well-controlled Crohn's disease presented with diarrhoea. He had undergone a terminal ileal resection for localized disease 2 years ago, and was not taking any regular medication.**

Investigations:

haemoglobin	134 g/L (130–180)
white cell count	9.7 x 10⁹/L (4.0–11.0)
platelet count	235 x 10⁹/L (150–400)
plasma thyroid-stimulating hormone	0.7 mU/L (0.4–5.0)
plasma free T_4	18 pmol/L (10.0–22.0)
serum vitamin B_{12}	127 ng/L (160–760)
serum ferritin	39 µg/L (15–300)
red cell folate	470 µg/L (160–640)
serum C-reactive protein	6 mg/L (< 10)
faecal elastase	280 µg/g (>200)
SeHCAT scan	5% (> 15%)

Which of the following statements regarding his diagnosis is most accurate?

A. Coeliac disease is commonly associated with this disorder

B. Pancreatic calcification on abdominal X-ray would be expected

C. Symptoms of IBS are unlikely to occur with this disorder

D. Small bowel bacterial overgrowth can give false-positive SeHCAT scan results

E. Treatment with colesevelam could be considered

3. **A 57-year-old man presented to hospital with persistent, non-bloody, watery diarrhoea. His GP had trialled management for irritable bowel syndrome, and there had been some improvement with a wheat- and dairy-free diet. He had had severe peptic ulcer disease for which he underwent a Billroth II procedure 10 years previously, after presenting in hypovolaemic shock.**

Investigations:

anti-tissue transglutaminase antibodies	12 U/mL (< 15)
faecal calprotectin	36 µg/g (< 50)
faecal elastase	356 µg/g (> 200)
stool microscopy and culture	negative
hydrogen breath test (see Figure 2.1)	

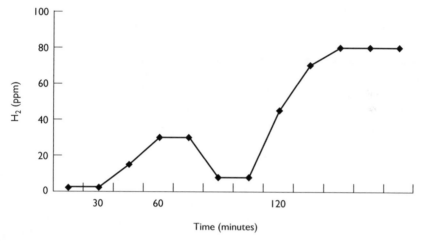

Figure 2.1 Hydrogen breath test

Reproduced from *Gut*, Simren M and Storzer P, 'Use and abuse of hydrogen breath tests', 55, 3, pp. 297–303. Copyright 2006, with permission from BMJ Publishing Group Ltd and British Society of Gastroenterology.

Which is the most likely diagnosis?

A. Bile salt malabsorption

B. Coeliac disease

C. Lactose intolerance

D. Pancreatic insufficiency

E. Small bowel bacterial overgrowth

4. **A 47-year-old man with a 25-year history of type I diabetes mellitus presented with intermittent, watery, largely nocturnal, non-bloody diarrhoea with a couple of episodes of faecal incontinence. He had no weight loss, abdominal pain, or fatigue.**

Investigations:

haemoglobin	134 g/L (130–180)
white cell count	9.7 x 10⁹/L (4.0–11.0)
platelet count	235 x 10⁹/L (150–400)
serum sodium	143 mmol/L (137–144)
serum potassium	4.6 mmol/L (3.5–4.9)
serum urea	6.8 mmol/L (2.5–7.0)
serum creatinine	123 µmol/L (60–110)
serum HbA1c	7.6% (< 6%)
hydrogen breath test	negative
colonoscopy	normal
colonic biopsy histology	normal

Which of the following neurotransmitters is most responsible for activating sensory neurones and thus the myenteric plexus, following stimulation of stretch receptors in the bowel?

A. Acetylcholine

B. Nitric oxide

C. Serotonin

D. Substance P

E. Vasoactive intestinal peptide

5. **A 19-year-old student was referred to clinic with persistent non-bloody diarrhoea, abdominal cramps, and bloating. She was in her first year at university, having returned from her gap year a month earlier. The symptoms started while she was travelling.**

Investigations:

haemoglobin	110 g/L (115–165)
white cell count	6.8 × 10⁹/L (4.0–11.0)
platelet count	415 × 10⁹/L (150–400)
MCV	88 fL (80–96)
serum albumin	37 g/L (37–49)
anti-tissue transglutaminase antibodies	11 U/mL (< 15)
plasma thyroid-stimulating hormone	1.7 mU/L (0.4–5.0)
stool microscopy and culture	negative
duodenal histopathology	villous flattening, deepening of the crypts, increased inflammatory infiltrate in the lamina propria. *Giardia lamblia* organisms seen

Which statement best describes the *Giardia lamblia* trophozoite cycle?

A. Trophozoites adhere to the mucosal surface, causing cytokine release and consequent fluid and electrolyte loss

B. Trophozoite colonization is limited to the upper small bowel

C. Trophozoites invade the mucosa and submucosa, causing cytokine release and consequent fluid and electrolyte loss

D. Trophozoites invade tissues and gain entry to the lymphatic system, facilitating systemic spread

E. Upon entry into the duodenum, intestinal bacteria break down the encapsulating cyst, releasing the trophozoite

6. **A 65-year-old woman presented to her GP with a 4-year history of watery diarrhoea. Her only comorbidity was depression, which was managed with sertraline.**

    Investigations:

haemoglobin	132 g/L (115–165)
white cell count	4.6 x 10⁹/L (4.0–11.0)
platelet count	470 x 10⁹/L (150–400)
MCV	88.1 fL (80–96)
serum sodium	137 mmol/L (137–144)
serum potassium	3.8 mmol/L (3.5–4.9)
serum urea	7.1 mmol/L (2.5–7.0)
serum creatinine	89 µmol/L (60–110)
anti-tissue transglutaminase antibodies	9 U/mL (< 15)
plasma thyroid-stimulating hormone	3.4 mU/L (0.4–5.0)
stool microscopy, culture, and sensitivities	negative
faecal elastase	405 µg/g (> 200)
colonoscopy	normal
colonic histopathology	pending

    Which of the following histological findings would be most in keeping with a diagnosis of collagenous colitis?

    A. > 20 eosinophils per high-powered field

    B. > 20 lymphocytes per 100 epithelial cells

    C. Focal active cryptitis

    D. Preservation of crypt architecture

    E. Subepithelial collagen layer 6 µm in thickness

7. **An 82-year-old diabetic woman was referred to the acute medical take with severe diarrhoea and abdominal pain. She was resident in a nursing home and had had a recent course of clindamycin for a chronic infection of her third metatarsal.**

    Which of the following is the gold standard method of determining clinically significant *Clostridium difficile*?

    A. Cell culture cytotoxicity assay

    B. Enzyme-linked immunosorbent assay

    C. Glutamate dehydrogenase antigen testing

    D. Polymerase chain reaction

    E. Stool microscopy and culture

8. **A 67-year-old man was referred to the gastroenterology clinic with diarrhoea, fresh rectal bleeding, lower abdominal pain, and pain on defecation. He had undergone chemoradiotherapy for rectal cancer, and radiotherapy was last carried out 12 months earlier. His bowel symptoms were getting worse and he had lost 8 kg in weight.**

    Investigations:

CT abdomen and pelvis	no evidence of recurrence of colorectal cancer
colonoscopy	no evidence of malignant recurrence; erythematous friable rectum

    Which of the following is the most appropriate first-line treatment?

    A. Corticosteroid enema
    B. Hyperbaric oxygen
    C. Mesalazine
    D. Metronidazole
    E. Sucralfate enema

9. **A 25-year-old girl with constipation-predominant irritable bowel syndrome (C-IBS) was referred to clinic with ongoing anal pain. She described excruciating pain on defecation with hard stools. On rectal examination her GP had identified an anal fissure. Treatment with warm baths, stool softeners, and topical anaesthetic gels had failed to provide relief.**

    What would be the next most appropriate treatment?

    A. Botulinum toxin injections
    B. Lateral sphincterotomy
    C. Topical diltiazem
    D. Topical glyceryl trinitrate
    E. Topical hydrocortisone

10. **A 39-year-old homosexual man was referred to clinic. He had a 6-month history of rectal pain, tenesmus, and a mucopurulent, occasionally bloody, anal discharge. He had lost 6 kg in weight and developed widespread lymphadenopathy. He had had three new sexual partners during the last year.**

    Investigations:

flexible sigmoidoscopy	distal proctitis, pus in rectum
colonic histopathology	possible Crohn's disease

    Which of the following most closely resembles Crohn's disease on histopathology specimens?

    A. *Chlamydia lymphogranuloma venereum* (LGV)
    B. *Chlamydia trachomatis*
    C. Herpes simplex virus
    D. *Neisseria gonorrhoeae*
    E. *Treponema pallidum*

11. **A 19-year-old British man spent July and August working at an American summer camp as a water-sports instructor. He was fit and well with no medical conditions.**

    He presented to his general practitioner the following April complaining of an intermittent patch of raised itchy skin, which appeared and disappeared in a matter of hours, at different sites on his back. He had had an area of inflamed skin between his toes while in the USA; he attributed this to a fungal infection. He had also suffered from travellers' diarrhoea while abroad.

    Investigations:

haemoglobin	156 g/L (130–180)
MCV	92 fL (80–96)
white cell count	10.2×10^9/L (4.0–11.0)
neutrophil count	6.5×10^9/L (1.5–7.0)
lymphocyte count	1.7×10^9/L (1.5–4.0)
eosinophil count	1.6×10^9/L (0.04–0.40)
basophil count	0.04×10^9/L (< 0.1)
platelet count	420×10^9/L (150–400)
stool microscopy and culture	negative x 3

    Which treatment is the most appropriate?

    A. Corticosteroids
    B. Filaricides
    C. Ivermectin
    D. Metronidazole
    E. Tiabendazole

12. **A 40-year-old man presented for the first time to your outpatient clinic. He had recurrent abdominal pain which improved with defecation, and mushy stools up to three times a day for the last 4 months. He denied weight loss, rectal bleeding, or a family history of colorectal cancer.**

    Investigations:
    stool microscopy, culture, and sensitivity   negative for ova, cysts, and parasites

    Which of the following is the next most appropriate management step?

    A. Abdominal ultrasound
    B. Colonoscopy
    C. Flexible sigmoidoscopy
    D. Thyroid function test
    E. Tissue transglutaminase

13. **A 38-year-old man presented to the gastroenterology outpatient clinic for the first time. He complained of recurrent abdominal pain, every other day, for the last 3 months.**

    Which of the following symptoms most favours a diagnosis of irritable bowel syndrome?

    A. Episodes of abdominal pain every 2 months
    B. Full sensation, even after a small meal
    C. Improvement with defecation
    D. Mucus discharge per rectum
    E. Nausea

14. **A 42-year-old male patient attended your outpatient clinic. He was diagnosed with acromegaly in his early twenties. He did not complain of any bowel symptoms, but has read about an increased risk of developing colorectal cancer.**

    His screening colonoscopy at age 40 years demonstrated one 3 mm hyperplastic polyp which was completely excised from the sigmoid colon. He is otherwise healthy and his body mass index is 25 kg/m².

    Investigations:
    thyroid-stimulating hormone   2.4 mU/L (0.4–5.0 mU/L)
    insulin-like growth factor-1   42.6 nmol/L (7.5–37.3 nmol/L)
    fasting plasma glucose   4.9 mmol/L (3.0–6.0 mmol/L)

    Which of the following is the most appropriate with regard to ongoing surveillance?

    A. Annual colonoscopy
    B. Colonoscopy at age 60 years on the national bowel cancer screening programme
    C. 5-yearly colonoscopy
    D. 10-yearly colonoscopy
    E. 3-yearly colonoscopy

15. **A 63-year-old patient underwent a colonoscopy to investigate a change in bowel habit. The colonoscopy report read as follows:**

    'The instrument was inserted to the terminal ileum, adequate bowel prep.
       In the rectum two 2 mm polyps were hot biopsied. A 4 mm rectal sessile polyp was excised and retrieved. In the sigmoid colon a pedunculated polyp of 15 mm was removed by snare polypectomy. A polyp of 7 mm and a polyp of 12 mm were found in the descending colon; these were snared and retrieved. Macroscopically all polyps were completely excised.'
       The histology report described four adenomatous polyps and two rectal hyperplastic polyps that were 2 mm in diameter.

    What is the most appropriate follow-up for this patient?

    A. Colonoscopy in 1 year's time
    B. Colonoscopy in 3 years' time
    D. Colonoscopy in 3 months' time
    C. Colonoscopy in 5 years' time
    E. Colonoscopy in 6 months' time

16. **A 35-year-old woman presented with a history of loose stools over the last 2 months. She was referred for a colonoscopy. Multiple polyps (around 50) were found in the ascending and transverse colon.**

    You asked about her family history and she revealed that her grandfather's brother died of bowel cancer, and her nephew recently had bowel surgery for polyps. Both of her parents, aged 65 and 70 years, and her two brothers, aged 45 and 42 years, are healthy.

    Which of the following is the most likely diagnosis?

    A. Familial adenomatous polyposis
    B. Juvenile polyposis syndrome
    C. Hereditary non-polyposis colorectal cancer
    D. MUTYH-associated polyposis
    E. Peutz–Jeghers syndrome

17. **A 20-year-old man presented to the gastroenterology outpatient clinic. He is an only child whose father was diagnosed with hereditary non-polyposis colorectal cancer at the age of 40 years, and died of colorectal cancer. No other family history is available. He is well and not complaining of any symptoms.**

    What is the next most appropriate step in his management?

    A. Colonoscopy and gastroduodenoscopy
    B. Colonoscopy from age 25 years
    C. Colonoscopy with dye spray
    D. 5-yearly colonoscopy from age 50 to 75 years
    E. Genetic testing

18. **A 23-year-old man attended the gastroenterology clinic for advice. His brother was recently diagnosed with familial adenomatous polyposis, and genetic testing identified a germ-line mutation. He asked for your advice on further management.**

    What would be the most appropriate next step?

    A. Colonoscopy

    B. Flexible sigmoidoscopy

    C. Genetic testing

    D. Oesophagogastroduodenoscopy and colonoscopy

    E. Prophylactic surgery

19. **A 40-year-old female patient presented to your outpatient clinic with a history of intermittent central abdominal pain. Examination revealed freckles on her lips, buccal mucosa, and eyelids. Her past medical history included breast cancer, which was diagnosed 1 year ago.**

    What would be the most appropriate next step?

    A. Colonoscopy and genetic testing for breast cancer susceptibility gene 1 and breast cancer susceptibility gene 2

    B. Colonoscopy and genetic testing for serine/threonine kinase 11 gene mutation

    C. Colonoscopy and mammogram

    D. Colonoscopy under the 2-week wait rule

    E. CT of the chest, abdomen, and pelvis

20. **A 20-year-old patient presented with iron-deficiency anaemia and intermittent abdominal pain. His brother had been diagnosed with juvenile polyposis syndrome.**

    Which investigation is the most appropriate next step?

    A. Colonoscopy and further surveillance

    B. CT colonography

    C. Genetic testing and colonoscopy

    D. Oesophagogastroduodenoscopy

    E. Video capsule endoscopy

21. **A 35-year-old woman complained of constipation for the last 8 months. She was treated with movicol and sodium docusate at the maximum doses; this did not improve her symptoms.**

    Which is the most appropriate next drug to try?

    A. Glycerol suppositories

    B. Lactulose

    C. Poloxamer drops

    D. Prucalopride

    E. Sodium phosphate enemas

22. **A 53-year-old woman was referred to your outpatient clinic. She complained of accidental leakage of solid and also liquid stools for the last 2 years. She denied any short-term diarrhoeal illness during that time. She was 167 cm tall and weighed 87 kg. There was no history of inflammatory bowel disease and she had been diagnosed with irritable bowel syndrome. She has smoked 20 cigarettes a day for 35 years. She had a vaginal forceps delivery at the age of 27 years and a cholecystectomy at the age of 40 years. On examination she was obese, but the physical examination was otherwise normal.**

    What is the weakest independent risk factor for faecal incontinence in this woman?

    A. Cholecystectomy
    B. Forceps-assisted delivery
    C. High body mass index
    D. Irritable bowel syndrome
    E. Smoking

23. A 72-year-old woman underwent a colonoscopy because of abdominal bloating and discomfort. The colonoscopy revealed brownish discoloration of the colonic wall. The histological finding is shown in Figure 2.2a/Colour Plate 1 and Figure 2.2b/Colour Plate 2.

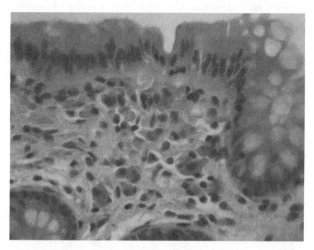

Figure 2.2a See also Plate 1. Permission granted by Dr N. Ryley, Torbay Hospital; slides from his personal collection.

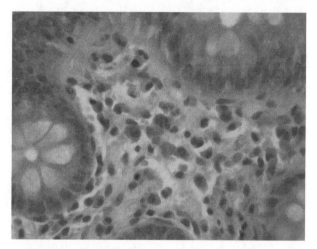

Figure 2.2b See also Plate 2. Permission granted by Dr N. Ryley, Torbay Hospital; slides from his personal collection.

The pigmentation found in the submucosa is most likely:

A. Haemosiderin
B. Iron sulphide
C. Lipofuscin
D. Melanin
E. Silicate

24. **This 51-year-old patient presented with a history of abdominal symptoms for 2 years. She opened her bowels every 4 to 5 days, passing hard and lumpy stool; she also complained of abdominal pain and bloating. She denied any weight loss, fever, or bloody stools. There was no family history of inflammatory bowel disease and she had no past medical history of note.**

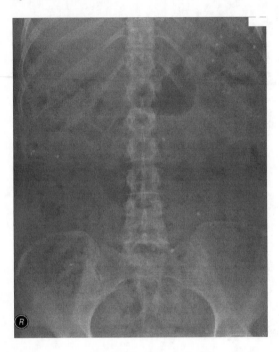

Figure 2.3 X-ray.

Investigations:

haemoglobin	125 g/L (115–165)
white cell count	5.6 x 10⁹/L (4.0–11.0)
platelet count	290 x 10⁹/L (150–400)
MCV	88.1 fL (80–96)
serum sodium	139 mmol/L (137–144)
serum potassium	3.9 mmol/L (3.5–4.9)
serum urea	6.7 mmol/L (2.5–7.0)
serum creatinine	89 µmol/L (60–110)
anti-tissue transglutaminase antibodies	9 U/mL (< 15)
plasma thyroid-stimulating hormone	3.4 mU/L (0.4–5.0)
stool microscopy, culture, and sensitivities	negative
faecal elastase	405 µg/g (> 200)
colonoscopy	normal
colonic histopathology	normal
ano-rectal manometry	normal

Which of the following is the most likely finding on a bowel transit study?

A. Constipation-predominant irritable bowel syndrome
B. Dyssynergic defecation
C. Normal-transit constipation
D. Slow-transit constipation
E. Slow-transit constipation and dyssynergic defecation

25. A 35-year-old woman is diagnosed with dyssynergic defecation. Which of the following is the most efficacious treatment modality?

A. Biofeedback therapy
B. Diet
C. Laxatives
D. Myectomy of the anal sphincter
E. Botulinum toxin injection

1. D. Coeliac disease is an inflammatory condition of the mucosa of the small intestine, caused by ingestion of gluten. It affects 1 in 100 of the UK adult population.

Patients may present with or without gastrointestinal symptoms and many will be anaemic at presentation. The commonest cause of this is iron deficiency followed by low folate; when combined this may result in a mixed picture. The blood film can show a hypochromic, microcytic, or dimorphic picture. Atypical presentations exist. Patients may have coeliac disease as part of a group of autoimmune conditions; they may also present with an itchy blistering rash suggestive of dermatitis herpetiformis, or a spectrum of neurological and psychological conditions.

A genetic predisposition exists, involving HLA class II molecules; approximately 95% of patients with coeliac disease express HLA-DQ2, and the remainder express DQ8. HLA typing indicating lack of DQ2 or DQ8 has a high negative predictive value for coeliac disease and may occasionally be helpful in excluding the diagnosis in ambiguous cases.

For either serological antibody or tissue diagnosis, there is a risk of a false-negative result if the patient is not consuming gluten at the time of investigation. Therefore in the case of this question, she should be advised to reintroduce gluten (at least 4 slices of gluten-containing bread per day for 2 to 6 weeks) before undergoing a gastroscopy.

Serological diagnosis involves positive ELISA detection of antibodies to the enzyme tissue transglutaminase (TTG). This enzyme is responsible for deamidation and subsequent increase in antigenicity of a specific peptide found in gliadin, which is the peptide to which the majority of coeliac patients react. Alternatively, IgA anti-endomysial antibodies (EMA) may be detected; although this test has a high sensitivity and specificity, it is more expensive and labour intensive. IgA deficiency must also be excluded to avoid a false-negative serological test.

The gold standard for the diagnosis of coeliac disease is biopsy of the mucosa of the second part of the duodenum. The table below describes the Marsh criteria for biopsy findings. With Marsh I and II, serology and symptomatology must be taken into account when making a diagnosis of coeliac disease, as lymphocyte infiltration alone is not diagnostic.

Complications of coeliac disease include the following:

- *Osteoporosis*. If untreated, 70% of patients with coeliac disease will have reduced bone density. All patients with coeliac disease should undergo DEXA scanning at presentation, and there are specific BSG guidelines regarding the treatment of osteoporosis.
- *Autoimmune diseases*. These may be co-diagnosed, and can improve when on a gluten-free diet.
- *Non-Hodgkin's lymphoma*, specifically enteropathy-associated T-cell lymphoma (EATL). Diagnosis is often delayed, and the majority are advanced and incurable at diagnosis and may require surgical intervention for perforation, haemorrhage, or obstruction.
- *Pneumococcal sepsis*. Patients with coeliac disease may suffer from hyposplenism, and vaccination against pneumococcus is recommended.

Classification	Histological features
Marsh I: infiltrative	Epithelial lymphocytic infiltration (IEL count > 40 per 100 surface enterocytes) Mucosal architecture is normal
Marsh II: hyperplastic	Lymphocytosis Crypt hyperplasia Increased mitotic activity Reduced villous height/crypt depth (VH/CD) ratio (normal VH/CD ratio is 3–5)
Marsh III: destructive	Villous atrophy IIIA = partial villous atrophy, VH/CD ratio < 1 IIIB = subtotal villous atrophy – some individual villi seen IIIC = total villous atrophy (resembles colonic mucosa)
Marsh IV: hypoplastic	Rare, may be irreversible Flat atrophic mucosa May be associated with development of enteropathy-associated T cell lymphoma

Data from Marsh M (1992) 'Gluten, major histocompatibility complex, and the small intestine. A molecular and immunobiologic approach to the spectrum of gluten sensitivity ("celiac sprue")', *Gastroenterology*, 102, 1, pp. 330–354.

Treatment involves strict adherence to a gluten-free diet, recovery may take months, and cases of refractory coeliac disease do exist. In these cases absolute adherence to a gluten-free diet must be confirmed, and there have been studies of the use of steroids, azathioprine, and ciclosporin. Elemental feeding may be required to overcome severe malnutrition, and regular screening for lymphoma is advised.

Refractory coeliac disease in the presence of a strictly compliant diet is challenging—investigation involves serial duodenal biopsies and exclusion of lymphoma. Immunosuppression may be required.

Ciclitira PJ, Dewar DH, McLaughlin SD et al. BSG Guidance on Coeliac Disease 2010. The management of adults with coeliac disease. www.bsg.org.uk/clinical-guidance/small-bowel-nutrition/bsg-guidance-on-coeliac-disease-2010.html (accessed 1 September 2011).

2. E. The primary bile acids cholic acid and chenoxydeoxycholic acid are synthesized from cholesterol in the liver, and are conjugated with glycine and taurine. These are stored in the gallbladder and then released into the small bowel in response to a meal, facilitating absorption of fats and fat-soluble vitamins. Around 95% of bile acids are usually resorbed in the terminal ileum and return to the liver via the portal system. However, those bile acids that transit into the colon are exposed to colonic bacteria causing dehydroxylation to form the secondary bile acids deoxycholic acid and lithocholic acid. These stimulate water and electrolyte release, resulting in the diarrhoea and other symptoms associated with bile acid malabsorption (BAM).

Figure 2.4 shows the recirculation of bile acids.

BAM is underdiagnosed, and is thought to affect up to 1% of the population. Causes of BAM can be primary—either idiopathic or due to other rare causes such as congenital deficiency of the sodium-dependent bile acid transporter. In the case of idiopathic BAM, some studies now suggest that the pathology may be due to overproduction of bile acids.

More commonly, BAM is a secondary diagnosis, as for example in Crohn's disease, ileal resection, post cholecystectomy, post infectious diarrhoea, ileal radiation enteritis, coeliac disease, and cystic fibrosis.

Symptoms are similar to those of D-IBS, namely bloating, abdominal discomfort, and diarrhoea. Patients may also suffer from steatorrhoea due to fat malabsorption, as there are fewer bile acids available in the small bowel. Gallstones may be a feature.

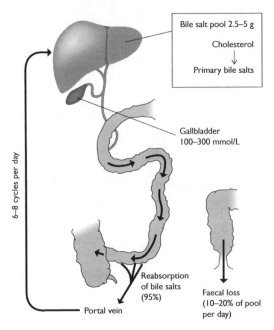

Figure 2.4 Recirculation of bile acids.

This article was published in *Clinical Medicine*, 4th edition, Kumar P and Clark M, Figure 5.5, p. 291. Copyright Elsevier 1998.

The BSG guidelines from 2003 suggest three options for assessing BAM:

- Measurement of the turnover of radiolabelled bile acids: this involves quantifying the faecal recovery of 14C-glycocholate in stool over a period of 48–72 hours after ingestion of an oral load of this marker
- Measurement of serum metabolites: this avoids the use of radiolabels and correlates with SeHCAT results
- Quantification of excreted bile acids by the selenium 75-labelled homotaurocholic acid test (SeHCAT): this involves ingestion of a synthetic analogue of the natural conjugated bile acid taurocholic acid. The retained fraction is assessed with a gamma camera 7 days after oral administration. Values of less than 15% are suggestive of BAM.

As some diagnostic modalities may be unavailable, a 3-day trial of cholestyramine, cholestipol, or colesevelam may give some indication as to whether BAM is the cause of the diarrhoea; occasionally cholestyramine may worsen the situation. The patient should be well hydrated to reduce oxalate gallstone formation. Supplementation of fat-soluble vitamins may be necessary.

Thomas PD, Forbes A, Green J et al. Guidelines for the investigation of chronic diarrhoea, 2nd edition. *Gut* 2003; 52 (Suppl. V): v1–15.

Bloom S, Webster G and Marks D. *Oxford Handbook of Gastroenterology and Hepatology*, 2nd edition. Oxford: Oxford University Press; 2012.

Walters RF and Pattni SS. Managing bile acid diarrhoea. *Therapeutic Advances in Gastroenterology* 2010; 3: 349–367.

Kumar P and Clark M. *Clinical Medicine*, 4th edition. Oxford: Bailliere Tindall; 1998. p. 291.

3. E. This patient has small bowel bacterial overgrowth (SBBO). There are very few CFU/ml of bacteria in the small bowel in the healthy state compared with the large bowel. This is thought to be due to a number of factors, including the ileocaecal valve, intestinal peristalsis, and gastric acidity. Factors that increase the risk of SBBO include intestinal dysmotility syndromes, which can be associated with systemic disease such as diabetes. Other factors include changes to anatomy, such as strictures, jejunal diverticulosis, or surgery. The risk is much higher if the post-surgical anatomy involves a blind-ended loop, such as a Billroth type 2 procedure.

Culture of small bowel aspirate is considered to be the most sensitive diagnostic test. However, there is poor standardization of results, and the test also identifies healthy individuals, as a positive result does not necessarily have clinical significance. Hydrogen breath tests are a non-invasive method of diagnosing SBBO. However, a number of bacterial flora, including *Staphylococcus aureus*, *Streptococcus viridans*, *Enterococci* species, *Serratia*, and *Pseudomonas* species, do not produce hydrogen, and therefore the result will be a false-negative. A trial of treatment with empirical antibiotics is the approach accepted in the BSG guidelines.

Thomas PD, Forbes A, Green J *et al*. Guidelines for the investigation of chronic diarrhoea, 2nd edition. *Gut* 2003; 52 (Suppl. V): v1–15.

Simren M and Storzer P. Use and abuse of hydrogen breath tests. *Gut* 2006; 55: 297–303.

4. C. Passage of food through the gastrointestinal tract is regulated by the enteric nervous system, which has two main networks—the myenteric plexus and the submucous plexus. The enteric nervous system is connected to the central nervous system by parasympathetic (cholinergic, increases intestinal smooth muscle activity) and sympathetic (noradrenergic, decreases intestinal smooth muscle activity) innervation. However, the gut does not need these connections to function: it can be autonomous.

Stretch receptors are responsible for the waves of peristalsis. Following stretch, serotonin is released, which stimulates sensory neurones that activate the myenteric plexus. This plexus contains cholinergic neurons which run in a retrograde direction and cause release of substance P and acetylcholine. These cause contraction of smooth muscle, so the contractile effect is behind the area of stretch, thus pushing the food further along the bowel. Distal relaxation is caused by cholinergic neurons running in an antegrade direction; these release ATP, vasoactive intestinal polypeptide, and nitric oxide, and so the wave continues.

The basic electrical rhythm (BER) is a pacemaker-like activity that coordinates peristaltic activity; it cannot cause a contraction but it can increase muscle tension. Contractions only occur as the BER wave is depolarizing.

Although patients with diabetes mellitus often have symptoms of delayed gastric emptying, and this is linked to chronic hyperglycaemia, they may also present with watery diarrhoea due to vagal and sympathetic nerve damage. Biofeedback training can improve continence. Clonidine can be used for gastroparesis, but is often not tolerated due to its adverse side-effect profile.

Duchen LW, Anjorin A, Watkins PJ *et al*. Pathology of autonomic neuropathy in diabetes mellitus. *Annals of Internal Medicine* 1980; 92(2 Pt 2): 301–303.

Ganong WF. Regulation of Gastrointestinal Function. In: *Review of Medical Physiology*, 19th Edition. Appleton and Lange; 1999. pp 459–467.

5. A. *Giardia lamblia* is a flagellate protozoan that exists worldwide and is spread by faeco-oral route. Chlorination does not eradicate the cysts, so water must be boiled or filtered. The cysts are ingested and, following excystation of the trophozoites, flat teardrop-shaped organisms are released. Excystation occurs after contact with gastric acid. The trophozoites undergo asexual reproduction in the gut and then colonize the upper small bowel using a sucking disc to adhere to, but not invade, the mucosa. In patients with achlorhydria they may colonize the stomach, and some patients have biliary involvement.

Adherence disrupts the brush border, causing cytokine release and water and electrolyte loss. The trophozoites will encyst as they pass through the large intestine, and cysts are passed in the faeces. The cysts are infectious and can survive outside the host; when ingested by the subsequent host they excyst again to form trophozoites.

Incubation times vary from a few days to several months. Symptoms include non-bloody diarrhoea, bloating, flatulence, and abdominal pain, and colonization can lead to malabsorption and weight loss.

Treatment is with a single dose of tinidazole or a short course of metronidazole. If the patient does not respond, consider treating them with higher doses of metronidazole and look for immunodeficiency or consider lactose intolerance, which can persist following treatment for giardiasis.

Gill GV and Beeching N. Giardiasis and other intestinal protozoal infections. In: *Lecture Notes in Tropical Medicine*, 6th edition. Chichester: Wiley-Blackwell; 2009. pp. 199–203.

6. D. Microscopic colitis can be divided into two subgroups—collagenous and lymphocytic colitis. There is also a mixed form in which there are histological features of both main subtypes. Presentation is with watery, secretory diarrhoea rather than bloody diarrhoea, and other non-specific symptoms such as mild abdominal pain and lethargy. Onset can be sudden or gradual. The cause is not always obvious. Iatrogenic causes include PPI, NSAIDs, and SSRIs, among others, and there is also an association with coeliac disease.

Diagnosis is based on histology; barium studies and macroscopic findings at colonoscopy will be normal. Biopsies need to be taken from throughout the colon, as there is a significant false-negative rate if only the sigmoid colon is biopsied. Right-sided and transverse colon biopsies give the highest yield.

Histological findings in microscopic colitis

- Collagenous colitis: increase in the colonic mucosal subepithelial collagen layer, a collagen band > 10 µm thick, usually type I or III collagen, rather than type IV
- Lymphocytic colitis: increased numbers of intraepithelial lymphocytes, > 20 lymphocytes per 100 epithelial cells. By comparison, the histological lymphocyte count in normal, IBD, and infectious colitis specimens is 4–5 lymphocytes per 100 epithelial cells.

Once a diagnosis has been made, first-line therapy is to consider withdrawal of potential causative medications and to investigate for and treat coexistent coeliac disease. For mild symptoms, anti-diarrhoeal agents such as loperamide or diphenoxylate can be used first, and if symptoms are moderate, consider other therapies such as bismuth salicylate, colestyramine, or aminosalicylates. If symptoms are severe, a course of budesonide may help. However, if corticosteroids are ineffective, other therapies such as azathioprine, 6-mercaptopurine, methotrexate or even surgery may be required. The patient can be reassured that although relapse may occur, there is no association with the development of malignancy; colonoscopic surveillance is not necessary.

Eosinophilic colitis is a rare diagnosis and a subset of the primary eosinophilic gastrointestinal diseases. Secondary eosinophilia may be induced by many factors, including parasites and drugs, but if these causes are eliminated, primary eosinophilia may be treated with steroids, antihistamines, leukotriene inhibitors, or possibly biological therapy. Diagnosis is based on history, serum and/or ascitic eosinophilia, endoscopy, and eosinophil count at histology. There is no consensus, but most authors use a threshold of > 20 eosinophils per high-power field.

Offner FA, Jao RV, Lewin KJ et al. Collagenous colitis: a study of the distribution of morphological abnormalities and their histological detection. *Human Pathology* 1999; 30: 451–457.

Bloom S, Webster G and Marks D. *Oxford Handbook of Gastroenterology and Hepatology*, 2nd edition. Oxford: Oxford University Press; 2012.

Yen EF and Pardi DS. Review article: Microscopic colitis—lymphocytic, collagenous and 'mast cell' colitis. *Alimentary Pharmacology and Therapeutics* 2011; 34: 21–32.

Okpara N, Aswad B and Baffy G. Eosinophilic colitis. *World Journal of Gastroenterology* 2009; 15: 2975–2979.

Fenoglio Preiser CM. *Gastrointestinal Pathology: an atlas and text*, 2nd edition. Philadelphia, PA: Lippincott-Raven; 1999. p. 863.

7. A. *Clostridium difficile* is a Gram-positive bacillus that colonizes the gut following transmission via the faeco–oral route and disruption of the gut flora, usually following a course of antibiotics. There is a relatively high carrier population, especially in hospitals or care institutions; there is no evidence that these patients should be treated for eradication.

The organism produces two exotoxins—toxin A (an enterotoxin) and toxin B (a cytotoxin). These are responsible for the development of inflammation leading to diarrhoea and possibly pseudomembranous colitis. Some strains may not produce toxin A, leading to false-negative results if only toxin A is tested for.

With regard to laboratory testing a variety of approaches are available, and hospitals will differ in their test sequence of choice. The options are as follows.

Glutamate dehydrogenase (GDH) antigen testing. GDH is an enzyme produced by all strains of *C. difficile*, whether toxin or non-toxin producing. This is a rapid test and it will determine whether or not a patient is colonized, so it could be used as a rapid screening test, if positive further analysis can be performed. Another initial screening test is the *nucleic acid amplification test (NAAT)*.

Cytotoxin testing. This can follow positive GDH antigen screening to determine whether or not the strain of *C. difficile* is toxin producing. This can be done by means of the following:

- *Cell culture cytotoxicity assay.* This is the gold standard for testing. However, it is expensive and time consuming. If positive it does not require a second confirmatory test
- *Enzyme immunoassay (EIA).* This uses reagents to detect toxins A and B. It is quicker and simpler than the cytotoxin assay, but has a higher rate of false negatives
- *Polymerase chain reaction (PCR).* This is a rapid test that has high sensitivity and specificity.

Anaerobic stool culture. This is not routinely used; it takes a long time to obtain results, and it does not differentiate between toxin- and non-toxin-producing strains.

The Department of Health updated guidance on the diagnosis and reporting of *Clostridium difficile*, published in March 2012, advises the use of the following diagnostic algorithm for interpretation of results:

- If GDH EIA (or NAAT) is positive, and toxin EIA is positive (PPV = 91.4%), *C. difficile* is most likely to be present and the case to be associated with a poor outcome
- If GDH EIA (or NAAT) is positive, and toxin EIA is negative, *C. difficile* could be present (i.e. potential *C. difficile* excretors)
- If GDH EIA is negative, and toxin EIA is negative (NPV = 98.9%), *C. difficile* or CDI is very unlikely to be present.

Health Protection Scotland supports the guidelines determined by the Scottish *Salmonella, Shigella, Clostridium difficile* Reference Laboratory and the Scottish Microbiology Forum, which advise initial and confirmatory testing as follows.

- *Initial test*: toxin immunoassay *or* PCR for toxin B gene *or* GDH test. A negative result can be established at this stage
- *Confirmatory test*: used if the initial test was positive, and using a different assay from the initial test. The test should be performed on the same faecal sample for all specimens testing positive on the initial screen—toxin immunoassay *or* PCR for toxin B gene *or* GDH test *or* cell-culture cytotoxin assay *or* C. *difficile* culture.

However, a positive cell-culture cytotoxin assay as a stand-alone test can confirm the diagnosis.

Other investigations of this patient may include an abdominal radiograph to look for toxic megacolon. Sigmoidoscopy and biopsy may be useful; insufflation should be done with caution, as the mucosa may be very friable. The classic appearance of pseudomembranous colitis at endoscopy is of white/yellow plaques, or a patchy or continuous pseudomembrane, with an oedematous and inflamed bowel wall.

Treatment is with oral metronidazole or oral vancomycin. If the patient is unable to take oral medications, intravenous metronidazole can be used. There is no role for intravenous vancomycin, as it is not excreted into the colon. In severe resistant cases, or when an ileus has occurred, there may be a role for rectal antibiotic enemas or surgery.

Loftus CG. Gastrointestinal infections, *Clostridium difficile*-associated disease, and diverticular disease. In: Hauser SC, Pardi DS and Poterucha JJ (eds). *Mayo Clinic Gastroenterology and Hepatology Board Review*, 3rd edition. New York: Mayo Clinic Scientific Press; 2008. pp. 193–204.

Advisory Committee on Antimicrobial Resistance and Healthcare Associated Infection (ARHAI), Department of Health. *Updated Guidance on the Diagnosis and Reporting of* Clostridium difficile. London: Department of Health; 2012. www.dh.gov.uk/prod_consum_dh/groups/dh_digitalassets/@ dh/@en/documents/digitalasset/dh_133016.pdf (accessed 29 April 2012).

Health Protection Scotland. *Recommended Protocol for Testing for* Clostridium difficile *and Subsequent Culture*. Glasgow: Health Protection Scotland; 2009. www.documents.hps.scot.nhs.uk/hai/sshaip/guidelines/clostridium-difficile/smf-recommended-protocol-testing-for-cdiff-2009–12.pdf (accessed 29 April 2012).

8. E. Radiation enteritis is damage to the bowel following radiotherapy directed to that region, most frequently affecting the rectum and sigmoid colon following radiotherapy to the rectum, cervix, prostate, bladder, or testis. The risk of developing enteritis is higher if concomitant chemotherapy is used. The risk can be reduced by insertion and subsequent removal of a tissue expander to push loops of bowel out of the radiotherapy field.

The onset of symptoms can be acute (within 6 weeks) or chronic, in which case it may not develop for years after the radiotherapy was administered. Symptoms include abdominal pain, rectal pain, diarrhoea, rectal bleeding, urgency, and weight loss. Patients may also develop symptoms associated with fistulating and structuring disease, as these are recognized complications.

Acute radiation enteritis is due to direct mucosal damage and may resolve when the course of radiation stops. Chronic radiation enteritis is related to atrophy and fibrosis of the epithelium, due to an obliterative arteritis leading to a chronically ischaemic segment of bowel.

Diagnosis is usually made on colonoscopy or flexible sigmoidoscopy; the findings include pallor with friability, and telangiectasias.

With regard to treatment there is very little evidence available, although sucralfate enemas have been shown in RCTs and case series to be useful. Hyperbaric oxygen has also been demonstrated in RCTs to be effective, but centres that offer it are limited, and the course of treatment is long. Some patients may not need treatment, but just simple symptom control measures, which may be medical (anti-diarrhoeal agents) or endoscopic (coagulation), although endoscopic measures are associated with risk.

Jervoise H, Andreyev N, Davidson S et al. Practice guidance on the management of acute and chronic gastrointestinal problems arising as a result of treatment for cancer. Gut 2012; 61: 179–192.

McKay GD, Wong K and Kozman DR. Laparoscopic insertion of pelvic tissue expander to prevent radiation enteritis prior to radiotherapy for prostate cancer. Radiation Oncology 2011; 6: 47.

O'Brien PC, Hamilton CS, Denham JW et al. Spontaneous improvement in late rectal mucosal changes after radiotherapy for prostate cancer. International Journal of Radiation Oncology, Biology, Physics 2004; 58: 75–80.

Kochhar R, Patel F, Dhar A et al. Radiation-induced proctosigmoiditis. Prospective, randomized, double-blind controlled trial of oral sulfasalazine plus rectal steroids versus rectal sucralfate. Digestive Diseases and Sciences 1991; 36: 103–107.

Chun M, Kang S, Kil HJ et al. Rectal bleeding and its management after irradiation for uterine cervical cancer. International Journal of Radiation Oncology, Biology, Physics 2004; 58: 98–105.

9. C. Following the initial development of an anal fissure, passage of subsequent stool will continue to irritate the area. The internal sphincter may be involved and can go into spasm, causing further pain. It also pulls the edges of the fissure further apart, impairing wound healing, leading to the development of a chronic fissure.

Although conservative treatment may be sufficient for some acute fissures, other patients will need medical or surgical therapy. Stool softeners may reduce the pain and progression of a fissure, warm baths may relax the sphincter, and topical anaesthetic gel can provide pain relief. The Association of Coloproctology of Great Britain and Ireland has provided a summary of treatment recommendations. It recommends diltiazem as the first-line treatment choice; this has the same efficacy as topical glyceryl trinitrate, with a better side-effect profile (25% of patients who use topical glyceryl trinitrate suffer from headache). Treatment with botulinum toxin has a similar efficacy to that of glyceryl trinitrate. However, it is more expensive and therefore may be used in patients whose fissures do not heal with topical (diltiazem or glyceryl trinitrate) therapy.

With regard to surgical treatment, lateral sphincterotomy is useful for healing fissures, with less recurrence than with medical therapy; however, there is a higher rate of incontinence following treatment. In general, sphincterotomy and the various alternative surgical techniques available should only be used if the patient does not respond to medical treatment.

Cross KLR, Massey EJD, Fowler AL et al. The management of anal fissure: ACPGBI Position Statement. Colorectal Disease 10 (Suppl. 3), 1– 7.

10. A. All of the infections in the table can cause proctitis, and often there will be coexisting infections. Patients should be tested for HIV, especially in cases of *Chlamydia lymphogranuloma venereum*, syphilis, and herpes simplex virus. Contact tracing should be instigated.

McMillan A, van Voorst Vadre PC and de Vries HJ. The 2007 European Guideline (International Union against Sexually Transmitted Infections/World Health Organization) on the management of proctitis, proctocolitis and enteritis caused by sexually transmissible pathogens. *International Journal of STD & AIDS* 2007; 18: 514–520.

Organism	Diagnostic test
Chlamydia trachomatis	Detection of specific DNA sequences by NAAT in rectal material
Chlamydia lymphogranuloma venereum	Genotyping of positive *C. trachomatis* NAAT material for LGV is advised. The histology of LGV proctitis may resemble Crohn's disease. Rectal PCR may detect chlamydial DNA that may not be identified on a swab sample. *C. trachomatis*-specific serology can help to support the LGV diagnosis when clinical features are present
Neisseria gonorrhoeae	Gram-negative diplococci may be seen within the cytoplasm of neutrophilic granulocytes. Material for culture of *Neisseria gonorrhoeae* should be obtained
Syphilis	Dark-field microscopy for treponemes. NAAT for *Treponema pallidum* DNA from biopsy material or exudate. IgG anti-treponemal antibody enzyme immunoassay with confirmation by another specific treponemal antibody test support a diagnosis of syphilitic proctitis
Herpes simplex virus	Nucleic acid amplification by PCR

11. C. This patient is suffering from strongyloidiasis due to infection with the nematode, *Strongyloides stercoralis*. This organism is not confined to the tropics or subtropics, but is also found in southern Europe and the USA. Many patients are asymptomatic during the acute infection stage, which usually occurs while walking barefoot on soil. The nematode larvae can cause an area of itchy skin at the site of entry, and this may be accompanied by non-specific abdominal pain, weight loss, and diarrhoea, and also rarely a cough and wheeze if the larvae migrate to the lungs.

The life cycle of *Strongyloides stercoralis* includes autoinfection via the colonic/rectal/perianal mucosa. Therefore a state of chronic strongyloidiasis can occur. The rash is described as larva currens—a creeping eruption thought to be pathognomonic for this condition. This rash is caused by subcutaneous migration of the larvae; it is raised and itchy like a wheal, transient, and usually develops on the trunk of the body. Other symptoms of chronic strongyloidiasis include vague abdominal pain, and intermittent diarrhoea and weight loss.

Diagnosis is difficult, as stool microscopy is often negative. Duodenal aspirate or biopsy and histology may be helpful, and a string-test may be used such as Entero-Test. A capsule contains a thread, the end of which is taped to the nose. As the capsule is swallowed and dissolves in the stomach, it releases the string, which passes through to the duodenum and 2 to 3 hours later is pulled back; the fluid is then examined. Serology ELISA tests are also available. However, in the presence of a typical rash, and eosinophilia with unexplained diarrhoea, a therapeutic trial of an anti-helminth agent may be successful. Tiabendazole can be used, but it is less well tolerated than ivermectin.

A rare complication of *Strongyloides stercoralis* is hyperinfection syndrome. This can be precipitated by immunosuppressive conditions, malnutrition, and other comorbidities, such as haematological malignancy, diabetic ketoacidosis, and (in the tropics) lepromatous leprosy. It can also be triggered by immunosuppressant treatment, especially corticosteroid use. These triggers can cause widespread dissemination of filariform larvae into tissues, with the risk of bacterial infection as they migrate through the bowel wall.

Features of hyperinfection syndrome

- Severe and often bloody diarrhoea
- Bowel perforation with multiple microperforations
- Bacterial peritonitis and paralytic ileus
- Gram-negative septicaemia
- Pulmonary exudates, haemoptysis, pleural effusions, and hypoxia
- Encephalitis and bacterial meningitis

Given the widespread dissemination of larvae, diagnosis with microscopy is easier in the hyperinfection state. Treatment is with anti-helminth agents and supportive therapy; in the UK, the anti-helminth agent of choice is ivermectin.

Gill GV and Beeching N. Strongyloidiasis. In: *Lecture Notes in Tropical Medicine*, 6th edition. Chichester: Wiley-Blackwell; 2009. pp. 322–325.

British Medical Association and the Royal Pharmaceutical Society of Great Britain. *British National Formulary 60*. London: BMJ Group and the Royal Pharmaceutical Society of Great Britain; 2010. pp. 415–417.

12. E. Irritable bowel syndrome is common; approximately 5–11% of the population are affected. Chronic abdominal pain, bloating, and altered bowel habit are the main characteristics. Irritable bowel syndrome cannot be cured, and treatment should focus on the relief of symptoms.

Diagnostic tests

If the patient meets the diagnostic criteria for irritable bowel syndrome, the following tests should be undertaken to exclude other diagnoses (blood tests would be expected to be normal in irritable bowel syndrome).

- Full blood count
- Erythrocyte sedimentation rate or plasma viscosity
- C-reactive protein
- Antibody testing for coeliac disease – endomysial antibodies or tissue transglutaminase.

The NICE guidelines suggest that the following tests are unnecessary in primary care to confirm the diagnosis of irritable bowel syndrome in people who meet the diagnostic criteria for this disorder:

- Ultrasound examination
- Rigid/flexible sigmoidoscopy
- Colonoscopy; barium enema
- Thyroid function test (however, the British Society of Gastroenterology suggests that testing should be undertaken in cases of chronic diarrhoea)
- Faecal ova and parasite testing
- Faecal occult blood
- Breath tests for lactose intolerance or bacterial overgrowth.

However, any woman aged 50 years or over who has experienced symptoms within the last 12 months that suggest irritable bowel syndrome should have appropriate tests to rule out ovarian cancer, following the NICE guidelines on ovarian cancer published in 2011.

- This includes a serum CA 125 and, if this is 35 IU/ml or higher, an ultrasound examination of the abdomen and pelvis.

Spiller R, Aziz Q, Creed F et al. Guidelines on the irritable bowel syndrome: mechanisms and practical management. *Gut* 2007; 56: 1770–1798.

National Institute for Health and Clinical Excellence. *Irritable Bowel Syndrome in Adults: diagnosis and management of irritable bowel syndrome in primary care*. NICE Clinical Guideline 61. London: NICE; 2008. www.nice.org.uk/CG061 (accessed 31 August 2011).

National Institute for Health and Clinical Excellence. *The Recognition and Initial Management of Ovarian Cancer*. NICE Clinical Guideline 122. www.nice.org.uk/CG122 (accessed 19 November 2011).

13. C. Improvement with defecation is one of the diagnostic criteria for irritable bowel syndrome; all of the others are 'supportive symptoms.'

Rome III diagnostic criteria for irritable bowel syndrome

Recurrent abdominal pain or discomfort at least 3 days per month in the last 3 months associated with two or more of the following, with symptom onset at least 6 months before diagnosis:

- Improvement with defecation
- Onset associated with a change in frequency of stool
- Onset associated with a change in form (appearance) of stool.

(Reproduced from *Gut*, Spiller R, Aziz Q, Creed F et al., 'Guidelines on the irritable bowel syndrome: mechanisms and practical management', 56, 12, pp. 1770–1798. Copyright 2007, with permission from BMJ Publishing Group Ltd.)

Supportive symptoms that are not part of the Rome III criteria include abnormal stool frequency ($\leq$ 3 bowel movements per week or > 3 bowel movements per day), abnormal stool form (lumpy/hard or loose/watery), defecation straining, urgency, or a feeling of incomplete bowel movement, passing mucus, and bloating or a feeling of abdominal distension.
Four subtypes of irritable bowel syndrome are recognized:

- Irritable bowel syndrome with constipation (hard or lumpy stools $\geq$ 25%/loose or watery stools < 25% of bowel movements)
- Irritable bowel syndrome with diarrhoea (loose or watery stools $\geq$ 25%/hard or lumpy stools < 5% of bowel movements)
- Mixed irritable bowel syndrome (hard or lumpy stools $\geq$ 25%/loose or watery stools $\geq$ 25% of bowel movements)
- Unsubtyped irritable bowel syndrome (insufficient abnormality of stool consistency to meet the above subtypes.).

All patients with possible irritable bowel syndrome should be screened for the following features which may suggest an alternative diagnosis:

- Age > 50 years
- Male gender
- Unintentional and unexplained weight loss
- Rectal bleeding
- Family history of bowel or ovarian cancer
- Change in bowel habit to looser and/or more frequent stools persisting for more than 6 weeks in a person aged over 60 years

- Nocturnal or progressive abdominal pain, which is not compatible with irritable bowel syndrome
- Short history of symptoms
- Nocturnal symptoms
- Anaemia
- Recent antibiotic use
- Abdominal or rectal masses
- Raised inflammatory markers
- Significant concern that symptoms may suggest ovarian cancer; a pelvic examination should also be considered.

National Institute for Health and Clinical Excellence. *Irritable Bowel Syndrome in Adults: diagnosis and management of irritable bowel syndrome in primary care.* NICE Clinical Guideline 61. London: NICE; 2008. www.nice.org.uk/CG061 (accessed 31 August 2011).

Spiller R, Aziz Q, Creed F *et al.* Guidelines on the irritable bowel syndrome: mechanisms and practical management. *Gut* 2007; 56: 1770–1798.

14. E. Patients with acromegaly:

- These patients are at increased risk of developing colorectal cancer
- Specific colorectal screening is required, which differs from other colorectal cancer screening programmes
- Colonoscopic screening should start at the age of 40 years (unless there are colonic symptoms at an earlier age)
- If an adenoma is found at first screening, or serum insulin-like growth factor-1 levels are elevated above the maximum of the age-corrected normal range, colonoscopic screening should be offered 3-yearly
- If the initial colonoscopy is negative, or hyperplastic polyps are found, or the growth hormone/insulin-like growth factor-1 levels are normal, screening should be offered every 5 to 10 years
- Colonoscopy is required rather than sigmoidoscopy, as a significant number of adenomas and carcinomas are right-sided
- Colonoscopy can be technically more difficult because of the increased bowel length, loop complexity, and poor bowel preparation. This can lead to a higher number of complications, and patients need to be counselled about this.

Cairns SR, Scholefield JH, Steele RJ *et al.* Guidelines for colorectal cancer screening and surveillance in moderate and high risk groups (update from 2002). *Gut* 2010; 59: 666–690.

Renehan AG, Painter JE, Duncan G *et al.* Determination of large bowel length and loop complexity in patients with acromegaly undergoing screening colonoscopy. *Clinical Endocrinology* 2005; 62: 323–330.

15. A. The British Society of Gastroenterology published guidelines in 2010 regarding surveillance following adenoma removal (see Figure 2.5).

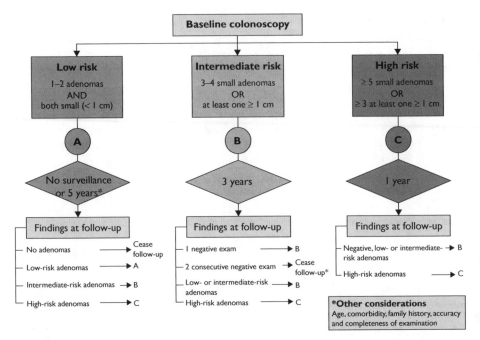

Figure 2.5 Surveillance following adenoma removal.

Reproduced from *Gut*, Atkin WS and Saunders BP, 51 (Supplement 5), pp. V6–V9. Copyright 2002 with permission from BMJ Publishing Group.

16. D. Cancer risk stratification for every patient should involve eliciting a family history of cancers, including the type of cancer, the age of onset, and a family history of colorectal adenomas.

Although there are rarer syndromes associated with excess colorectal cancer risk, the BSG guidance restricts the discussion to those listed above. All except MUTYH-associated polyposis are due to dominant transmission of a gene defect associated with a susceptibility to colorectal cancer and other cancer types.

MUTYH-associated polyposis (MAP)

- MYH is located on chromosome 1p and is one of three identified genes involved in base-excision repair (BER)
- The MutY human homologue (MYH) gene, which was discovered in 2002, encodes for MUTYH glycosylase, which is involved in oxidative DNA damage repair
- MUTYH-associated polyposis (MAP) is inherited in an autosomal-recessive pattern.
- It accounts for less than 0.4–3% of all colorectal cancers
- The lifetime risk of a homozygous person developing colon cancer is estimated to be 100% at 60 years
- The number of colonic polyps found in MUTYH-associated polyposis can vary significantly, from thousands to less than 100

- Upper gastrointestinal polyps (fundic and duodenal) have been seen, albeit rarely
- An increased incidence of breast cancer has been seen in female bi-allelic mutation carriers
- The population prevalence of heterozygotes is 1:100
- Heterozygotes may have a slightly increased risk of colorectal cancer compared with the general population
- Genetic screening should be offered to the partner and first-degree relatives of homozygotes.

Management

- Colonoscopy surveillance should start at 25 years on a 2- to 3-yearly basis using dye-spray colonoscopy for patients who are bi-allelic MUTYH carriers
- It is recommended that upper gastrointestinal surveillance is started at age 30 years and continued 3- to 5-yearly
- Depending on the number of polyps found and the degree of dysplasia, prophylactic colectomy should be considered
- Breast screening should be considered, as there may be an increased risk of developing breast cancer.

Clark S. *A Guide to Cancer Genetics in Clinical Practice.* Shrewsbury: TFM Publishing Ltd; 2009. pp. 75–84.

Cairns SR, Scholefield JH, Steele RJ et al. Guidelines for colorectal cancer screening and surveillance in moderate and high risk groups (update from 2002). *Gut* 2010; 59: 666–690.

17. E. Hereditary non-polyposis colorectal cancer (HNPCC)

- This is also known as Lynch syndrome
- It is the most common hereditary colorectal cancer syndrome; around 3–5% of all colorectal cancers are due to HNPCC
- The incidence of HNPCC is 1 in 3100 in the general population and up to 1 in 100 in patients with colorectal cancer
- It is an autosomal-dominant colorectal cancer syndrome with 80% penetrance for the development of colorectal cancer and 13–20% penetrance for the development of gastric cancer
- The onset of gastrointestinal cancer is early (mean age 44 years)
- Genetic testing is helpful in affected families, to predict whether relatives are affected
- The mutations accounting for HNPCC can be found in any one of four DNA mismatch repair (MMR) genes:
  - MSH2
  - MLH1 (MSH2 and MLH1 account for more than 80% of the identified MMR gene alterations in HNPCC families)
  - MSH6 (in 10% of HNPCC families)
  - PMS2 (infrequently)
- Microsatellite instability (MSI) occurs in most cancers and adenomas detected in patients with HNPCC.

Colonic manifestations

- Right-sided colorectal cancers (60–80% proximal to the splenic flexure), but many patients develop tumours in the left colon and rectum
- Colorectal cancers develop more rapidly than sporadic colorectal cancers

- Synchronous tumours (two or more tumours present at the same time) or metachronous tumours (where the first tumour is followed by a second one at a later date) are common, and any individual who is diagnosed with two primary colon cancers needs to be evaluated for HNPCC.

Extracolonic manifestations

- In patients with HNPCC, there is a significantly raised incidence of extracolonic cancers, such as malignancies of the gastrointestinal, female reproductive (endometrial and ovarian), and urinary tract, and neoplasms of the skin
- Female patients have a 27–71% lifetime risk of developing endometrial cancer, and a 3–13% risk of developing ovarian cancer.

Diagnosis

- Diagnosis is difficult, as there is no specific phenotype
- A strong family history of colorectal cancer or HNPCC-associated extra-intestinal cancers, or a history of colorectal cancer at a young age, should lead to a high level of clinical suspicion.

There are two main diagnostic guidelines which are used to identify patients with HNPCC in the western world:

- The revised Amsterdam criteria (Amsterdam II criteria) (1998) to identify families with a high risk of developing an autosomal-dominant-inherited cancer
- The Bethesda guidelines (1997) for patients with colorectal cancer at increased risk of developing HNPCC.

Amsterdam II criteria

- At least three relatives with colorectal cancer or a Lynch-syndrome associated cancer (endometrium, small bowel, or urinary tract)
- One relative should be a first-degree relative of the other two
- At least two successive generations should be affected
- At least one tumour should be diagnosed before the age of 50 years
- Familial adenomatous polyposis should be excluded in the colorectal cancer case
- Tumours should be verified by pathological examination.

(Reprinted from *Gastroenterology*, 116, 6, Hans F.A. Vasen *et al.*, 'New clinical criteria for hereditary nonpolyposis colorectal cancer (HNPCC, Lynch syndrome) proposed by the International Collaborative Group on HNPCC', pp. 1453–1456. Copyright 1999, with permission from Elsevier.)

Revised Bethesda criteria

- Colorectal cancer diagnosed in a patient under 50 years of age
- The presence of synchronous or metachronous colorectal or other HNPCC-related tumours, regardless of age
- Colorectal cancer with histology suggestive of microsatellite instability diagnosed in a patient under 60 years of age
- Patient with colorectal cancer with a first-degree relative with a Lynch HNPCC-associated tumour, with one cancer diagnosed under the age of 50 years
- Patient with colorectal cancer with two or more first-degree relatives or second-degree relatives with an HNPCC-related tumour, regardless of age.

(Reproduced from Asad Umar, C. *et al.* 'Revised Bethesda Guidelines for Hereditary Nonpolyposis Colorectal Cancer (Lynch Syndrome) and Microsatellite Instability', *Journal of the National Cancer Institute*, 2004, 96, 4, pp. 261–268, by permission of Oxford University Press.)

Management

Colonoscopic surveillance

- This should commence at 25 years of age, or 5 years less than the first colorectal cancer case in the family, whichever is earlier
- Colonoscopies should be repeated every 18 months up to the age of 70–75 years, or until comorbidity makes them clinically inappropriate
- Once a culprit mutation is found in a relative and the patient is confirmed to be a non-carrier, the colonoscopic surveillance can stop
- The patient is then followed up in the national colorectal cancer surveillance programme.

Upper gastrointestinal surveillance for HNPCC family members and/or MMR gene carriers

- In families where there are cases of gastric cancer, biennial upper gastrointestinal endoscopy should commence at 50 years of age, or 5 years less than the first gastric cancer case in the family, whichever is earlier
- Surveillance should continue up to 75 years of age, or until the causative mutation in that family has been excluded.

Endometrial and ovarian cancer surveillance

- Transvaginal ultrasound and aspiration cytology from 30–35 years of age may be useful for detecting early cancer.

Surgery

- The decision as to whether to perform segmental or subtotal colectomy with ileorectal anastomosis needs to be discussed with each patient individually
- An ileorectal anastomosis is advantageous, as it reduces the risk associated with the high rate of development of metachronous colorectal cancer
- Segmental resection leads to a better functional outcome, but with an increased risk of developing metachronous cancer, and therefore requires ongoing surveillance colonoscopy
- Chemotherapy needs to be discussed on an individual basis.

Clark S. *A Guide to Cancer Genetics in Clinical Practice*. Shrewsbury: TFM Publishing Ltd; 2009. pp. 85–98.

Cairns SR, Scholefield JH, Steele RJ *et al.* Guidelines for colorectal cancer screening and surveillance in moderate and high risk groups (update from 2002). *Gut* 2010; 59: 666–690.

18. C. Familial adenomatous polyposis (FAP)

- This is the second commonest inherited colorectal cancer syndrome
- It accounts for approximately 0.07% of colorectal cancer cases; the incidence of FAP is approximately 1 in 14 000 individuals
- There is autosomal-dominant inheritance with almost 100% penetrance
- The responsible adenomatous polyposis coli (APC) gene is located on 5q21 in up to 85% in patients with a clinical phenotype of FAP
- Approximately 30% of cases develop new gene mutations in the APC gene
- Lack of a family history of polyposis does not exclude FAP
- The classic FAP phenotype is characterized by hundreds to thousands of adenomatous polyps in the colon; these usually appear after puberty and increase in number with age

- The risk of developing colorectal cancer is nearly 100% by the time the patient reaches middle age, if not treated
- Around 90% of patients with FAP develop adenomatous polyps in the duodenum, particularly in the ampullary region
- Other extracolonic malignancies associated with FAP include papillary thyroid cancer, adrenal carcinomas, hepatoblastoma, central nervous system tumours, and desmoid tumours; cutaneous non-malignant lesions are seen more frequently
- Congenital hypertrophy of the retinal pigment epithelium (CHRPE) is more common in FAP.

Diagnosis

- Identification of a classical phenotype
- Genetic testing for APC gene mutations on chromosome 5q21.

Differential diagnosis

- FAP-like phenotype but no APC gene mutation found—consider MYH-associated polyposis
- Very strong family history of autosomal-dominant-inherited colorectal cancer, but no significant adenomatous polyposis—consider HNPCC.

Genetic testing

- If a culprit mutation for FAP has been identified in a patient, at-risk relatives should be tested for the specific mutation as well
- If the mutation cannot be found, they can be discharged from follow-up
- If the mutation is found, surveillance and prophylactic surgery should be offered to these individuals.

Management

Surveillance

- The initial entry age for entering bowel surveillance programme varies between endoscopy units.
- St Mark's Hospital in London starts annual flexible sigmoidoscopies at the age of 14 years
- At the age of 20 years the surveillance changes to a colonoscopy instead of a flexible sigmoidoscopy every fifth year
- Surveillance should not cease before the age of 50 years
- Once colorectal adenomas have been seen, upper endoscopy surveillance is recommended, starting at age 25 years and 3-yearly thereafter, to assess for adenomas in the duodenum and ampulla
- If large duodenal polyps are found, yearly endoscopic surveillance is recommended.

Surgery

- After confirmation of FAP, surgical removal of the colon is a life-saving management approach, and is the treatment of choice, as colorectal adenomas are too numerous to be removed endoscopically
- Total proctocolectomy with ileoanal anastomosis is one option, and requires annual pouchoscopy
- If less extensive surgery, such as subtotal colectomy with ileorectal anastomosis, is performed, the risk of neoplastic transformation requires 6- to 12-monthly flexible sigmoidoscopy
- If the rectum is preserved, surveillance is required every 6 months to 1 year for life.

Chemoprevention

- Although not considered a treatment for FAP, non-steroidal anti-inflammatory drugs and cyclooxygenase-2-inhibitors have been shown to decrease adenoma size and number in the large bowel.

Clark S. *A Guide to Cancer Genetics in Clinical Practice.* Shrewsbury: TFM Publishing Ltd; 2009. pp. 57–74.

Cairns SR, Scholefield JH, Steele RJ *et al.* Guidelines for colorectal cancer screening and surveillance in moderate and high risk groups (update from 2002). *Gut* 2010; 59: 666–690.

19. B. The hamartomatous polyposis syndromes include:

- Juvenile polyposis syndrome
- Peutz–Jeghers syndrome
- PTEN hamartoma tumour syndrome, including Cowden syndrome, Bannayan–Riley–Ruvalcaba syndrome and Proteus syndrome.

Peutz–Jeghers syndrome (PJS)

- This is an autosomal-dominant syndrome with high penetrance
- Its prevalence is 1 in 25 000 to 1 in 280 000 live births
- It is characterized by hamartomatous polyps throughout the gastrointestinal tract, but mainly in the small bowel, colon, stomach, and rectum
- Usually less than 20 polyps are found
- Mucocutaneous pigmentation occurs around the mouth, nostrils, perianal and genital area, hands, and feet
- PJS is associated with a substantial risk of colon, stomach, pancreatic, and breast cancers
- PJS is associated with an increased risk of colorectal, gastric, small bowel, pancreas, breast, ovary, lung, cervix, uterus, and testicular cancers.

Genetics of PJS

- Germline mutation – serine/threonine kinase 11 (STK11), also known as liver kinase B1 (LKB1) – associated with PJS is located on chromosome 19p13.3
- Approximately 40–80% of patients with PJS have no detectable mutation in serine/threonine kinase 11.

Diagnosis of PJS

This is based on any of the following:

- More than two hamartomatous polyps seen and histologically confirmed as Peutz–Jeghers polyps, *or*
- A single polyp seen in a patient with a close relative with PJS, *or*
- A patient with the classic pigmentation with a close relative with PJS, *or*
- A patient with any number of Peutz–Jeghers polyps and also the characteristic mucocutaneous pigmentation.

Genetic testing for PJS

- Features such as hamartomatous polyps or classic pigmentation should lead to genetic evaluation
- All first-degree relatives should be tested.

Colorectal surveillance for PJS

- This is not currently evidence based, because of the rarity of the disease
- On the one hand it detects polyp-related complications such as intussusceptions, obstruction, or bleeding; on the other it detects cancer early
- Colonoscopy and upper gastrointestinal endoscopy is indicated at 8 years of age
- Where significant polyps are seen, 3-yearly endoscopy is to be repeated
- If the baseline endoscopies show no significant polyps, routine surveillance should be repeated at 18 years of age and 3-yearly thereafter
- At the age of 50 years the surveillance frequency should be 1- to 2-yearly
- Small bowel screening in the form of video capsule endoscopy should be performed 3-yearly if polyps are found at the initial examination, from the age of 8 years, or if symptoms appear earlier
- If no polyps are found initially, commence screening with capsule endoscopy.

Clark S. *A Guide to Cancer Genetics in Clinical Practice*. Shrewsbury: TFM Publishing Ltd; 2009. pp. 203–224.

Cairns SR, Scholefield JH, Steele RJ et al. Guidelines for colorectal cancer screening and surveillance in moderate and high risk groups (update from 2002). *Gut* 2010; 59: 666–690.

Beggs AD, Latchford AR, Vasen HFA et al. Peutz–Jeghers syndrome: a systematic review and recommendations for management. *Gut* 2010; 59: 975–986.

20. C. Juvenile polyposis syndrome (JPS)

- This is a rare autosomal-dominant disorder (its prevalence ranges from 1 in 50 000 to 1 in 120 000) with full penetrance with variable expression
- Around 60% of cases are familial and 40% occur sporadically
- JPS is associated with a colorectal cancer risk of around 10–38% and a gastric cancer risk of 15–21%
- Hamartomatous polyps can be found throughout the gastrointestinal tract, but predominantly in the colon and rectum
- Cancers appear to arise from adenomatous components present in some juvenile polyps.

Genetics of JPS

- Mutations can be found in three genes—*SMAD4/DPC4* located on chromosome 18q21.2, *BMPR1A* on chromosome 10q22.3, and ENG1 on chromosome 9q33-q34.1.

Colorectal surveillance using colonoscopy for at-risk individuals and mutation carriers

- It is recommended that surveillance should start at age 15–18 years and be repeated 1- to 2-yearly thereafter
- It should continue until the age of 70 years
- Upper gastrointestinal surveillance should be undertaken every 1 to 2 years from the age of 25 years.

Clark S. *A Guide to Cancer Genetics in Clinical Practice.* Shrewsbury: TFM Publishing Ltd; 2009. pp. 203–224.

Cairns SR, Scholefield JH, Steele RJ et al. Guidelines for colorectal cancer screening and surveillance in moderate and high risk groups (update from 2002). *Gut* 2010; 59: 666–690.

21. D. Prucalopride is a selective 5-hydroxytryptamine type 4 receptor agonist; it has a stimulating effect on colonic motility. It is recommended for the treatment of chronic constipation in women who have been treated with at least two different classes of laxatives at the highest tolerated dose for at least 6 months, and in whom this treatment has failed to provide adequate relief, and invasive treatment for constipation is being considered. If it is not effective after 4 weeks, re-examination and the benefit of continuing treatment need to be considered.

The most common side-effects are headaches, abdominal pain, nausea, and diarrhoea, and they seem to appear early after starting treatment with prucalopride.

National Institute for Health and Clinical Excellence. *Prucalopride for the Treatment of Chronic Constipation in Women.* NICE Technology Appraisal 211. London: NICE; 2010. http://guidance.nice.org.uk/TA211 (accessed 19 November 2011).

22. B. Faecal incontinence is defined as any involuntary loss of faeces that causes a social or hygienic problem. It is a common symptom which is often under-reported due to social stigma. Around 0.5–1.0% of adults suffer from regular faecal incontinence which affects their quality of life. A common error is to assume that a single cause is responsible for the patient's symptoms.

Baseline assessment

- Take a relevant medical history
- Discuss the patient's bowel habit
- Consider faecal loading or treatable causes of diarrhoea (e.g. infective causes, inflammatory bowel disease, and irritable bowel syndrome)
- Red Flag symptoms for gastrointestinal cancer
- Perform a general examination and assess for disc prolapse/cauda equina syndrome
- Perform an anorectal examination, and assess for rectal prolapse, third-degree haemorrhoids, and acute anal sphincter injury, including obstetric and other trauma
- If appropriate, perform a cognitive assessment.

According to a population-based case–control study conducted by the Mayo Clinic, diarrhoea, IBS, and prior cholecystectomy are the strongest independent risk factors for faecal incontinence in middle-aged women in the community. The mean age of onset of faecal incontinence in this group was 55 years. Less strong risk factors are a high BMI, current smoking, rectocoele, and urinary stress incontinence. In contrast to being a risk factor for postpartum faecal incontinence, obstetric events on their own, such as vaginal delivery, forceps-assisted delivery, and episiotomy, did not predict delayed faecal incontinence.

National Institute for Health and Clinical Excellence. *Faecal Incontinence: the management of faecal incontinence in adults.* NICE Clinical Guideline 49. London: NICE; 2007. www.nice.org.uk/CG49 (accessed 18 November 2011).

Bharucha AE, Zinsmeister AR, Schleck CD et al. Bowel disturbances are the most important risk factors for late-onset fecal incontinence: a population-based case–control study in women. *Gastroenterology* 2010; 139: 1559–1566.

23. C. The pigment in melanosis coli is lipofuscin. Long-term use of laxatives such as senna and cascara causes damage to intracellular components, which are phagolysed. The products of this phagolysis are then found within the cells as lipofuscin. These cells are phagocytosed by macrophages which can later be found in the mucosa and submucosa of the colon.

Brown bowel syndrome is also a brown discoloration of the colon due to lipofuscin deposition. Unlike melanosis coli, the lipofuscin deposits are found in the tunica muscularis but not in the mucosa. An association between brown bowel syndrome, malabsorptive conditions, and hypovitaminosis E has been reported.

Aluminium, silicon, and magnesium are found in Peyer's patches in melanosis ilei. Haemosiderin in the lamina propria of the ileum has been found in a patient with melanosis ilei after chronic ingestion of iron.

Ghadially FN and Walley VM. Melanoses of the gastrointestinal tract. *Histopathology* 1994; 25: 197–207.

Cha JM, Lee JL, Joo KR *et al*. Melanosis ilei associated with chronic ingestion of oral iron. *Gut and Liver* 2009; 3: 315–317.

24. D. Colon transit time can be measured by any of three methods:

1. Ingestion of radio-opaque markers followed by abdominal X-ray
2. Radioisotopes and scintigraphy
3. Ingestion of a pressure and pH capsule (wireless motility capsule) and tracking its movement.

Using radio-opaque markers, the measurement of whole gut transit time (primarily colon transit time) is inexpensive, simple, and safe. The test is typically performed by administering a single capsule containing 24 plastic markers on day 1, followed by a plain abdominal X-ray on day 6 (120 hours later). In patients with normal transit time, less than 5 markers remain in the colon. The presence of 6 or more markers scattered throughout the colon is diagnostic of slow bowel transit. In dyssynergic defecation, 6 or more markers are found in the rectosigmoid region, with near normal transit of markers through the rest of the colon.

Primary or functional constipation

Constipation is common and polysymptomatic. The prevalence of chronic constipation ranges from 2% to 28%. Constipation is more common in women, with an estimated female: male ratio of 2.2:1. Its prevalence increases with advancing age. Chronic constipation has a significant impact on quality of life, and is a major cause of psychological distress.

Three subtypes of primary or functional constipation are known (of which slow-transit constipation and dyssynergic defecation are discussed in more detail here), and overlaps exist.

- *Slow-transit constipation* is characterized by prolonged delay of the transit time of stool through the colon
- *Dyssynergic defecation* (also known as anismus, pelvic floor dyssynergia, or outlet obstruction) is difficulty in expelling or inability to expel stool from the anorectum
- *Constipation-predominant irritable bowel syndrome* is characterized by symptoms of constipation, with discomfort or pain as a prominent feature.

Secondary causes of constipation

These include the following:

- Colonic pathology (e.g. stricture, cancer, anal fissure, proctitis, rectocoele)
- Metabolic pathology (e.g. hypercalcaemia, hypothyroidism, diabetes mellitus)

- Neurological disorders (e.g. parkinsonism, spinal cord lesions)
- Psychiatric disorders
- Drugs
- Diet and behavioural lifestyle.

Pathophysiology of dyssynergic defecation

- This is either an acquired behavioural disorder of defecation, or the process of defecation may not have been learned in childhood
- Normally, when an individual attempts to defecate, the rectal pressure rises. In addition, the anal sphincter pressure falls, mainly due to relaxation of the external anal sphincter. This manoeuvre is under voluntary control and is primarily a learned response
- The failure of rectoanal coordination in dyssynergic defecation consists of either impaired rectal contraction (61%), paradoxical anal contraction (78%), or inadequate anal relaxation.
- This incoordination or dyssynergia is primarily responsible for this condition
- Around 50–60% of patients also demonstrate an impaired rectal sensation
- In many patients there is an overlap with slow-transit constipation, because colonic transit is delayed in two-thirds of patients with difficult defecation
- Patients with defecation disorders often have several psychological abnormalities, such as such as obsessive-compulsive disorder, phobia with regard to stool impaction, or bulimia or anorexia nervosa, and often a history of physical or sexual abuse is found.

Pathophysiology of slow-transit constipation

- This is caused by a primary dysfunction of the colonic smooth muscle (myopathy) or its nerve innervations (neuropathy), or an evacuation disorder, such as dyssynergic defecation
- Colonic manometry shows significant impairment of the phasic colonic motor activity
- There is a significant decrease in the high amplitude and velocity of infrequent forceful propulsive waves known as high-amplitude propagated contractions (HAPCs)
- There is a significant reduction in the gastrocolonic responses following a meal and the morning waking responses after sleep, but preservation of the diurnal variation of colonic motor activity
- There is a significant increase in periodic rectal motor activity—a 3-cycles-per-minute activity that predominantly occurs in the rectum and rectosigmoid region and is invariably seen at night-time.

Diagnosis of functional constipation

Constipated patients present with a multitude of symptoms, and a detailed medical, surgical, dietary, and drug history is important in pointing towards the diagnosis of constipation. Alarm symptoms such as weight loss, bleeding, recent change in bowel habit, and significant abdominal pain need to be ruled out. The history should also include an assessment of stool frequency, stool consistency, and stool size. The Bristol Stool Scale is an invaluable tool in the assessment of constipation.

The Rome III diagnostic criteria distinguish between functional constipation and constipation-predominant irritable bowel syndrome (symptoms ≥ 3 months; onset ≥ 6 months prior to diagnosis).

Functional constipation	Constipation-predominant irritable bowel syndrome

• Must include at least two of the following:
   ✦ Straining*
   ✦ Lumpy or hard stools*
   ✦ Sensation of incomplete evacuation*
   ✦ Sensation of anorectal
   ✦ obstruction/blockage*
   ✦ Manual manoeuvres to facilitate defecation (e.g. digital evacuation, support of the pelvic floor)*
   ✦ < 3 defecations/week
• Loose stool rarely present without the use of laxatives
• Insufficient criteria for IBS-C
	• Irritable bowel syndrome: recurrent abdominal pain/discomfort
	   ✦ ≥3 days/month for the past 3 month, associated with ≥2 of the following:
	   ✦ Improvement with defecation
	   ✦ Onset associated with change in stool frequency
	   ✦ Onset associated with change in stool form
	• Hard or lumpy stools† ≥25% of defecations

* ≥ 25% of defecations.
† Bristol Stool Form Scale Type 1 (separate hard lumps, like nuts; difficult to pass) or Type 2 (lumpy, sausage-shaped stool).
Reprinted from *Gastroenterology*, 130, 5, Longstreth GF, Thompson WG, Chey WD, *et al.*, 'Functional bowel disorders', pp. 1480–1491. Copyright 2006, with permission from Elsevier.

Additional diagnostic criteria for dyssynergic defecation

1. Patients must satisfy the diagnostic criteria for functional chronic constipation (Rome III), *and*
2. Patients must demonstrate dyssynergia during repeated attempts to defecate.

In a normal pattern of defecation there is an increase in intrarectal pressure and simultaneously a relaxation of the anal sphincter. In patients with dyssynergic defecation, one of four abnormal patterns of defecation can be found:

- *Type I dyssynergia*—a rise in intrarectal pressure (≥ 40 mmHg) together with a paradoxical increase in anal sphincter pressure
- *Type II dyssynergia*—inadequate propulsive force with paradoxical anal contraction
- *Type III dyssynergia*—adequate propulsive force but either absent relaxation (a flat line) or incomplete (≤ 20%) relaxation of the anal sphincter
- *Type IV dyssynergia*—inadequate propulsive force together with absent or incomplete relaxation of the anal sphincter.

One or more of the following criteria during repeated attempts to defecate:

1. Inability to expel an artificial stool (a 50-mL water-filled balloon) within 1 minute
2. A prolonged colonic transit time, as demonstrated by more than 5 markers (≥ 20% marker retention) on a plain abdominal X-ray taken 120 hours after ingestion of one Sitzmark® capsule containing 24 radio-opaque markers
3. Inability to evacuate or ≥ 50% retention of barium during defecography.

(Reprinted from *Gastroenterology Clinics of North America*, 30, 1, Satish SC Rao, 'Dyssynergic defecation', pp. 97–114. Copyright 2001, with permission from Elsevier.)

Assessment

- Physical examination, including perianal/anal and digital rectal examination, observed simulated defecation, and neurological examination
- Blood tests, including full blood count, urea and electrolytes, liver function test, serum calcium, glucose levels, and thyroid function tests. If there is a high index of clinical suspicion, serum

protein electrophoresis, urine porphyrins, serum parathyroid hormone, and serum cortisol levels should be evaluated

- Imaging and manometry:
  - Abdominal X-ray
  - Endoscopic evaluation of the colon may be justified for patients aged 50 years or over with new symptoms, or for patients with alarm features, or a family history of colon cancer
  - Colonic transit study
  - Anorectal manometry (which is essential for a diagnosis of dyssynergic defecation).

Rao SSC. Constipation: evaluation and treatment of colonic and anorectal motility disorders. *Gastroenterology Clinics of North America* 2007; 36: 687–711.

Longstreth GF, Thompson WG, Chey WD et al. Functional bowel disorders. *Gastroenterology* 2006; 130: 1480–1491.

25. A. Biofeedback therapy is not only efficacious but also superior to other treatment modalities in dyssynergic defecation. Other modalities include:

- Avoiding constipating medications
- Increasing fibre (optimal intake is 20–30 g daily) and fluid intake
- Exercise
- Timed toilet training
- Laxatives
- Myectomy of the anal sphincter helps only 10–30% of patients
- Using botulinum toxin injections to paralyse the anal sphincter muscle and reverse the anal spasm shows no improvement.

In constipation that is refractory to medical therapy, surgery can be an option, including colectomy, ileostomy, or ileorectal anastomosis.

Rao SSC. Constipation: evaluation and treatment of colonic and anorectal motility disorders. *Gastroenterology Clinics of North America* 2007; 36: 687–711.

1. **A 26-year-old woman was admitted under the surgical team with abdominal pains, which were worsening over the last week. She has a past medical history of endometriosis, treated laparoscopically 3 weeks ago, for which she takes ibuprofen intermittently. Which of the following makes Crohn's disease the most likely diagnosis?**

    A. Abdominal fistula on examination
    B. Bright red blood per rectum and family history of inflammatory bowel disease
    C. Patchy rectal erythema on proctoscopy
    D. Small bowel stricturing on CT abdomen
    E. Terminal ileal ulceration at colonoscopy

2. **A 34-year-old man attended clinic with a new confirmed diagnosis of ulcerative colitis. In the outpatient clinic he had several questions about ulcerative colitis.**

    Regarding ulcerative colitis, which of the following statements is most accurate?

    A. Around 25% of patients with pancolitis eventually have a colectomy
    B. At 10 years, disease extent progresses in less than 10% of patients with proctitis
    C. The incidence of colorectal cancer is 20% at 20 years, and 40% at 30 years
    D. Maintenance 5-ASA therapy reduces colorectal cancer by 10%
    E. The relapse rate is 20% per year

3. **A 47-year-old man attended the gastroenterology clinic frustrated with changes to the surveillance interval for his long-standing ulcerative colitis. Both his grandfathers died from colorectal cancer in their sixties.**

    He was diagnosed 15 years ago and initially had left-sided disease; a year later he had a severe flare and intravenous steroids. A flexible sigmoidoscopy was performed during the flare, which demonstrated dysplasia in one of several post-inflammatory polyps; this polyp was completely excised and the patient declined colectomy at this time.

    A colonoscopy performed 10 years after diagnosis for screening was macroscopically normal, but biopsies demonstrated pancolitis, with mild activity.

    A month ago, 15 years after diagnosis, azathioprine was commenced, when a colonoscopic biopsy series demonstrated persistent mild colitis activity.

    When planning his surveillance, which of the following is most accurate?

    A. Annual surveillance is warranted, as dysplasia has been previously documented
    B. Colonoscopy is annual in the presence of post-inflammatory polyps
    C. Colorectal cancer in two relatives aged over 50 years warrants 3-yearly surveillance
    D. Left-sided colitis at diagnosis warrants 5-yearly colonic surveillance
    E. Surveillance should have occurred 2 years earlier according to guidelines

4. **A 36-year-old woman presented with rectal bleeding, tenesmus, and mucus discharge 3 years after a temporary loop ileostomy for refractory colonic Crohn's disease. After surgery she was managed in the community without further symptoms or medical therapy. She underwent stomoscopy, at which the mucosa was macroscopically normal. At flexible sigmoidoscopy, a diagnosis of diversion colitis was made.**

    What is the most appropriate next step?

    A. 5-ASA enemas
    B. Acetarsol suppositories
    C. Corticosteroid enemas
    D. Referral to surgeons
    E. Short-chain fatty acid enemas

5. **A 70-year-old woman presented to the gastroenterology outpatient clinic with a new diagnosis of inflammatory bowel disease unclassified (IBDU) on histology. Her general practitioner had performed rigid sigmoidoscopy for a long history of rectal bleeding, abdominal pain, and intermittent diarrhoea. The patient had a long history of arthralgia.**

    Which of the following extraintestinal manifestations of IBD is most likely to improve when a flare is successfully treated?

    A. Ankylosing spondylitis
    B. Episcleritis
    C. Primary sclerosing cholangitis
    D. pyoderma gangrenosum
    E. Scleritis

6. **A 41-year-old man with Crohn's disease underwent ileocaecal resection 2 months ago. His background medical history included type 2 diabetes mellitus, hypothyroidism, gastro-oesophageal reflux disease, and cholecystectomy. His long-standing medications included lansoprazole, aspirin, metformin, mesalazine, and co-codamol 30/500. He presented to the outpatient clinic complaining of loose stools 10 to 12 times daily and weight loss.**

    Investigations:

haemoglobin	112 g/L (130–180)
white cell count	7.6×10^9/L (4.0–11.0)
platelet count	202×10^9/L (150–400)
plasma thyroid-stimulating hormone	0.5 mU/L (0.4–5.0)
plasma free T_4	21.6 pmol/L (10.0–22.0)
haemoglobin A1c	9.0% (4.0–6.0)
serum vitamin B_{12}	127 ng/L (160–760)
red cell folate	770 µg/L (160–640)
serum C-reactive protein	9 mg/L (< 10)

    What is the most likely cause of the diarrhoea?

    A. Bile salt malabsorption
    B. Crohn's disease recurrence
    C. Metformin
    D. Over-treatment of hypothyroidism
    E. Small bowel bacterial overgrowth

7. **A 57-year-old man with pan-ulcerative colitis was admitted to hospital with 15 loose, bloody stools per day. On the third day of intravenous corticosteroids, his stool chart showed 9 bloody stools in the last 24 hours, his temperature was 37.6°C, and he had no abdominal pain. Abdominal X-ray excluded toxic megacolon. His blood pressure was 205/106 mmHg, his pulse was 86 beats/minute, and his urine output was 1 mL/kg/hour. His previous medical history included treatment for tuberculosis, hypertension, previous alcohol excess, and evidence of fatty liver disease.**

Investigations:

haemoglobin	98 g/L (130–180)
white cell count	12.0 x 10⁹/L (4.0–11.0)
platelet count	455 x 10⁹/L (150–400)
serum C-reactive protein	40 mg/L (< 10)
serum cholesterol	2.6 mmol/L (< 5.2)
serum magnesium	0.8 mmol/L (0.75–1.05)
serum alanine aminotransferase	35 U/L (5–35)
serum alkaline phosphatase	104 U/L (45–105)

What is the most appropriate plan?

A. Continue intravenous steroids for a further 3 days

B. Infliximab 5 mg/kg intravenous induction regime

C. Intravenous ciclosporin at a dose of 4 mg/kg per day

D. Oral ciclosporin at a dose of 2 mg/kg per day in divided doses

E. Subtotal colectomy

8. **A 35-year-old woman with ulcerative colitis was reviewed in the outpatient clinic. Her bowels were open one to three times per day, with soft brown stool. She did not report any symptoms and her weight was stable. She was diagnosed at the age of 18 years; she last had a colonoscopy at the age of 28 years, which showed evidence of quiescent inflammatory bowel disease consistent with pan-ulcerative colitis.**

Investigations:

haemoglobin	105 g/L (130–180)
MCV	77 fL (80–96)
serum ferritin	9 µg/L (15–300)
white cell count	12.0 × 10⁹/L (4.0–11.0)
platelet count	299 × 10⁹/L (150–400)
serum C-reactive protein	40 mg/L (< 10)
serum total bilirubin	26 µmol/L (1–22)
serum alanine aminotransferase	82 U/L (5–35)
serum alkaline phosphatase	167 U/L (45–105)
international normalized ratio	1.1 (< 1.4)
serum albumin	33 g/L (37–49)

Which of the following would be the most important investigation?

A. Colonoscopy

B. Gastroscopy (with duodenal biopsies)

C. Magnetic resonance cholangiopancreatogram

D. Ultrasound of the liver

E. Video capsule endoscopy

9. **A 26-year-old-woman attended the specialist nurse inflammatory bowel disease outpatient clinic, and the nurse contacted you for advice. The patient had left-sided ulcerative colitis diagnosed 5 years ago, which was confirmed as inactive on colonoscopy 6 months earlier. Having previously been in remission on mesalazine 1200 mg twice daily, despite good compliance, the patient's bowel frequency had increased to five times a day and there had been some rectal bleeding. Her GP had increased the mesalazine to 2400 mg twice daily 1 week ago, but without benefit. She was apyrexial, her pulse was 56 beats/minute, and her blood pressure was 120/70 mmHg.**

Investigations:

haemoglobin	134 g/L (130–180)
white cell count	9.0×10^9/L (4.0–11.0)
platelet count	320×10^9/L (150–400)
serum C-reactive protein	40 mg/L (< 10)
serum alanine aminotransferase	26 U/L (5–35)
serum alkaline phosphatase	96 U/L (45–105)

What should you recommend?

A. Azathioprine

B. Mesalazine enema

C. Mesalazine suppository

D. Oral prednisolone reducing course

E. Steroid enema

10. **A 66-year-old woman, who was previously well, presented with a 2-week history of abdominal pains, fevers, malaise, and increasing frequency, passing bloody stools 6 times per day. She had a regular pulse of 104 beats/minute. She has a sister with ulcerative colitis, and she is suspected of having inflammatory bowel disease.**

What is the best diagnostic investigation in this case?

A. Colonoscopy

B. Computed tomographic (CT) colonography

C. Faecal calprotectin

D. Stool testing for microscopy, culture, and sensitivity

E. Unprepared flexible sigmoidoscopy

11. **A 17-year-old man presented to the adult gastroenterology outpatient department as a direct referral from a paediatric clinic. He had a 4-year history of joint pains on a background of Crohn's disease diagnosed at the age of 6 years.**

    With regard to arthropathy associated with Crohn's disease, which of the following statements is most accurate?

    A. Axial arthropathies including ankylosing spondylitis and sacroiliitis present as lower back pain and stiffness, usually throughout the day

    B. Axial arthropathies often run a course concurrent with intestinal inflammation

    C. Biologics are recommended first-line treatment for an acute flare of Crohn's-associated arthropathy

    D. Large joint arthropathy associated with Crohn's disease usually occurs during remission

    E. Musculoskeletal extra-intestinal manifestations (EIMs) occur in up to 30% of IBD patients

12. **A 57-year-old local councillor, who was also a member of the National Association for Colitis and Crohn's Disease (NACC), attended the outpatient clinic to discuss the implications of NHS budget cuts both for his own healthcare and for that of his constituents.**

    Which of the following statements about the impact of inflammatory bowel disease (IBD) on patients and healthcare is most accurate?

    A. Costs to the health service are similar for IBD and heart disease

    B. The impact of IBD on society is disproportionately low, due to the young age of patients and the resulting good tolerance of symptoms

    C. The lifetime risk of surgery is around 70–80% for Crohn's disease and 40–50% for ulcerative colitis

    D. The majority of IBD patients in the UK are under hospital follow-up

    E. Ulcerative colitis accounts for over 75% of IBD patients in the UK

13. **A 27-year-old woman attended clinic with a background of ileocaecal Crohn's disease. After becoming steroid dependent, she had infliximab induction and achieved remission 15 months ago. She was maintained on azathioprine 2 mg/kg, and 3 months earlier she had stopped infliximab 5 mg/kg 8-weekly. She was keen to have a child in the near future.**

Investigations:

haemoglobin	120 g/L (130–180)
white cell count	5.8 x 10^9/L (4.0–11.0)
platelet count	200 x 10^9/L (150–400)
serum ferritin	61 µg/L (15–300)
serum folate	2.1 µg/L (2.0–11.0)
serum C-reactive protein	9 mg/L (< 10)

What would be the most appropriate advice?

A. Advise against pregnancy, due to the risk of congenital malformations after infliximab treatment
B. Advise that her medications are safe for breastfeeding
C. Recommend high-dose folate replacement prior to conception
D. Recommend stopping azathioprine for 3 months prior to conception
E. Suggest localized resection to facilitate pregnancy off medication

14. **A 34-year-old woman with proctitis presented to an outpatient clinic in early pregnancy with nausea and vomiting.**

Which is the recommended first-line treatment?

A. Domperidone
B. Ginger and P6 acupressure
C. Metoclopramide
D. Ondansetron
E. Pyridoxine

15. **A 27-year-old woman with perianal Crohn's disease presented during a 4-month flare at 13 weeks pregnancy. She had been off all medication for 8 months.**

Investigations:

haemoglobin	104 g/L (130–180)
white cell count	8.8 x 10^9/L (4.0–11.0)
platelet count	430 x 10^9/L (150–400)
serum ferritin	109 µg/L (15–300)
red cell folate	217 µg/L (160–640)
serum C-reactive protein	89 mg/L (< 10)

Which of the following statements is the most accurate?

A. A conservative approach should be adopted
B. Biological therapy can be considered
C. Caesarean section should be avoided due to the risk of Crohn's disease in the wound
D. Corticosteroids are contraindicated
E. In acute severe colonic disease, abdominal X-ray and flexible sigmoidoscopy should be avoided

16. **A 35-year-old patient with long-standing inflammatory bowel disease attended clinic; she was 17 weeks pregnant. She had a poor relationship with her general practitioner and sought advice about symptomatic control of her colitis and other symptoms.**

    Of the following, which is considered most safe in pregnancy?

    A. Aspirin for headaches and abdominal pain
    B. Cholestyramine for diarrhoea after ileal resection
    C. Ibuprofen for arthropathy and backache
    D. Loperamide for diarrhoea in ulcerative colitis
    E. Osmotic or softener laxatives for constipation

17. **One month following a normal vaginal delivery of her first child, a 26-year-old woman with inflammatory bowel disease asked to discuss her medications.**

    Which of the following is contraindicated when breastfeeding?

    A. Mesalazine for ulcerative colitis maintenance
    B. Metronidazole for perianal abscess
    C. Prednisolone for postpartum ulcerative colitis flare
    D. Sulphasalazine for Crohn's and axial arthropathy
    E. Thiopurines for post-operative recurrence in ileal Crohn's disease

18. **A paediatric gastroenterologist wrote to you, asking you to take over the care of a 16-year-old with two previous resections for small bowel Crohn's disease. He is maintained on azathioprine and infliximab.**

    Which of the following statements is most accurate?

    A. A transition coordinator is only necessary for inter-hospital transfers
    B. Consultations with teenage patients should focus on disease and its treatment, in order to avoid creating uncomfortable discussions about physical, emotional, educational, and sexual development
    C. Reportedly, one of the most difficult challenges for young patients and their families is the changing expectations of their gastroenterologist
    D. Transfer of care is best achieved through a formal written handover
    E. Transition should occur on completion of education

19. **A 43-year-old man with inflammatory bowel disease attended the outpatient clinic asking if he could manage his disease with nutritional measures.**

    Which of the following statements is most accurate?

    A. Evidence supports dietary strategies in mild ulcerative colitis
    B. Good evidence supports a low-residue diet and avoiding insoluble fibre in stricturing Crohn's disease
    C. Probiotics in the management of inflammatory bowel disease have no evidence base
    D. The evidence base for elemental feed and polymeric diet is similar in Crohn's disease
    E. Total parenteral nutrition and complete bowel rest are a useful adjunct to medical therapy in resistant Crohn's disease

20. **A 45-year-old woman attended the outpatient clinic, having recently developed extra-intestinal manifestations of Crohn's disease despite azathioprine maintenance.**

    Which of the following extra-intestinal manifestations most benefit from biological treatment in Crohn's disease?

    A. Aphthous ulcers
    B. Episcleritis
    C. Primary sclerosing cholangitis
    D. Pyoderma gangrenosum
    E. Small joint peripheral arthropathy

21. **An 18-year-old woman with a 3-month history of vague abdominal discomfort and unintentional weight loss presented with right-sided abdominal pain and vomiting. Her blood pressure was 110/70 mmHg and her pulse was 110 beats/minute.**

    Investigations:

haemoglobin	104 g/L (130–180)
white cell count	13.1 x 10^9/L (4.0–11.0)
platelet count	430 x 10^9/L (150–400)
serum C-reactive protein	112 mg/L (< 10)
CT abdomen and pelvis	There is a 12 cm length of terminal ileal stricturing with an adjacent intra-abdominal collection. There are loops of dilated small bowel. Three closely spaced mid-ileal strictures, each about 3 cm, are demonstrated proximal to the dilated loops. Appearances are compatible with active Crohn's disease

    What is the most likely surgical procedure?

    A. Defunctioning loop ileostomy proximal to the mid-ileal strictures
    B. Defunctioning loop ileostomy proximal to the terminal ileal stricture
    C. Ileocaecal resection
    D. Ileocaecal resection and en bloc mid-ileal stricture resection
    E. Ileocaecal resection and three mid-ileal stricturoplasties

22. **A 35-year-old woman with colonic Crohn's disease presented complaining of perianal pain and rectal discharge.**

Investigations:

haemoglobin	145 g/L (130–180)
white cell count	10.9 x 10⁹/L (4.0–11.0)
platelet count	534 x 10⁹/L (150–400)
serum C-reactive protein	67 mg/L (< 10)

Which of the following statements is the most accurate?

A. Ileocolonic Crohn's disease has a higher rate of perianal disease

B. Perianal disease presents late in the course of Crohn's disease

C. Perianal pain commonly occurs in fistulae

D. Routine assessment of perianal fistulae includes pelvic MRI, examination under anaesthesia (EUA), and anorectal ultrasound

E. Sigmoidoscopy is useful in determining the management of perianal fistulae

23. **A 63-year-old lorry driver with a previous diagnosis of ileal Crohn's disease and a perianal fistula attended the outpatient clinic of your specialist nurse. They reported that his fistula was producing a significant volume of exudate.**

Investigations:

haemoglobin	178 g/L (130–180)
white cell count	8.9 x 10⁹/L (4.0–11.0)
platelet count	145 x 10⁹/L (150–400)
serum C-reactive protein	35 mg/L (< 10)
pelvic magnetic resonance imaging	inter-sphincteric perianal fistula; no abscess was demonstrated
flexible sigmoidoscopy	quiescent disease

Which of the following treatments is the most appropriate?

A. Infliximab induction 5 mg/kg intravenously at weeks 0, 2, and 6

B. Intravenous ciclosporin 4–5 mg/kg/day

C. Laparoscopic surgical resection

D. Seton suture and antibiotics

E. Total parenteral nutrition

24. **A 50-year-old woman with ulcerative colitis was seen for routine follow-up in an outpatient clinic. She had a slight worsening of symptoms with looser stools, bowels opening three times a day, and occasional dark blood. She had been on mesalazine 2 g twice daily for the last 3 years.**

    A colonoscopy report with histopathological assessment of biopsies was available. It was concluded that she had active mild to moderate left-sided ulcerative colitis.

    What is the best choice of medication?

    A. Aminosalicylate suppositories
    B. Corticosteroid suppositories
    C. Oral budesonide
    D. Oral hydrocortisone
    E. Oral prednisolone

25. **A 40-year-old patient on mesalazine for pan-ulcerative colitis has had three flares in the last year requiring prednisolone to achieve disease control. Immunosuppressive drugs were considered in clinic, and the patient was counselled about starting azathioprine.**

    Which of the following statements most closely adheres to guidelines with regard to thiopurine use in inflammatory bowel disease?

    A. Azathioprine is metabolized to mercaptopurine; therefore the side-effect profiles are the same for the dose equivalent of each drug
    B. After 5 years azathioprine withdrawal should be considered, as risks may outweigh benefits
    C. Patients on thiopurines have a higher risk of post-operative complications; therefore stopping thiopurines prior to surgery should be considered
    D. There is an increased risk of non-melanoma skin cancer in patients treated with thiopurines, so the use of high-strength sun block should be advised
    E. Thiopurine doses should be reduced in renal impairment, or when the mean corpuscular volume rises

26. **A 19-year-old student with Crohn's disease is discussed with you following an examination under anaesthesia which demonstrated an extra-sphincteric fistula. The surgical team placed a seton and requested guidance regarding additional therapy.**

    Investigations:

haemoglobin	124 g/L (130–180)
white cell count	14.9 x 10⁹/L (4.0–11.0)
platelet count	456 x 10⁹/L (150–400)
serum C-reactive protein	70 mg/L (< 10)
pelvic magnetic resonance imaging	no abscess
flexible sigmoidoscopy	active colitis

    Which of the following treatments is the most appropriate?

    A. Azathioprine and ciprofloxacin
    B. Fistulectomy and metronidazole
    C. Infliximab and co-amoxiclav
    D. Mercaptopurine and infliximab
    E. Methotrexate and infliximab

27. **A 24-year-old girl was recently diagnosed with terminal ileal Crohn's disease. Her mother is a complementary therapist and she asked you in clinic for more information on alternative therapies.**

    Which of the following therapies is most likely to be of benefit to the girl's symptoms?

    A. Acupuncture
    B. Aloe vera gel
    C. *Boswellia serrata* extract
    D. Omega-3 free fatty acids
    E. Wheatgrass juice

28. **A 36-year-old man was seen in the outpatient clinic having undergone restorative pouch surgery 1 year ago. This followed a subtotal colectomy and end ileostomy 8 years ago for acute severe ulcerative colitis. He complained of increased stool frequency and liquidity, urgency, abdominal cramps, and incontinence, and was diagnosed with pouchitis. After a course of metronidazole he relapsed, and the option of rotating antibiotics was discussed. The patient asked whether antibiotics could be avoided.**

    Which of the following would be most appropriate?

    A. *Bifidobacterium* and *Saccharomyces boulardii*
    B. *Escherichia coli* Nissle 1917
    C. *Lactobacillus rhamnosus* GG
    D. *Saccharomyces boulardii*
    E. *Streptococcus thermophilus, Lactobacilli* and *Bifidobacterium*

29. **A 37-year-old man with Crohn's disease presented to the Emergency Department with right iliac fossa pain and pyrexia. He had had three ileal resections for stricturing disease in the last 10 years. On admission he was taking azathioprine 1 mg/kg OD and an oral 5-ASA.**

    Investigations:

haemoglobin	113 g/L (130–180)
white cell count	18 x 10⁹/L (4.0–11.0)
platelet count	556 x 10⁹/L (150–400)
serum C-reactive protein	358 mg/L (< 10)
serum albumin	24 g/L (37–49)
CT abdomen	tethered loops of small bowel in the right iliac fossa with evidence of active disease and a 1 x 1 cm abscess in the region of the ileocaecal valve

    What is the most appropriate next management step?

    A. Cessation of azathioprine and prescribing of intravenous antibiotics
    B. Intravenous antibiotics and infliximab induction regime
    C. Intravenous antibiotics and azathioprine 2 mg/kg OD
    D. Laparotomy, ileocaecal resection, and end ileostomy
    E. Radiologically guided percutaneous drainage and intravenous antibiotics

30. **A 33-year-old woman with a 15-year-history of ileocolonic Crohn's disease attended clinic for a follow-up appointment. She had no family history of CD; her husband's older brother and his father both had CD. She was 33 weeks pregnant and concerned about the risk of CD in her child.**

    Which of the following percentages most accurately reflects the child's likelihood of developing Crohn's disease?

    A. 1%
    B. 10%
    C. 25%
    D. 30%
    E. 45%

31. A 32-year-old black, African-born man presented with a 12-week history of bloody diarrhoea and weight loss. He had migrated to the UK at the age of 4 years and had been living there ever since. He last visited Africa 20 years ago.

Investigations:

stool MC&S	negative
flexible sigmoidoscopy	patchy inflammation and ulcers in the left colon
histology	crypt architectural distortion, increased lamina propria cellularity, cryptitis, and granulomas

Which of the following statements is most accurate regarding the epidemiology of IBD?

A. Black people are more commonly affected by UC and less commonly affected by CD than white people

B. Both UC and CD are less common in black people than white people

C. British-born black people are less commonly affected by IBD than African-born black people

D. CD is more common in males, whereas UC is more common in females

E. Geographically, there is a decreasing gradient in the prevalence of IBD from south to north and from east to west

32. A 40-year-old man with a 5-year history of Crohn's colitis was admitted to hospital with a severe flare of the disease. Despite 3 days of treatment with intravenous hydrocortisone, his disease remained active. He was commenced on infliximab with a satisfactory response.

Which of the following most accurately reflects the cytokines responsible for the pro-inflammatory effects in IBD?

A. IL-1 and IL-6

B. IL-4 and TNF-α

C. IL-6 and IL-10

D. IL-10 and IL-23

E. IL-17 and TGF

33. A 34-year-old man presented with abdominal pain and vomiting. He had a previous diagnosis of ileocolonic CD, which was controlled with azathioprine.

Investigations:

haemoglobin	109 g/L (130–180)
white cell count	16.9 x 10^9/L (4.0–11.0)
platelet count	502 x 10^9/L (150–400)
serum C-reactive protein	87 mg/L (< 10)
flexible sigmoidoscopy	normal rectum with areas of focal serpiginous ulceration of the sigmoid

With regard to the immunological changes in Crohn's disease, which of the following statements is most accurate?

A. Adaptive immunity is responsible for cytokine production

B. Environmental factors affect both innate and adaptive immunity

C. IL-6 and IL-10 are anti-inflammatory cytokines

D. Type 1 helper T cells (T$_h$1) produce IL-2, IL-6, and tissue necrosis factor (TNF)

E. T$_h$2 cells produce TNF, causing tissue inflammation

34. A 35-year-old Caucasian woman with colonic and terminal ileal Crohn's disease was admitted with worsening abdominal pain and diarrhoea. She was previously controlled on azathioprine and 5-ASAs. After a partial response to corticosteroids she was commenced on infliximab (IFX); she showed a good response after the second dose and was maintained on 8-weekly doses.

She was seen urgently in clinic with a 5-month history of worsening symptoms, despite maintenance IFX.

Investigations:

serum C-reactive protein	57 mg/L (< 10)
faecal calprotectin	256 µg/g (< 50)
human anti-chimeric antibody (HACA)	positive
IFX level	subtherapeutic

What is the next most appropriate management step?

A. Continue azathioprine and change IFX to adalimumab

B. Continue azathioprine and increase the dosage of IFX infusions

C. Continue azathioprine and increase the frequency of IFX infusions

D. Continue IFX and increase azathioprine dose

E. Stop IFX and increase the dose of azathioprine

35. **A 21-year-old student with a 7-month history of intermittent postprandial abdominal pain and fatigue was referred with worsening of symptoms during her final exams. On further enquiry, she reported 3 kg of weight loss with no diarrhoea or anorexia. She had a previous history of irritable bowel syndrome, is a non-smoker, and had no family history of inflammatory bowel disease. Colonoscopy to the terminal ileum was normal, and a small bowel follow-through did not reveal a small bowel stricture.**

    Investigations:

haemoglobin	109 g/L (115–165)
serum albumin	33 g/L (37–49)
serum C-reactive protein	18 mg/L (< 10)

    Which of the following would have the highest diagnostic yield for small bowel Crohn's disease?

    A. CT enteroclysis

    B. Capsule endoscopy

    C. Double-balloon enteroscopy

    D. Faecal calprotectin

    E. Small bowel MRI

36. **A 35-year-old man was recently diagnosed with ulcerative colitis. He had stopped smoking 6 weeks earlier after smoking for 12 years, and had taken ibuprofen and paracetamol for chronic back pain for the last 6 months. His grandfather had Crohn's disease; none of his siblings had IBD. He had lived in Cardiff for the past 15 years, working as a solicitor, and he was a vegetarian.**

    Which of the following risk factors most strongly predispose him to developing ulcerative colitis?

    A. Chronic intake of non-steroidal anti-inflammatory drugs (NSAIDs)

    B. Family history of IBD

    C. Smoking cessation

    D. Urban lifestyle

    E. Vegetarian diet

37. **A 66-year-old woman with a 15-year history of Crohn's colitis attended the outpatient clinic with worsening back and hip pain. A recent X-ray showed evidence of sacroiliitis. Her Crohn's colitis had been maintained in clinical remission for the last 2 years on mesalazine and azathioprine. She had a normal surveillance colonoscopy with normal colonic biopsies 8 months ago.**

    Investigations:
haemoglobin	136 g/L (115–165)
serum albumin	38 g/L (37–49)
serum C-reactive protein	26 mg/L (< 10)

    Which of the following statements is most accurate with regard to the extra-intestinal manifestations (EIMs) in Crohn's disease?

    A. Anti-tumour necrosis factor alpha (anti-TNF-α) drugs are effective in most patients with inflammatory bowel disease who have sacroiliitis and/or ankylosing spondylitis

    B. In this case, the sacroiliitis is unrelated to the Crohn's disease and represents a separate pathology

    C. Sacroiliitis, peripheral arthropathy, and erythema nodosum are EIMs of inflammatory bowel disease which are unrelated to disease activity

    D. Patients with EIMs will have a poor prognosis for their IBD

    E. The presence of EIMs increases the risk of colorectal carcinoma

38. **A 52-year-old African American man with a 12-year history of Crohn's colitis underwent a gastroscopy and colonoscopy. Gastroscopy was macroscopically and microscopically normal. Colonic biopsies showed changes consistent with mild disease activity in the descending and sigmoid colon. Ileal biopsies were unremarkable. His disease was controlled on azathioprine at a standard dose. His father had colorectal cancer at the age of 63 years.**

    Which of the following most accurately represents this patient's Vienna classification?

    A. A1 L1 B1

    B. A1 L4 B3

    C. A2 L2 B1

    D. A2 L2 B3

    E. A2 L3 B2

39. **A 22-year-old Caucasian woman attended the outpatient clinic with a 6-week history of worsening bloody diarrhoea with a frequency of 8 stools per day, abdominal discomfort, and feeling unwell. She had no family history of inflammatory bowel disease.**

    On examination, her pulse was 96 beats/minute, her temperature was 38.5°C, and her blood pressure was 110/54 mmHg. Abdominal examination was unremarkable.

    Which of the following is the most appropriate investigation?

    A. Barium enema with oral bowel preparation
    B. Colonoscopy with oral bowel preparation
    C. Flexible sigmoidoscopy and phosphate enema
    D. Flexible sigmoidoscopy with no preparation
    E. Flexible sigmoidoscopy with oral bowel preparation

40. **A 35-year-old male patient was admitted with acute severe ulcerative colitis. He had been on a reducing dose of steroids while at home, but failed to respond. After 5 days of treatment with intravenous hydrocortisone he became tachycardic and complained of abdominal pain.**

    Investigations:
haemoglobin	136 g/L (115–165)
serum albumin	31 g/L (37–49)
serum C-reactive protein	68 mg/L (< 10)

    What is the next most appropriate investigation?

    A. CMV serum PCR
    B. CT abdomen
    C. Faecal calprotectin
    D. Stool for *Clostridium difficile*
    E. Unprepared flexible sigmoidoscopy and biopsy

41. **A 35-year-old patient with acute severe Crohn's colitis, who was on intravenous hydrocortisone, developed worsening abdominal pain, distension, and shock. He was treated with intravenous fluids, and an abdominal X-ray was performed.**

    With regard to toxic megacolon and its treatment, which of the following statements is most accurate?

    A. It is diagnosed when the caecum is dilated to more than 5.5 cm
    B. Opiate analgesia is appropriate
    C. Perforation occurs in approximately 35% of patients
    D. Surgery is advisable if the patient is fit for anaesthesia
    E. The knee–elbow rolling position has been shown to relieve colonic dilatation

42. **A 46-year-old woman with a long history of Crohn's colitis attended the outpatient clinic 7 months after a diversion ileostomy. At her stoma site a small pustule had rapidly developed into a painful serpiginous ulcer.**

    Which of the following treatments is most appropriate?

    A. Intralesional infliximab
    B. Intravenous infliximab
    C. Surgical referral
    D. Topical corticosteroids
    E. Topical tacrolimus

43. **A 56-year-old woman with long-standing ulcerative colitis telephoned the inflammatory bowel disease nurse specialist due to a flare in her colitis symptoms. She was on a maximum dose of 5-aminosalicylate treatment. Outpatient clinic review was arranged, and multiple bilateral nodules were noted on the patient's face. These were found to be warm and tender on examination.**

    What is the most appropriate treatment of this woman's rash?

    A. Induction and maintenance with infliximab
    B. Oral corticosteroids
    C. Topical emollient
    D. Topical ibuprofen
    E. Topical potassium iodide

44. A 59-year-old woman with quiescent Crohn's disease, asthma, and hypertension presented to the Emergency Department with an acute febrile illness following her annual influenza vaccination. She complained of fever, malaise, headache, mouth ulcers, and arthralgia. The Emergency Department doctor noted the development of multiple erythematous and tender papules on her neck and at her immunization site.

Investigations:

haemoglobin	156 g/L (115–165)
white cell count	15.9 × 10⁹/L (4.0–11.0)
platelet count	365 × 10⁹/L (150–400)
serum albumin	35 g/L (37–49)
serum C-reactive protein	67 mg/L (< 10)
anti-neutrophil cytoplasmic antibodies:	
c-ANCA	negative
p-ANCA	weakly positive
PR3-ANCA	8 U/mL (< 10)
MPO-ANCA	4 U/mL (< 10)

Which of the following is the most likely diagnosis?

A. Dermatitis herpetiformis

B. Erythema nodosum

C. *Mycobacterium tuberculosis*

D. Pyoderma gangrenosum

E. Sweet's syndrome

45. A 78-year-old man with a long history of quiescent ulcerative colitis attended his annual gastroenterology clinic review. His colitis control had deteriorated since he stopped his medications, as he had been concerned by the polypharmacy he was experiencing after a recent inpatient stay with an acute coronary syndrome.

Following the hospital stay his district nurse had documented poor oral intake and an 8 kg weight loss. The patient reported severe oral pain on eating, and had avoided oral intake as a result.

Examination revealed angular stomatitis and multiple aphthous ulcers.

What is the most appropriate management?

A. Difflam oral wash (benzydamine hydrochloride)

B. Iron supplementation

C. Oral corticosteroids

D. Topical corticosteroids

E. Topical non-steroidal anti-inflammatory drugs

46. **An 18-year-old man with a childhood diagnosis of small bowel Crohn's disease attended the eye hospital Emergency Department with a painless, erythematous right eye. His vision was reported to be unchanged.**

    What is the most likely diagnosis?

    A. Anterior uveitis
    B. Episcleritis
    C. Intermediate uveitis
    D. Posterior uveitis
    E. Scleritis

47. **A 47-year-old man with small bowel and colonic Crohn's disease was reviewed in the gastroenterology outpatient clinic. He was in remission on low-dose corticosteroid treatment maintenance, having had multiple courses of oral corticosteroids in the past. He was asymptomatic and reported no new medications.**

    His background medical history included glaucoma, morbid obesity, diverticular disease, and hypertension.

    Investigations:

serum total protein	65 g/L (61–76)
serum albumin	39 g/L (37–49)
serum globulin	25 g/L (24–27)
serum total bilirubin	14 µmol/L (1–22)
serum conjugated bilirubin	3.0 µmol/L (< 3.4)
serum alanine aminotransferase	78 U/L (5–35)
serum aspartate aminotransferase	35 U/L (1–31)
serum alkaline phosphatase	116 U/L (45–105)
serum gamma glutamyl transferase	44 U/L (< 50)

    Which is the most likely diagnosis?

    A. Autoimmune hepatitis associated with IBD
    B. Autoimmune pancreatitis associated with IBD
    C. Gallstones complicating Crohn's disease
    D. Non-alcoholic steatohepatitis secondary to obesity
    E. Primary sclerosing cholangitis associated with IBD

48. A 37-year-old man was in remission on corticosteroid maintenance. He had had multiple courses of oral corticosteroids in the past for ulcerative colitis. He had developed bloody diarrhoea whenever prednisolone doses were reduced below 15 mg; azathioprine treatment was recommended.

Investigations:

haemoglobin	146 g/L (115–165)
white cell count	13.6 x 10⁹/L (4.0–11.0)
platelet count	423 x 10⁹/L (150–400)
serum albumin	38 g/L (37–49)
thiopurine methyltransferase	16 U/L (> 25)

Which of the following statements about thiopurine methyltransferase (TPMT) levels prior to azathioprine prescription is most accurate?

A. Concurrent TPMT deficiency and leukaemia increase the risk of leucopenia
B. Normal TPMT levels predict clinical response to thiopurines
C. TPMT activity is absent in 1% of the population
D. TPMT activity is normal in 50% of the population
E. TPMT levels accurately predict the risk of leucopenia

49. A 79-year-old man presented to the outpatient clinic with his second flare of ulcerative colitis in a year. He was maintained on mesalazine 1200 mg twice daily. His bowels opened five times daily, with minimal blood and no abdominal pain. His pulse rate was 70 beats/minute, he was afebrile, and he complained of a chronic cough.

He had a long history of recurrent chest infections relating to bronchiectasis.

Investigations:

haemoglobin	151 g/L (115–165)
white cell count	10.9 x 10⁹/L (4.0–11.0)
platelet count	412 x 10⁹/L (150–400)
serum albumin	40 g/L (37–49)
serum C-reactive protein	17 mg/L (< 10)
thiopurine methyltransferase	78 U/L (> 25)

Which of the following is the best option for controlling his ulcerative colitis?

A. Azathioprine 2.5 mg/kg orally daily
B. Infliximab induction and maintenance
C. Mesalazine 2400 mg twice daily
D. Prednisolone 40 mg daily reducing by 5 mg weekly
E. Subtotal colectomy

1. D. All of these may herald a diagnosis of Crohn's disease (CD), but the case is complicated by the recent laparoscopic surgery. This is the likely cause of her abdominal fistula, although in the absence of surgery, CD is far more likely than the other differentials for abdominal fistulae (gastrointestinal obstruction, abdominal radiation such as radiotherapy, and penetrating trauma).

Bright red blood per rectum in the absence of colonic symptoms in an age group < 40 years would favour haemorrhoids or an anal fissure, but this woman's chances of developing CD would be increased by a family history. Despite this, her likelihood of developing CD is still less than if she has small bowel stricturing, which is most commonly caused by CD. Rarer causes of small bowel stricturing include non-steroidal anti-inflammatory drugs (NSAIDs) (conceivably the cause in this case), enteric-coated potassium chloride solutions, radiotherapy, tumours (carcinoid, lymphoma, carcinoma), and mesenteric ischaemia.

Patchy red rectal erythema and terminal ileal ulceration can both lend weight to a diagnosis of CD, but not as much as small bowel stricturing. Patchy rectal erythema may be non-specific, or related to constipation with or without digitation for this. NSAIDs are a common cause of terminal ileal ulceration.

The BSG 2011 guidelines state that the diagnosis of IBD is confirmed by clinical evaluation and a combination of biochemical, endoscopic, radiological, histological, or nuclear medicine-based investigations.

- History—to rule out drug-induced injury (NSAIDs), a classical IBS history, and features more in keeping with an alternative diagnosis such as microscopic colitis, Behçet's disease, or other vasculitis
- Initial investigation—FBC, U&Es, LFTs, and ESR or CRP
- Microbiological testing for infectious diarrhoea, including *Clostridium difficile* toxin. Amoebic infection should be considered when travel to the developing world has taken place. CMV may also be a differential in those who are immunocompromised
- Abdominal radiography for patients with suspected severe IBD
- Endoscopic investigation—sigmoidoscopy for acute diarrhoea, with full colonoscopy for symptoms that are mild to moderate
- Laparoscopy can be considered if intestinal tuberculosis is suspected
- In UC the 'diagnosis should be made on the basis of clinical suspicion supported by appropriate macroscopic findings on sigmoidoscopy or colonoscopy, typical histological findings on biopsy and negative stool examinations for infectious agents'
- For CD the 'diagnosis depends on demonstrating focal, asymmetric and often granulomatous inflammation, but the investigations selected vary according to the presenting manifestations, physical findings and complications.'

Mowat C, Cole A, Windsor A *et al*. Guidelines for the management of inflammatory bowel disease in adults. *Gut* 2011; 60: 571–607.

2. A. Among individuals with ulcerative colitis, around 50% have a flare each year. Around 25% of patients with pancolitis will eventually have a colectomy. Progression beyond the rectosigmoid occurs in 16% of patients at 5 years and 31% at 10 years. The cumulative incidence of colorectal cancer or dysplasia is 8% at 20 years, and 16% at 30 years. A meta-analysis suggests a 50% risk reduction for colorectal cancer in patients taking 5-ASAs.

Mowat C, Cole A, Windsor A et al. Guidelines for the management of inflammatory bowel disease in adults. Gut 2011; 60: 571–607.

3. E. The BSG guidelines recommend a screening colonoscopy, with pan-colonic dye spray, at 10 years of disease, ideally while in remission. If dye spray is unavailable, two to four random biopsies should be performed every 10 cm. After each procedure, the surveillance interval is determined by the latest endoscopic and histological findings (not those at the index 10-year screening colonoscopy). Consideration should be given to the patient's preferences, age, comorbidities, and the quality of the examination; medications do not affect surveillance intervals.

Five-yearly surveillance

- Extensive colitis with no macroscopic or microscopic activity
- Left-sided colitis
- Crohn's colitis affecting less than half of the colon
- Pouch surveillance post-colectomy unless there are high-risk features (detailed in annual surveillance).

Three-yearly surveillance

- Extensive colitis with mild macroscopic or microscopic activity
- Pseudo-polyps/post-inflammatory polyps
- Colorectal cancer in a first-degree relative over 50 years of age.

Annual surveillance

- Extensive colitis with moderate/severe macroscopic or microscopic activity
- History of stricture or dysplasia declining surgery in the last 5 years
- Colorectal cancer in a first-degree relative under 50 years of age
- Primary sclerosing cholangitis (PSC) including post-transplant for PSC and those with a pouch
- Pouch with dysplasia previously in the rectum or colon at the time of resection
- Pouch in previous colorectal cancer
- Atrophic and severely inflamed (type C) pouch mucosa.

This patient's interval should be calculated from his 10-year surveillance colonoscopy (5 years earlier). He has not had dysplasia for over 5 years, so does not need annual surveillance on these grounds. At his 10-year screening colonoscopy he was found to have mild histological disease activity with extensive disease (pancolitis), and he has had previous post-inflammatory polyps. Therefore a 3-year surveillance colonoscopy interval was appropriate after his 10-year screening colonoscopy—hence this surveillance is 2 years late. His family history does not affect his surveillance interval, as they are not first-degree relatives.

Cairns SR, Scholefield JH, Steele RJ et al. Guidelines for colorectal cancer screening and surveillance in moderate and high risk groups (update from 2002). Gut 2010; 59: 666–690.

4. E. The diagnosis of diversion colitis can occur within a few months or after a long delay following diversion. The majority of patients have histological evidence, but it is not mandatory for the diagnosis. Of those with histological evidence, only up to one-third have symptoms. *Clostridium difficile* is an important differential, but is not causative.

Diversion colitis is thought to occur as a result of deficiency of short-chain fatty acids (SCFAs). Unabsorbed carbohydrates entering the colon are metabolized by bacteria to SFCAs that provide nutrition for the colonic mucosa. Diversion colitis may respond to SCFA enema treatment; corticosteroid enemas and mesalazine also have a role. Treatment is not urgent, as many cases resolve spontaneously. This patient has quiescent Crohn's disease; therefore medical therapy is not indicated. Surgical options should also be discussed to restore faecal flow and provide definitive treatment.

Glotzer DJ, Glick ME, Goldman H. Proctitis and colitis following diversion of the fecal stream. *Gastroenterology* 1981; 80: 438–441.

Harig JM, Soergel KH, Komorowski RA et al. Treatment of diversion colitis with short-chain fatty acid irrigation. *New England Journal of Medicine* 1989; 320: 23–28.

5. B. About one-third of patients with IBD develop EIMs (extra-intestinal manifestations). Erythema nodosum, oral aphthous ulcers, peripheral arthritis, and episcleritis activity run concurrent with active IBD. Importantly, EIMs whose activity is concurrent with active IBD respond to anti-TNF therapy. Ankylosing spondylitis, primary sclerosing cholangitis, pyoderma gangrenosum, and scleritis are independent of disease activity.

Musculoskeletal EIMs occur in 30% of IBD patients.

- Type 1 peripheral arthropathy affects less than five large joints; it is an acute, self-limiting arthropathy, which is strongly associated with other EIMs, and occurs alongside intestinal inflammation
- Type 2 peripheral arthropathy affects more than five peripheral joints; it runs a prolonged course independent of gut inflammation, and is associated with uveitis only
- Axial arthropathies, including ankylosing spondylitis and sacroiliitis, present as lower back pain and stiffness in the morning; they improve with exercise, are commoner in smokers, and are often independent of intestinal inflammation.

Treatment of musculoskeletal EIMs is with NSAIDs and COX-2 inhibitors, but these may exacerbate IBD. Sulphasalazine, steroids, and methotrexate are often used; infliximab and adalimumab have an emerging role.

Trost LB and McDonnell JK. Important cutaneous manifestations of inflammatory bowel disease. *Postgraduate Medical Journal* 2005; 81: 580–585.

Barrie A and Reguiero M. Biologic therapy in the management of extra-intestinal manifestations of inflammatory bowel disease. *Inflammatory Bowel Disease* 2007; 13: 1424–1429.

Kaufman I, Caspi D, Yeshurun D et al. The effect of infliximab on extra-intestinal manifestations of Crohn's disease. *Rheumatology International* 2005; 25: 406–410.

Mehta TA and Probert CSJ. Which extra-intestinal manifestations of IBD respond to biologics? In: Irving PM, Siegel CA, Rampton DS et al. (eds) *Clinical Dilemmas in Inflammatory Bowel Disease: new challenges*, 2nd edition. Oxford: Wiley-Blackwell; 2011. doi: 10.1002/9781444342574.ch28.

6. E. All of these are potential causes, but the combination of low vitamin B_{12} and high folate levels favours small bowel bacterial overgrowth (although folate levels can be low in small bowel bacterial overgrowth). Metformin is a common cause of diarrhoea, but unlikely in this case, as it is a long-term drug. CD recurrence would be unlikely as early as 2 months, particularly without supporting inflammatory marker elevation. A negative SeHCAT scan has a high negative predictive value for bile salt malabsorption, with a sensitivity of 80–90% and a specificity of 70–100%.

Pattni S and Walters JRF. Recent advances in the understanding of bile acid malabsorption. http://bmb. oxfordjournals.org/content/92/1/79.full.pdf (accessed 29 February 2012).

7. E. Severe colitis fulfils the Truelove and Witts criteria, namely bloody stool frequency of ≥ 6 per day and any of:

- Tachycardia (> 90 beats/minute)
- Temperature (> 37.8°C)
- Anaemia (haemoglobin < 10.5 g/dL)
- Elevated erythrocyte sedimentation rate (ESR) (> 30 mm/hour).

There is no evidence that prolonged intravenous steroids are helpful; those cases that meet the Travis criteria have an 85% chance of requiring colectomy. The Travis criteria for predicting failure to respond to intravenous corticosteroids on the third day of treatment are:

- Stool frequency ≥ 6, *or*
- CRP ≥ 45 mg/L and a stool frequency of ≥ 3 per 24 hours.

This case meets the Travis criteria and needs consideration of second-line therapy. Intravenous ciclosporin is prescribed at a dose of 2 mg/kg, and is not appropriate for individuals with uncontrolled hypertension. Oral ciclosporin is also contraindicated in uncontrolled hypertension. Other contraindications include a serum magnesium level of < 0.5 mmol/L or a serum cholesterol level of < 3.0 mmol/L. Infliximab is relatively contraindicated in patients with prior tuberculosis, due to the risk of reactivation. Of the options that are given, surgery is the safest. Indications for emergency surgery in acute severe ulcerative colitis include toxic megacolon, perforation, massive haemorrhage, and obstruction.

Travis S, Satsangi J and Lemann M. Predicting the need for colectomy in severe ulcerative colitis: a critical appraisal of clinical parameters and currently available biomarkers. *Gut* 2001; 60: 3–9.

Truelove SC and Witts LJ. Cortisone in ulcerative colitis: final report on a therapeutic trial. *British Medical Journal* 1955; 2: 1041–1048.

Mowat C, Cole A, Windsor A *et al.* Guidelines for the management of inflammatory bowel disease in adults. *Gut* 2011; 60: 571–607.

8. A. This woman is at risk of colonic carcinoma; the gold standard for this diagnosis is colonoscopy. Coeliac testing with tissue transglutaminase (TTG) is indicated in new iron-deficiency anaemia. Gastroscopy and duodenal biopsies are indicated except in the case of asymptomatic menstruating women. Due to the recognized risk of colonic cancer, colonoscopy would be the first-choice investigation. Autoimmune testing, including anti-neutrophil cytoplasmic antibodies and magnetic resonance cholangiopancreatography (MRCP), would be reasonable given the risk of primary sclerosing cholangitis (PSC), but not more important than colonoscopy. Capsule endoscopy or other small bowel imaging may be considered in cases of normal gastroscopy and colonoscopy with unresponsive iron-deficiency anaemia.

Mowat C, Cole A, Windsor A et al. Guidelines for the management of inflammatory bowel disease in adults. Gut 2011; 60: 571–607.

Goddard AF, James MW, McIntyre AS et al. Guidelines for the management of iron deficiency anaemia. Gut 2011; 60: 1309–1316.

9. B. Combined therapy has been shown to work more rapidly and effectively than oral or topical mesalazine therapy alone. In left-sided disease, enemas are more appropriate; in proctitis, suppositories may be sufficient. If mesalazine treatment fails to resolve rectal bleeding within 10–14 days, treatment with corticosteroids should be considered. Although controlled trial evidence exists for the use of the probiotic VSL#3 in mild to moderate ulcerative colitis, it has not yet found favour in international guidelines. Azathioprine (AZA) and mercaptopurine (MCP) are thiopurines indicated in corticosteroid-refractory disease or steroid-intolerant patients. They have a slow onset of action and therefore are not useful for acute therapy.

One in five patients who are treated with AZA or MCP will develop an adverse event. Early effects include an allergic response such as fever, arthralgia, or a rash that resolve on withdrawal of treatment. Around 3% develop profound leucopenia, mostly commonly early on, but it can occur after many years. Therefore all sore throats and infections should be reported, and blood monitoring should continue long term. Hepatotoxicity or pancreatitis occurs in less than 5% of cases. When initiating therapy, the patient should be warned about common early side effects such as nausea and vomiting, and should be fully informed about potential adverse events. If the first 3 weeks of therapy are tolerated, long-term treatment is likely to be beneficial.

Thiopurines are immunosuppressants, as is methotrexate. As such, when initiating therapy it is advisable to consider opportunistic infections as described in the guidelines published by the European Crohn's and Colitis Organisation (ECCO) in 2009. Malnutrition, severe disease, increasing age, concurrent immunosuppression, and comorbidities may increase the risk of infection. Prednisolone dosages higher than 20 mg per day for more than 2 weeks are considered to be a risk factor. The ECCO guidelines on opportunistic infections have yet to be universally adopted, and are summarized below.

- *Hepatitis A*: vaccination should be given as per population travel guidelines
- *Hepatitis B*: vaccination is recommended in all patients with IBD. To avoid flares, HBsAg-positive carriers should receive antivirals prior to and during treatment with immunomodulators. Immunomodulators should be delayed until acute hepatitis B has been treated. Crohn's disease may be exacerbated by interferon treatment
- *Hepatitis C*: acute hepatitis C can be treated on immunomodulators, and screening is not mandatory
- *HIV*: testing should be considered before treating the patient with immunomodulators
- *CMV*: screening prior to immunomodulators is not essential; latent or sub-clinical CMV is not a contraindication. Once the patient is on immunomodulators, screening should be undertaken before increasing immunosuppression. In severe colitis, patients should be screened with endoscopic biopsies for CMV. CMV colitis is managed with 3 weeks of antiviral treatment (intravenous ganciclovir for 3 to 5 days, then oral valganciclovir), while withholding immunomodulators. Systemic CMV is a contraindication for immunomodulators

- *HSV*: screening is not necessary. In recurrent genital or labial infection, antivirals should be prescribed concurrently with immunomodulators. Once the patient is on immunomodulators, screening should be undertaken before increasing immunosuppression. In severe colitis, the patient should be screened with endoscopic biopsies for HSV; treatment is with antivirals and withholding immunomodulators

- *VZV*: pre-immunomodulator screening with history of previous illness, immunization, and, if necessary, VZV IgG is recommended. VZV vaccination should be undertaken at least 3 weeks before immunomodulator treatment. Immunomodulators should not be initiated, and should be withheld during acute infection; once acute symptoms have resolved, immunomodulators can be used

- *EBV*: screening is not necessary. Severe acute EBV is managed with antivirals and withholding immunomodulators. If EBV-associated lymphoma occurs, stop treatment with immunomodulators, and if spontaneous regression does not occur, refer the patient for chemotherapy

- *HPV*: all female IBD patients should have regular cervical cancer screening and prophylactic HPV vaccination. Past HPV is not a contraindication to immunomodulators, but they should be stopped if there are extensive cutaneous warts

- *PML*: progressive multifocal leukoencephalopathy from reactivation of JC polyomavirus (JCV) has been associated with natalizumab—hence its withdrawal

- *Influenza*: annual vaccination with trivalent inactive influenza vaccine is indicated. Seroconversion may be reduced with thiopurines and ciclosporin. Antivirals are recommended within 36 hours of illness during an epidemic

- *Parasitic and fungal*: no screening is recommended, although infections can be severe, need specialist input, and require withholding of immunomodulators if severe. Secondary chemoprophylaxis may allow reintroduction of immunomodulators after an acute infection has resolved

- *Tuberculosis*: screening should be undertaken for TB by chest X-ray or tuberculin skin testing prior to anti-TNF treatment. Latent TB should be treated with a full course of treatment and anti-TNF postponed for at least 3 weeks. If TB occurs during immunomodulator therapy, only anti-TNF must be discontinued, and it can be reintroduced 2 months later. All other immunomodulators can be continued except in multi-drug-resistant TB

- Streptococcus pneumoniae: vaccinate against pneumococcus at least 2 weeks before immunomodulator therapy, with revaccination at 3 to 5 years if the patient is still on immunosuppression. Methotrexate reduces vaccine-induced seroconversion. Immunomodulators should be withheld during acute infection

- Legionella pneumophila: legionella testing should be arranged for patients with pneumonia; immunomodulators should be withheld during acute infection

- Salmonella: immunomodulators should be withheld during acute infection

- Listeria monocytogenes: anti-TNF is a higher risk than other immunomodulators. Anti-TNF should be withheld during infection, perhaps permanently

- Nocardia: patients on anti-TNF, particularly with corticosteroids, are at risk; anti-TNF should be discontinued after infection

- Clostridium difficile: screening is recommended during flares. Metronidazole or vancomycin can be used for mild to moderate flares. Vancomycin is preferred for severe disease, with pulsed vancomycin for recurrence. Concomitant immunomodulators remain controversial.

Travel vaccinations are not affected by IBD; vaccinations are best given before immunomodulators. Non-live vaccines are safe in patients on immunomodulators, but may be less effective. Live vaccines are contraindicated, except with less than 2 weeks of corticosteroids or less than 20 mg of prednisolone. For live vaccination to be given, immunomodulators should be omitted for 3 months, and corticosteroids for 1 month. Three weeks after live vaccines have been administered, immunomodulators may be given. Traveller's diarrhoea should be treated early with quinolones or azithromycin in IBD, and if there is no improvement within 48 hours, specialist advice should be sought.

Mowat C, Cole A, Windsor A et al. Guidelines for the management of inflammatory bowel disease in adults. *Gut* 2011; 60: 571–607.

Rahier JF, Ben-Horin S and Chowers Y. European evidence-based Consensus on the prevention, diagnosis and management of opportunistic infections in inflammatory bowel disease. *Journal of Crohn's and Colitis* 2009; 3: 47–91.

10. E. Colonoscopy is relatively contraindicated when there is a clinical suspicion of acute severe colitis. Faecal calprotectin or faecal lactoferrin markers are useful for discriminating IBD from IBS. This patient does not have clinical features favouring IBS. CT colonography is primarily used for polyp/tumour detection, and is less useful in IBD diagnosis.

Histology is key in diagnosis; features may be suggestive of IBD or of an alternative diagnosis.

IBD histology

- Mucosal architecture abnormality: surface irregularity, decreased crypt density, crypt architectural distortion, branching and shortening
- Lamina propria cellularity: plasma cells, lymphocytes, histiocytes, and eosinophils are increased, and giant cells may be present
- Neutrophil polymorph infiltration: present in the lamina propria, cryptitis (in crypt epithelium), crypt abscesses (crypt lumina), and the surface epithelium
- Epithelial abnormality: mucin depletion, surface epithelial damage, and paneth cell metaplasia.

Ulcerative colitis features

- Severe crypt architectural distortion and decreased crypt density
- Villous surface appearance
- Heavy, diffuse transmucosal lamina propria cell increase
- Severe mucin depletion.

Crohn's features

- Epithelioid granulomas
- Discontinuous inflammation and crypt distortion
- Focal cryptitis.

Non-IBD features on histology

- Intra-epithelial lymphocytes: lymphocytic colitis and coeliac disease
- Apoptosis in crypt epithelium or increased in surface epithelium: NSAIDs induced, graft vs. host disease, HIV and AIDS
- Sub-epithelial collagen: collagenous colitis
- Normal architecture, superficial increase in lamina propria cellularity, neutrophil polymorph infiltration, mucin depletion, discontinuous inflammation, and focal cryptitis: acute infection.

Jenkins D, Balsitis M, Gallivan S et al. Guidelines for the initial biopsy diagnosis of suspected chronic idiopathic inflammatory bowel disease. The British Society of Gastroenterology Initiative. *Journal of Clinical Pathology* 1997: 50: 93–105.

11. E. Musculoskeletal manifestations of Crohn's disease can be divided into peripheral arthropathies, sacroiliitis, and ankylosing spondylitis.

Peripheral arthropathies can be divided into two types.
- Type 1 affects less than five large joints, and is an acute self-limiting arthropathy strongly associated with other EIMs; it occurs alongside intestinal inflammation
- Type 2 affects more than five peripheral joints, runs a prolonged independent course, and is associated with uveitis only.

Axial arthropathies are commoner in smokers, and present with predominantly morning symptoms, improving with exercise; they often run a course independent of intestinal inflammation. Traditionally, NSAIDs and COX-2 inhibitors have been used as treatment, but these may exacerbate IBD. Sulphasalazine, corticosteroids, and methotrexate are often used to treat arthropathy. There is emerging evidence, although no RCT data, for the use of adalimumab and infliximab. Etanercept is effective in ankylosis but not in IBD.

Mehta TA and Probert CSJ. Which extra-intestinal manifestations of IBD respond to biologics? In: Irving PM, Siegel CA, Rampton DS et al. (eds) *Clinical Dilemmas in Inflammatory Bowel Disease: new challenges*, 2nd edition. Oxford: Wiley-Blackwell; 2011. doi: 10.1002/9781444342574.ch28.

12. A. IBD has a disproportionately high impact on society, as young patients have a prolonged disease course, which affects their potential for education and employment. IBD can also affect childhood growth and sexual development, it can have a psychological impact, and there may be treatment side effects from medical therapy and surgery, such as infertility. Only around 30% of IBD patients in the UK are under hospital follow-up. Two-thirds of IBD patients in the UK have ulcerative colitis. The lifetime risk of surgery is around 70–80% for Crohn's disease, but is 20–30% for ulcerative colitis.

Mowat C, Cole A, Windsor A et al. Guidelines for the management of inflammatory bowel disease in adults. *Gut* 2011; 60: 571–607.

13. B. Fertility
- Around 25% of female patients become pregnant after diagnosis
- Unlike inactive Crohn's disease, active disease reduces fertility
- Previous surgery for CD is associated with a risk of tubular dysfunction in women
- Rectal excision is associated with a risk of impotence or ejaculatory problems in men
- Sulphasalazine reduces sperm motility and count, causing reversible infertility
- Limited data suggest that infliximab is safe for fathering children.

Planning pregnancy
- It is recommended that women conceive during remission, continuing maintenance medication (except methotrexate) to optimize maternal and fetal outcomes
- It is important to optimize nutritional state. Advise standard (400 µg once/day) folate supplementation, and measure and correct vitamin B_{12}, ferritin, and folate levels
- Sulphasalazine interferes with folate absorption. Therefore supplementation should be increased to 2 mg daily
- Preterm delivery and low birth weight are more common in Crohn's disease
- Congenital malformations have been associated with infliximab use. Most commonly these are heart defects. Anomalies on the VACTERL spectrum have been demonstrated to be increased in women on etanercept and infliximab. No events have been demonstrated with adalimumab

- It is not yet known whether antibodies develop in the fetus, but it is possible for maternal antibodies to cross the placenta. Placental transfer of infliximab has been demonstrated; infliximab in breast milk has not been demonstrated
- Azathioprine can be continued during pregnancy, as risks to the fetus from disease activity are greater than those from continued therapy.

Women planning pregnancy in prolonged remission may reasonably choose to stop therapy, but that is not the case here. In this case the folate level is normal, and the patient can have normal folate supplementation. Although surgery for localized disease is a reasonable therapeutic option, it may increase the risk of tubular dysfunction. Options should be discussed thoroughly. It may be best to continue maintenance therapy, optimize the patient's nutritional state, supplement folate (5 mg/day), and measure and correct vitamin B_{12}/ferritin levels.

Carter JD, Ladhani A, Ricca LR et al. A safety assessment of tumour necrosis factor antagonists during pregnancy: a review of the Food and Drug Administration database. Journal of Rheumatology 2009; 36: 635–641.

Vasailiauskas EA, Church JA, Silverman N et al. Case report: evidence for transplacental transfer of maternally administered infliximab to the newborn. Clinical Gastroenterology and Hepatology 2006; 4: 1255–1258.

Cavagnaro JA. Preclinical Safety Evaluation of Biopharmaceuticals: a science-based approach to facilitating clinical trials. Chichester: Wiley-Blackwell; 2008.

Mowat C, Cole A, Windsor A et al. Guidelines for the management of inflammatory bowel disease in adults. Gut 2011; 60: 571–607.

14. B. Metoclopramide, ondansetron, and pyridoxine are all safe anti-emetics in pregnancy. NICE guidelines recommend trialling non-pharmacological therapy such as ginger and P6 (wrist) acupressure. H_2-receptor antagonists and sucralfate are safe antacids; however, this woman is not reporting heartburn. PPIs are used with caution in pregnancy, as although no adverse events have been reported, they are teratogenic in animals; they are only used if all other antacids fail.

National Institute for Health and Clinical Excellence. Antenatal Care: routine care for the healthy pregnant woman. NICE Clinical Guideline 62. London: NICE; 2008. www.nice.org.uk/nicemedia/live/11947/40110/40110.pdf (accessed 10 November 2011).

15. B. Relapse during pregnancy
- If disease is quiescent, the relapse risk of one-third in 9 months is not altered by pregnancy
- If disease is active at the time of pregnancy, one-third of cases improve and two-thirds have ongoing activity, of which two-thirds deteriorate
- Ensure gastroenterological and obstetric monitoring during pregnancy, particularly in the third trimester
- Treat flares appropriately
- Pregnancy should not alter the management of acute severe colitis or other life-threatening complications of disease
- To aid treatment decisions, endoscopic procedures may be performed; flexible sigmoidoscopy is safe.

Mode of delivery

- Obstetric review and advice should be sought
- In perianal or rectal CD disease and ileoanal pouch, Caesarean section is recommended, to avoid damage to the anal sphincter. Colostomy and ileostomy patients can deliver vaginally
- Perineal CD can occur after episiotomy and tears.

5-ASA therapy and pregnancy

- Sulphasalazine is safe in pregnancy, but should be stopped in suspected neonatal haemolysis
- Up to 3 g daily of mesalazine is safe; data are lacking for higher doses.

Corticosteroids and pregnancy

- In active disease, corticosteroids can be used; low fetal blood levels occur
- The risks of increased oral cleft malformations and prematurity are less than the risks from active disease
- Prednisolone is recommended; data on budesonide are lacking.

Antibiotic therapy and pregnancy

- Avoid metronidazole in the first trimester, but thereafter it may be used with caution as it can increase the risk of prematurity
- Short courses of co-amoxiclav, amoxicillin, and quinolones are safe
- Avoid tetracyclines and sulphonamides.

Immunosuppression and pregnancy

- Thiopurines can be continued during pregnancy, as risks to the fetus from disease activity are greater than the risks from continued therapy; babies may have lower birth weight
- Mothers in prolonged remission may reasonably choose to stop therapy
- Men on thiopurines should be advised to stop therapy for 3 months prior to conception, to reduce pregnancy complications
- Ciclosporin use is associated with low birth weight and prematurity
- Tacrolimus use is associated with prematurity only
- Methotrexate is absolutely contraindicated in pregnancy; abortion should be discussed
- A 6-week period without methotrexate is advised for men and women prior to conception; women should have high-dose folate replacement.

Biologics in pregnancy

- Infliximab has been associated with congenital malformations, particularly cardiac ones and those on the VACTERL spectrum
- Adalimumab appears to be safe in pregnancy
- Placental transfer occurs; fetal antibody formation has not been examined. Anti-TNF antibodies may cross the placenta in the third trimester.

Surgery in pregnancy

- Life-saving emergency surgery is not contraindicated
- If fetal maturation is critical, prolonged aggressive medical therapy may be employed
- After intestinal resection, temporary ileostomy reduces complications.

With active disease, this patient had a 66% chance of further deterioration. Corticosteroids could be used for active disease; the risks from disease activity outweigh the risks of therapy. There is no current evidence that adalimumab is unsafe in pregnancy. However, there is emerging evidence of congenital abnormalities with infliximab and etanercept. The fetus is best served by optimal management of the mother, including abdominal radiograph.

Van Assche G, Dignass A, Reinisch W et al. The second European evidence-based Consensus on the diagnosis and management of Crohn's disease: special situations. Journal of Crohn's and Colitis 2010; 4: 63–101.

Carter JD, Ladhani A, Ricca LR et al. A safety assessment of tumour necrosis factor antagonists during pregnancy: a review of the Food and Drug Administration database. Journal of Rheumatology 2009; 36: 635–641.

Vasailiauskas EA, Church JA, Silverman N et al. Case report: evidence for transplacental transfer of maternally administered infliximab to the newborn. Clinical Gastroenterology and Hepatology 2006; 4: 1255–1258.

Cavagnaro JA. Preclinical Safety Evaluation of Biopharmaceuticals: a science-based approach to facilitating clinical trials. Chichester: Wiley-Blackwell; 2008.

16. B. Aspirin can cause both prematurity and prolonged gestation, and an increased risk of bleeding during labour. NSAIDs have been inadequately studied. For constipation, NICE recommends fibre supplements as first-line treatment, and stimulant laxatives as second line. They report that evidence for safety and effectiveness of osmotic and softener laxatives is lacking. Loperamide is probably safe in pregnancy, although congenital malformations have been reported; also it is not therapeutic in ulcerative colitis.

National Collaborating Centre for Women's and Children's Health, National Institute for Health and Clinical Excellence. Antenatal Care: routine care for the healthy pregnant woman. London: NICE; 2008. www.nice.org.uk/nicemedia/live/11947/40145/40145.pdf (accessed 27 July 2011).

17. B. Sulphasalazine, mesalazine, thiopurines, and infliximab are considered safe. Mesalazine safety has been demonstrated, and although sulphasalazine is present in breast milk, levels in infants are negligible. Infliximab is undetectable in breast milk. Tiny (nanomolar) concentrations of thiopurine metabolite are detected in breast milk, but are not detectable in neonates. Metronidazole and ciprofloxacin are not recommended, as they are excreted in breast milk. Breastfeeding should be delayed for 4 hours after taking prednisolone.

Van Assche G, Dignass A, Panes J et al. The second European evidence-based Consensus on the diagnosis and management of Crohn's disease: special situations. Journal of Crohn's and Colitis 2010; 4: 63–101.

Esbjorner E, Jarnerot G and Wranne L. Sulphasalazine and sulphapyridine serum levels in children to mothers treated with sulphasalazine during pregnancy and lactation. Acta Paediatrica Scandinavica 1987; 76: 137–142.

18. C. Paediatric and adult notes may be separated by hospital and location, and a copy of the paediatric notes and/or a written summary from the paediatric team is a vital resource. However, this 'transfer' does not equate to 'transition of care.' It is recommended that all trusts have a coordinator for planning transitional care, and a defined protocol and policy. Transition should be a process that occurs gradually over time, and at a time determined to be appropriate on an individual case-by-case basis. In adult services, patients are expected to take responsibility for their own healthcare, and will be expected to ask questions and represent themselves. This can be a challenge for patients and parents alike, and should be managed sensitively.

Personal development is a key element of paediatric care and is often overlooked by adult gastroenterologists. Discussion regarding the impact of IBD on young people's development should be made available in adult services.

National Association for Colitis and Crohn's Disease. *Inflammatory Bowel Disease. Transition to adult health care: advice for parents.* Brighton: Oyster Healthcare Communications; 2008. www.ibdtransition. org.uk/downloads/IBD_Transition_Guide_Parents.pdf (accessed 7 July 2011).

19. D. There is no evidence for dietary strategies in ulcerative colitis. Evidence for a low-residue diet in stricturing Crohn's disease is lacking, although it is a safe and common-sense measure. The efficacy of elemental feed and a polymeric diet in Crohn's disease is similar. There is evidence for the use of the probiotic VSL#3 in pouchitis, and some evidence for its role in the maintenance and treatment of ulcerative colitis (UC). *E. coli* Nissle 1917 has a similar efficacy to mesalazine for UC remission maintenance. There is no evidence for total parenteral nutrition to induce remission in Crohn's disease as a sole therapy or adjunct.

The prescription of calcium and vitamin D is advisable with corticosteroid courses. Additional bisphosphonates should be prescribed for all patients over 65 years of age, and those under 65 years having corticosteroids for longer than 3 months.

Van Assche G, Dignass A, Reinisch W *et al.* The second European evidence-based Consensus on the diagnosis and management of Crohn's disease: special situations. *Journal of Crohn's and Colitis* 2010; 4: 63–101.

20. D. Biologics with benefit in Crohn's disease

- Infliximab, a chimeric anti-TNF-alpha monoclonal antibody, is licensed for use in Crohn's disease, ulcerative colitis, and fistulating Crohn's disease
- Adalimumab, an anti-TNF-alpha recombinant human IgG1 monoclonal antibody, is licensed for use in Crohn's disease that is unresponsive to standard immunosuppression
- Natalizumab, a humanized monoclonal antibody against alpha-4 integrin, was withdrawn due to associated progressive multifocal leukoencephalopathy from JC virus.

Biologics without benefit in Crohn's disease

- Etanercept, a recombinant human TNF receptor fusion protein, has a role in the management of ankylosis, but not of IBD
- Rituximab, a B-cell-depleting anti-CD20 antibody, has a deleterious effect.

The extra-intestinal manifestations (EIMs) of Crohn's disease, whose activity is concurrent with active IBD (erythema nodosum, peripheral arthritis, and episcleritis), generally respond to anti-TNF therapy. There are exceptions, including pyoderma gangrenosum, where there is RCT evidence for the use of infliximab. There is no established efficacy for biologics in primary sclerosing cholangitis.

EIMs in which biological therapy is efficacious

Extra-intestinal manifestation		Course parallel to IBD	Recommended treatments
Joints	Sacroiliitis		
	Ankylosing spondylitis	No	Physiotherapy Sulphasalazine Methotrexate Infliximab Adalimumab
	Type 1 large joint peripheral arthropathy	Yes	Steroids (oral or intra-articular) Sulphasalazine Immunomodulators Infliximab
	Type 2 small joint peripheral arthropathy	No	
Skin	Pyoderma gangrenosum	No	Oral steroids Ciclosporin Infliximab
	Erythema nodosum	Yes	Treatment of IBD flare Infliximab
	Sweet's syndrome		Steroids Infliximab
	Aphthous ulcers		Topical steroids Oral steroids Infliximab
Liver	PSC	No	Transplant
Eyes	Uveitis	No	Steroids Ciclosporin Infliximab
	Episcleritis	Yes	Topical steroids

Mehta TA and Probert CSJ. Which extra-intestinal manifestations of IBD respond to biologics? In: Irving PM, Siegel CA, Rampton DS et al. (eds) *Clinical Dilemmas in Inflammatory Bowel Disease: new challenges*, 2nd edition. Oxford: Wiley-Blackwell; 2011. doi: 10.1002/9781444342574.ch28.

21. D. The patient has an apparent perforation with raised inflammatory markers, so surgery rather than medical therapy is indicated. The length of stricture at the terminal ileum is such that future obstruction is likely, although not inevitable, even after successful medical management.

The mid-ileal strictures are causing symptomatic subacute small bowel obstruction. Although medical management post ileocaecal resection is a possibility, the patient would probably be advised to have the strictures treated surgically in this case. Stricturoplasty would be recommended if the strictures were separated, but is not possible with closely spaced strictures.

Surgery and IBD

Medical therapy is the mainstay of IBD management with immunomodulatory and biological therapies. However, surgery still has an important role, and the 2010 syllabus emphasizes that:

- Early surgical liaison is important when a patient is admitted with active disease
- Involvement of surgeons is important with difficult chronically active disease or complex cases.

Pre-operative considerations

Clearly, a medically optimized patient is less likely to have complications.

- Optimize anaemia, Na^+, K^+, phosphate, Mg^{2+} and Ca^{2+}
- Treat concurrent infections
- Consider oral nutrition or intravenous nutrition
- Anticoagulate with low-molecular-weight heparin
- Involve a stoma nurse if the patient is at risk of, or likely to require, a temporary or permanent stoma. If sepsis and malnutrition are present, primary anastomosis must not be performed.

Surgery for CD

Symptomatic small bowel disease and perianal disease are the most common reasons for surgical involvement, followed by Crohn's colitis. Bowel-sparing surgery is advised, leaving other diseased bowel *in situ* for medical treatment to avoid short bowel syndrome.

Colonic resections for Crohn's colitis can be segmental, just as for small bowel. Colonic resections are usually for strictures in CD and only rarely for toxic megacolon. Pouch formation should be avoided in Crohn's disease. Repair of fistulas may be appropriate in selected cases with absent or minimal rectal disease.

Anal disease should only be managed surgically if it is symptomatic. Surgical treatment for perianal IBD is for the purpose of drainage and control of sepsis, rather than curing the condition, which may recur regardless. Abscesses should be opened, and fistula tracks drained with loose seton sutures. These can be left long term, and they help to prevent further abscess formation, spreading sepsis, and multiple fistula openings. Sepsis must be drained before contemplation of treatment with biological agents.

Surgery for ulcerative colitis

Surgery should be advised for disease that is not responding to intensive medical therapy. It should be considered in the following cases:

- Patients with dysplasia (not amenable to complete endoscopic removal) or carcinoma
- Poorly controlled disease, including recurrent acute or chronic episodes of UC
- Those with a retained rectal stump following previous colectomy
- Acute severe colitis with complications (e.g. toxic megacolon, massive haemorrhage, perforation, failure to respond to medical therapy, or deterioration on optimal medical therapy).

Segmental colonic resection and anastomosis is not undertaken for any reason in a patient with active symptomatic or medically maintained ulcerative colitis, as the UC flares post-operatively, and further surgery is usually required within a short time frame.

Emergency cases should ideally be dealt with by a surgeon experienced in ileoanal pouch reconstruction, so that the anatomy can be left ready for pouch formation. The initial operation is a total colectomy with end ileostomy, and closure of the rectal stump (or it is brought out to a mucous fistula). If the stump is left without a mucous fistula, a large rectal catheter should be sutured in place for about 5 days; some surgeons advocate daily irrigation. The next stage is a completion proctectomy and ileal pouch–anal anastomosis (IPAA) at least 3 months later. IPAA is done in one or two stages. In the two-stage procedure, pouch construction with a temporary loop ileostomy is performed, and the ileostomy is then closed about 2 months later. Even if the patient is unlikely to want or be suitable for a pouch, acute colitis surgery should be limited to colectomy and the rectum left for excision after the patient has been restored to health. IBD centres now routinely offer elective (and, in some cases, emergency) colectomies and ileoanal pouch formation as a laparoscopic procedure. This reduces the risk of future adhesions and incisional hernias.

For elective cases, a one-stage panproctocolectomy and ileoanal pouch reconstruction (laparoscopically or open) can be performed. More often this is a two-stage procedure with a diverting loop ileostomy for the first stage. An ileoanal pouch is a neo-rectum fashioned from ileum, creating a larger lumen, which is often referred to as a J-pouch, although it may be J-, W- or S-shaped. This is then either stapled to a rectal stump with a short cuff of rectal mucosa, or alternatively a mucosectomy (removal of the cuff) is undertaken, and a hand-sewn true ileoanal anastomosis from below is performed. A stapled rectal stump is technically easier and may benefit function, but leaves the possibility of 'cuffitis.' A mucosectomy might be advised in cases of rectal cancer or dysplasia complicating colitis, or in FAP. Despite this, the risk of dysplasia or rectal cancer is very low in the remaining mucosa, and in any event, cases of dysplasia or cancer under the pouch–anal anastomosis after mucosectomy have been recorded. In young women who have not completed their family, pouch formation may be delayed to avoid the risk of infertility.

Pouch formation may not be possible or appropriate in some cases—for example, frail patients, those with poor anal sphincter control, or those with rectal cancer, for whom a panproctocolectomy and permanent ileostomy is the best option. Where this is planned, and the rectum and anal canal are removed, the latter should be excised in the intersphincteric plane to maximize the integrity of the closed pelvic floor and avoid perineal hernia formation.

Panproctocolectomy and Kock pouch formation is now rare, as it is fraught with complications. A reservoir is formed from small bowel and brought out to the abdominal wall. Ileum protrudes into the pouch creating a 'nipple valve', which prevents waste from exiting or water from entering. Because of the continence afforded, a collection bag is not required, so the ileostomy can be formed flush with the skin. The stoma can be covered with a dressing (to absorb mucus), and the Kock pouch catheterized/intubated three to five times a day to empty it.

Perianal disease generally occurs with Crohn's disease, but can be found in patients with histologically proven UC. In this latter group the disease is more likely to behave as for Crohn's rather than UC, and ileoanal pouches are best avoided.

Dignass A, Van Assche G, Lindsay JO et al. The second European evidence-based Consensus on the diagnosis and management of Crohn's disease: current management. *Journal of Crohn's and Colitis* 2010; 4: 28–62.

Mowat C, Cole A, Windsor A et al. on behalf of the IBD Section of the British Society of Gastroenterology. *Guidelines for the Management of Inflammatory Bowel Disease in Adults.* London: British Society of Gastroenterology; 2011. www.bsg.org.uk/images/stories/docs/clinical/guidelines/ibd/ibd_2011.pdf (accessed 7 May 2012).

22. E. Perianal fistulae affect up to half of Crohn's disease patients, and are commonest in colonic disease affecting the rectum, where rates exceed 90%. Perianal disease can occur before, with, or after intestinal Crohn's disease. Perianal pain is strongly predictive of the presence of an abscess.

The management of fistulae in Crohn's disease should include the following:

- Mapping the fistula, including which organs are affected
- Assessing concurrent active disease and stricturing
- Imaging to identify abscesses
- General status, such as nutrition and quality of life.

Pelvic MRI is a useful first-line investigation, as it is non-invasive. It is not always necessary, as simple fistulae may not require imaging. EUA is the gold standard investigation; it requires a specialist surgeon, and allows therapeutics management to be undertaken. Anorectal ultrasound is equivalent to pelvic MRI, and is a useful alternative modality. Endoscopy is essential for determining whether concurrent medical management is required with surgical management of fistulae, as treatment is rarely successful in untreated active Crohn's disease.

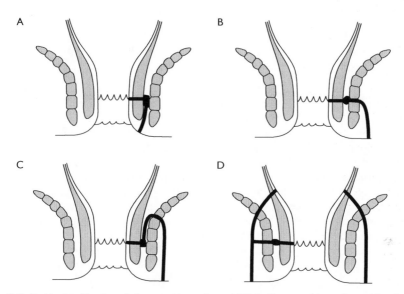

Figure 3.1 Park's classification. A, inter-sphincteric anal fistula; B, transphincteric anal fistula; C, supra-sphincteric anal fistula; D, extra-sphincteric anal fistula.

Reproduced from Parks AG, Gordon PH and Hardcastle JD, 'A classification of fistula-in-ano', *British Journal of Surgery*, 63, pp. 1–12, 1976, with permission from Wiley and British Journal of Surgery Society Ltd. doi: 10.1002/bjs.1800630102.

Van Assche G, Dignass A, Reinisch W *et al*. The second European evidence-based Consensus on the diagnosis and management of Crohn's disease: special situations. *Journal of Crohn's and Colitis* 2010; 4: 63–101.

23. D. The ECCO consensus is that first-line management of simple fistulae should be treatment with antibiotics, with thiopurines as second-line and anti-TNF treatment as third-line management. In symptomatic patients a combined approach with surgical intervention is warranted.

Classification of fistulae

Simple fistula	Complex fistula
Superficial perianal or ano-vaginal	Trans-sphincteric perianal
Inter-sphincteric perianal or ano-vaginal	Supra-sphincteric perianal
	Extra-sphincteric perianal
	Enterocutaneous
	Entero-enteric
	Enterovesical
	Recto-vaginal

Limited evidence exists for ciclosporin. Total parenteral nutrition can be a useful adjunct in the management of complex fistulae. Abscesses due to internal fistulae mandate early surgical intervention. The presence of fistulae predicts a high risk of conversion of gastrointestinal laparoscopic surgery to open laparotomy. Infliximab does not have a good evidence base in simple fistulae, but can be considered when other treatments fail.

Van Assche G, Dignass A, Reinisch W et al. The second European evidence-based Consensus on the diagnosis and management of Crohn's disease: special situations. Journal of Crohn's and Colitis 2010; 4: 63–101.

24. C. Colonic-release preparations of budesonide are as effective as prednisolone for mild to moderate left-sided or extensive colitis, but with high first-pass metabolism in the liver and fewer side effects. Intravenous hydrocortisone is used in moderate to severe active ulcerative colitis to achieve remission. Rectal aminosalicylates or corticosteroids are useful in mild to moderate disease in proctitis or distal disease, but are generally insufficient for left-sided disease. Aminosalicylates are available in suppository, liquid enema, or foam enema preparations. Suppositories do not reach much further than the rectum, but are the best choice for proctitis. Some patients find retaining liquid enemas difficult, although these and foam preparations usually reach the sigmoid or even descending colon. A combination of oral and rectal corticosteroids is better than either alone. Rectal corticosteroids are effective additional treatments to oral aminosalicylates in mild distal disease, but appear to be less effective than topical aminosalicylates.

Lee FI, Jewell DP, Mani V et al. A randomised trial comparing mesalazine and prednisolone foam enemas in patients with acute distal ulcerative colitis. Gut 1996; 38: 229–233.

Cohen RD, Woseth DM, Thisted RA et al. A meta-analysis and overview of the literature on treatment options for left-sided ulcerative colitis and ulcerative proctitis. American Journal of Gastroenterology 2000; 95: 1263–1276.

25. D. Thiopurines (azathioprine and 6-mercaptopurine) can potentially cause serious side effects, and formal drug counselling should be undertaken prior to initiating them. Patients need to be aware of the following:

- Slow onset of action (typically 3 months)
- The requirement for regular blood monitoring for leucopenia and myelotoxicity, which can be sudden and severe. Local policies on frequency may vary, but monitoring is usually every 2–4 weeks for 2 months, and then every 8–12 weeks
- The fact that the mean corpuscular volume is expected to rise on thiopurines
- Allergic reactions such as fever, arthralgia, and rashes, which usually resolve with cessation of thiopurines
- The need to report infections or sore throat
- The need to avoid co-prescription of allopurinol (unless under specialist supervision)
- The risk of liver disease or pancreatitis (uncommon)
- Evidence of a small risk of lymphoma, and concerns about lymphoproliferative disease. The absolute risk in the largest data analysis is small (< 1% after 10 years), and the benefits are considered to outweigh any risks
- The need to avoid prolonged sun exposure and to use high-strength sun block; thiopurines increase the risk of non-melanoma skin cancer.

Thiopurines should be considered in patients who have either a severe relapse of IBD, or at least two relapses within 1 year that require steroids ('steroid-refractory' disease). They should also be considered as 'steroid-dependent' if symptoms flare as the prednisolone dose drops below 15 mg, or if symptoms recur within 6 weeks of stopping steroids. Azathioprine has a long duration of action, and therefore stopping it prior to surgery is rarely indicated.

The target dose of azathioprine is 2–2.5 mg/kg and that of 6-mercaptopurine is 1–1.5 mg/kg. Azathioprine is metabolized to mercaptopurine, with the loss of a nitro-imidazole side chain; therefore the side-effect profile differs. The BSG guidelines state that recent evidence favours indefinite use of thiopurines once remission has been established.

Mowat C, Cole A, Windsor A et al. Guidelines for the management of inflammatory bowel disease in adults. Gut 2011; 60: 571–607.

Siegal CA. Risk of lymphoma in inflammatory bowel disease. Gastroenterology & Hepatology 2009; 5: 784–790.

26. A. Complex fistulae require a joint medical and surgical approach, with drainage of abscesses and placement of seton. Evidence is limited, but the ECCO consensus currently recommends antibiotics and thiopurines as first-line medical therapy, and anti-TNF treatment as second-line treatment. Thiopurines or methotrexate can be added to anti-TNF if there is an inadequate response, with antibiotics as a useful adjunct. Maintenance medical therapy is recommended for at least 1 year after fistula drainage ceases, with the treatment that achieved remission.

Medical treatments of fistulae

- 5-ASA has no benefit
- Corticosteroids have no benefit, and possibly increase the risk of abscess
- Antibiotics are commonly used. There is no good evidence for fistula healing. However, they provide symptomatic benefit, and relapse often occurs on their cessation
- Thiopurines are commonly used as first-line treatment. Limited RCT evidence demonstrates a benefit in fistula closure and maintenance of closure
- Methotrexate has case series evidence only
- Ciclosporin has 10 case series reporting reasonable outcomes, with no RCT evidence
- Tacrolimus has one RCT reporting reasonable outcomes in reducing fistulae, but not full closure of fistulae
- Infliximab and adalimumab have RCT evidence of some benefit in fistula closure and maintenance
- Combined infliximab and thiopurines had good outcomes in an uncontrolled pilot study
- Infliximab induction and methotrexate maintenance have had good outcomes in a small prospective study (33% complete closure, and 25% partial closure over a period of more than 6 months).

Emerging therapies

- Topical injection of infliximab can be considered in patients who do not respond to infliximab or who are intolerant of intravenous infliximab
- Adipose-derived stem cells
- Fistula plugs
- Fibrin glue
- Thalidomide
- Granulocyte colony-stimulating factor
- Hyperbaric oxygen.

Surgical therapy for fistulae

- Abscess drainage
- Seton placement
- Fistulectomy and fistulotomy are associated with a risk of incontinence, and are performed selectively
- In unresponsive disease, a diverting stoma is a useful therapeutic strategy
- Proctectomy may be performed if other management fails.

Enterocutaneous and enterogynaecological fistulae

- There is limited RCT evidence for infliximab effectiveness from a subgroup analysis of the ACCENT II trial, showing 45% closure of rectovaginal fistulae at 14 weeks
- An RCT of 120 patients with Crohn's disease assessed single or multiple, abdominal or perianal fistula closure. This demonstrated 55% closure with infliximab 5 mg/kg, 38% with 10 mg/kg and closure in 13% on placebo
- Surgery should be delayed until nutrition has been optimized, to avoid complications or recurrence
- No treatment is mandatory for asymptomatic low anal–introital fistula
- If enterogynaecological fistulae are symptomatic, surgery is required with resection of the affected bowel, including diversion
- Ongoing thiopurine or anti-TNF treatment is safe during surgery for enterogynaecological fistulae; corticosteroids should be tapered prior to surgery to reduce the risk of sepsis.

Mowat C, Cole A, Windsor A et al. Guidelines for the management of inflammatory bowel disease in adults. *Gut* 2011; 60: 571–607.

Van Assche G, Dignass A, Reinisch W et al. The second European evidence-based Consensus on the diagnosis and management of Crohn's disease: special situations. *Journal of Crohn's and Colitis* 2010; 4: 63–101.

Present DH, Rutgeerts P, Targan S et al. Infliximab for the treatment of fistulas in patients with Crohn's disease. *New England Journal of Medicine* 1999; 340: 1398–1405.

27. A. Complementary therapy refers to therapy that is used in conjunction with conventional medicine, whereas alternative therapy is used in place of conventional medicine. Evidence with regard to efficacy and safety is lacking for complementary and alternative medicine (CAM), as there are only a small number of controlled trials assessing these therapies in IBD. In addition, CAM therapies are unregulated.

Confounding factors in the trials of CAM include the following:

- The effects of CAM therapies may coincide with natural periods of disease remission
- Placebo success rates are as high as 50% in IBD trials
- When there is improvement after both alternative and medical treatment, the CAM therapy often gets a disproportionate share of the credit from patients, IBD groups, or organizations with vested interests.

All CAM therapies should be supported by scientific evidence of efficacy in the same way as conventional therapy. Inadequate symptom control is the primary reason for turning to complementary therapy. The commonest complementary therapies are diet (45%), herbal (17%), exercise (15%), prayer (11%), and relaxation therapy (10%). Acupuncture has shown a significant decrease in the CDAI score (–87 points) compared with penetrating sham acupuncture

(−39 points), but did not reach the −100 point threshold of benefit to achieve adoption into best practice. Trials have been carried out looking at the use of aloe vera gel, *Boswellia serrata* extract, and wheatgrass juice in ulcerative colitis; evidence is lacking due to limited trial size, lack of randomization, and controls. There is no significant benefit to the use of omega-3 free fatty acids compared with placebo in the treatment of CD.

Most patients attribute 'significant benefits' to CAM therapy, and up to 60% make use of them. Therefore physicians should enquire about their use, if only to identify those patients who want more information about therapeutic options and the reasons for, or efficacy of, conventional therapy.

Van Assche G, Dignass A, Reinisch W *et al*. The second European evidence-based Consensus on the diagnosis and management of Crohn's disease: special situations. *Journal of Crohn's and Colitis* 2010; 4: 63–101.

Joos S, Brinkhaus B, Maluche C *et al*. Acupuncture and moxibustion in the treatment of active Crohn's disease: a randomized controlled study. *Digestion* 2004; 69: 131–139.

28. E. There is evidence for the efficacy of the probiotic combination that is commercially known as VSL#3 in pouchitis. It contains the following:

- *Streptococcus thermophilus*
- *Bifidobacterium breve*
- *Bifidobacterium longum*
- *Bifidobacterium infantis*
- *Lactobacillus acidophilus*
- *Lactobacillus plantarum*
- *Lactobacillus paracasei*
- *Lactobacillus delbrueckii* subsp. *bulgaricus*.

Mowat C, Cole A, Windsor A *et al*. Guidelines for the management of inflammatory bowel disease in adults. *Gut* 2011; 60: 571–607.

29. A. The ECCO guidelines state that this patient should be managed with IV antibiotics and percutaneous or surgical drainage (if amenable), followed by consideration of a delayed surgical resection. In this case it is likely that the abscess is too small to drain, even percutaneously.

This patient has active disease which requires treatment. However, there is no consensus as to when it is safe to start further immunosuppression. The ECCO guidelines support withholding immunosuppression until the resolution of bacterial infections.

Dignass A, Van Assche G, Lindsay JO *et al*. The second European evidence-based Consensus on the diagnosis and management of Crohn's disease: current management. *Journal of Crohn's and Colitis* 2010; 4: 28–62.

Rahier JF, Ben-Horin S, Chower Y *et al*. European evidence-based Consensus on the prevention, diagnosis and management of opportunistic infections in inflammatory bowel disease. *Journal of Crohn's and Colitis* 2009; 3: 47–91.

30. B. There is strong evidence that genetic factors play an important role in determining susceptibility to IBD.

- The risk of disease in the offspring of patients remains difficult to calculate accurately
- Observations of temporal trends and geographical distribution of IBD point to the risks associated with a western lifestyle, such as diet and urbanization
- Smoking in Crohn's disease and smoking cessation in ulcerative colitis are established risk factors for the manifestation of the disease. As a result, smoking may affect management decisions, particularly as cessation achieves a 65% reduction in the risk of a relapse (similar to immunosuppression)
- The greatest risk factor is an affected first-degree relative; siblings of an affected individual are at highest risk
- Genetic susceptibility is more frequently identified in patients with Crohn's disease (9–15%) than in those with ulcerative colitis (6–9%)
- Genetic factors are more common in patients with early disease onset, and in those of Jewish descent
- In Crohn's disease, the rate of concordance for identical twins has been reported to be as high as 53%; in ulcerative colitis the concordance rate is in the range 6–17%
- Nucleotide-binding oligomerization domain-containing protein 2 (NOD2), also known as caspase recruitment domain-containing protein 15 (CARD15), has shown the greatest association with Crohn's disease
- Recent studies suggest that offspring of couples who are both affected by IBD (either CD, UC, or 'mixed', i.e. one parent with CD and the other with UC) have about a 30% chance of developing disease by 30 years of age
- If only one parent has IBD, the risk is much less (9% in parental CD and 6% in parental UC).

Sandler RS and Loftus EV Jr. Epidemiology of inflammatory bowel disease. In: Sartor RB and Sandborn WJ (eds) *Kirsner's Inflammatory Bowel Diseases*, 6th edition. New Delhi: Elsevier; 2005. pp. 245–262.

Van der Heide F, Dijkstra A, Weersma RK et al. Effects of active and passive smoking on disease course of Crohn's disease and ulcerative colitis. *Inflammatory Bowel Diseases* 2009; 15: 1199–1207.

Duerr RH. The genetics of inflammatory bowel disease. *Gastroenterology Clinics of North America* 2002; 31: 63–76.

Halfvarson J, Bodin L, Tysk C et al. Inflammatory bowel disease in a Swedish twin cohort: a long-term follow-up of concordance and clinical characteristics. *Gastroenterology* 2003; 124: 1767–1773.

Newman B and Siminovitch KA. Recent advances in the genetics of inflammatory bowel disease. *Current Opinion in Gastroenterology* 2005: 21: 401–407.

31. B.

- The incidence and prevalence of IBD varies across the world
- The UK incidence of ulcerative colitis is 10–20 per 100 000
- The UK incidence of Crohn's disease is 5–10 per 100 000
- The peak incidence of IBD is between the ages of 20 and 40 years.
- Gender-related differences in IBD show a slight predominance of females with Crohn's disease and of males with ulcerative colitis.
- IBD is traditionally considered to be most common in western countries and least common in the Asia-Pacific region.

- There is a decreasing gradient in the prevalence of the disease from north to south and, to a lesser extent, from west to east
- Racial and ethnic observations in different populations and immigration studies point towards genetic, inherited, environmental, and behavioural factors
- There is a racial–ethnic distribution. Black people are less affected by IBD than white people, although Crohn's disease is more common than ulcerative colitis in blacks, and the Jewish population is highly susceptible to IBD.

Shivanada S and Logan R. Incidence of IBD across Europe: is there a difference between north and south? *Gut* 1996; 39: 690–697.

Ahuja V and Tandon RK. Inflammatory bowel disease in the Asia-Pacific area: a comparison with developed countries and regional differences. *Journal of Digestive Disease* 2010; 11: 134–147.

Loftus JEV, Silverstein MD, Sandborn WJ et al. Crohn's disease in Olmsted County, Minnesota, 1940–1993: incidence, prevalence and survival. *Gastroenterology* 1998; 114: 1161–1168.

32. A. Immunological factors play an important role in the aetiology of IBD. Dysregulated and inappropriately exaggerated mucosal response to luminal antigens leads to an imbalance between regulatory and effector T cells. Antigenic exposure leads to activation of naive CD4$^+$ cells, leading to their differentiation into either T$_h$1 cells (which secrete IL-1, IL-2, IL-6, IL-12, IL-18, IFN, and TNF-α), T$_h$2 cells (which secrete IL-4, IL-5, and IL-13), or T$_h$17 cells (which secrete IL-6, IL-22, and IL-17).

T$_h$1 cells mount an immune reaction through production of pro-inflammatory cytokines such as IL-1 and IL-6, expression of adhesion molecules, and proliferation of fibroblasts.

TGF, IL-4, and IL-10 are regulatory or anti-inflammatory cytokines which play their role through the inhibition of activated macrophages and monocytes. IL-10 levels are found to be reduced in both Crohn's disease and ulcerative colitis. The role of IL-4 and TGF in IBD is less well characterized.

IL-17 and IL-22 are produced by T$_h$17 and are pro-inflammatory cytokines.

Kakazu T, Hara J, Matsumoto T et al. Type 1 T-helper cell predominance in granuloma of Crohn's disease. *American Journal of Gastroenterology* 1999; 94: 2149–2155.

Rogler G, Brand K, Vogal D et al. Nuclear factor kappa B is activated in macrophages and epithelial cells of inflamed intestinal mucosa. *Gastroenterology* 1998; 115: 357–369.

Bouma G and Strober W. The immunological and genetic basis of inflammatory bowel disease. *Nature Reviews. Immunology* 2003; 3: 521–533.

33. D. Both the innate and adaptive immune responses are the naturally occurring immune mechanisms in the human body. During health, gut microbiota and food antigens are in balance with the mucosal immune system, which is in a state of controlled inflammation called innate immunity. Innate immunity is genetically determined and can be affected by gut microbiota, whereas environmental factors such as diet and smoking affect adaptive immunity only.

Exposure to foreign antigen leads to activation of naïve CD4$^+$ cells which differentiate into either T$_h$1 cells, T$_h$2 cells, or T$_h$17 cells. T$_h$1 cells produce IL-2, IL-6, and tissue necrosis factor (TNF), which are pro-inflammatory cytokines and play a key role in IBD aetiology by mounting mucosal inflammation. Many studies have demonstrated elevated levels of IL-1 and IL-6 in both Crohn's disease and ulcerative colitis. In addition, IL-18 and IL-12 have also been shown to induce gut inflammation through production of IFN-α in animal models.

T$_h$17 cells participate in the inflammatory response by producing IL-17 in conjunction with IL-23. IL-17 leads to the induction of pro-inflammatory cytokines such as TNF-α, IL-6, and IL-1, which play an important role in the amplification of inflammation. The role of other anti-inflammatory cytokines, such as IL-4 and TGF, is less well characterized.

Kakazu T, Hara J, Matsumoto T et al. Type 1 T-helper cell predominance in granuloma of Crohn's disease. American Journal of Gastroenterology 1999; 94: 2149–2155.

Bouma G and Strober W. The immunological and genetic basis of inflammatory bowel disease. Nature Reviews. Immunology 2003; 3: 521–533.

34. A. Management of a patient who becomes symptomatic after an initial response to anti-TNF therapy is a challenging task. The first step is to determine whether the symptoms are due to active disease or functional in nature. Infliximab (IFX) is licensed in the UK for the treatment of patients with both active Crohn's disease and ulcerative colitis who fail to respond to first-line therapy such as corticosteroids and immunosuppressants.

IFX is a chimeric monoclonal antibody to TNF which has potential of immunogenicity leading to the formation of human anti-chimeric antibodies (HACA), or antibodies to infliximab (ATIs). Factors that increase the risk of immunogenicity are episodic IFX therapy and monotherapy (as opposed to scheduled treatment with IFX and combination treatment with immunosuppressant). Testing for IFX level and the presence of HACA (ATI) has a significant impact on further management decisions in patients who lose response despite being on maintenance doses of IFX.

A retrospective study of 150 patients with IBD treated with IFX found that one-third of them had sub-therapeutic IFX concentrations and an equal number had therapeutic levels, while 23% of patients developed HACA (ATI). Studies have shown that if patients have sub-therapeutic IFX levels and positive HACA (ATI), an increase in infliximab dose/frequency will only result in complete and partial response in 17%, while a switch to a different anti-TNF will achieve a clinical response in 92%. In contrast, 86% of those who have a sub-therapeutic IFX level and negative HACA (ATI) will respond to an increase in dosage/frequency of IFX.

Afif W, Loftus EV Jr, Faubion WA et al. Clinical utility of measuring infliximab and human anti-chimeric antibody concentrations in patients with inflammatory bowel disease. American Journal of Gastroenterology 2010;105:1133–1139.

35. B. Currently, the diagnosis of Crohn's disease involves an analysis of clinical, radiological, endoscopic, pathological, and stool specimen results. Contrast-enhanced radiography is used to localize the extent, severity, and contiguity of disease. CT scanning provides cross-sectional images for assessing mural and extramural involvement. Endoscopy enables direct visualization of the mucosa and enables a biopsy specimen to be obtained for histopathological correlation. Ultrasonography and MRI are adjuncts that provide alternative cross-sectional images in populations in whom radiation exposure is a concern.

Capsule endoscopy (CE) has emerged successfully as a non-invasive test in the diagnostic armamentarium of IBD, and may be considered to be the gold standard for diagnosing small bowel IBD. It has demonstrated superior performance compared with other modalities in its ability to detect early small bowel CD, especially when ileoscopy is negative or unsuccessful. It has a 30% incremental yield over other imaging modalities in non-stricturing CD. A recent meta-analysis also found a high incremental yield of capsule endoscopy over other modalities, both in patients with suspected symptoms of CD, and in those with established non-stricturing CD being evaluated for small bowel recurrence.

Triester S, Leighton JA, Leontiadis GI et al. A meta-analysis of the yield of capsule endoscopy compared to other diagnostic modalities in patients with non-stricturing small bowel Crohn's disease. American Journal of Gastroenterology 2006; 101: 954–964.

Dignass A, Van Assche G, Lindsay JO et al. The second European evidence-based Consensus on the diagnosis and management of Crohn's disease: current management. Journal of Crohn's and Colitis 2010; 4: 28–62.

36. C. The exact aetiology of IBD remains elusive, and it is postulated that there is chronic activation of immune and inflammatory cascade in genetically susceptible individuals.

Environmental factors play a significant role in its aetiology, as indicated by a rapid increase in its incidence in developed countries, the occurrence of Crohn's disease in spouses, and a lack of complete concordance in monozygotic twins.

Smoking in Crohn's disease and smoking cessation in ulcerative colitis are considered to be established risk factors. There are significant data showing the protective effect of smoking with regard to ulcerative colitis. The incidence of UC is lower in current and ex-smokers and the disease runs a more benign course with fewer flares, hospitalizations, and courses of oral steroids, and a lower colectomy rate, compared with those who have never smoked. Patients with ulcerative colitis have also noticed an exacerbation of symptoms on quitting smoking, and relief of symptoms on restarting it. In contrast, smoking increases the risk of developing Crohn's disease, and is associated with more frequent relapses and penetrating complications, and an increased need for steroids and immunosuppressant therapy.

Diet has been a major suspect in the aetiopathology of IBD, but the current level of evidence is unpersuasive. Studies have shown that high sugar intake, fast food and low consumption of fruit, vegetables, and fibre pose some risk for the development of IBD, but the data are limited.

Boyko EJ, Perera DR and Inui TS. Risk of ulcerative colitis among former and current smokers. New England Journal of Medicine 1987; 316: 707–710.

Lindberg E and Huitfeldt B. Smoking in Crohn's disease: effect on localization and clinical course. Gut 1992; 33: 779–782.

Geerling BJ, Dagnelie PC, Badart-Smook A et al. Diet as a risk factor for the development of ulcerative colitis. American Journal of Gastroenterology 2008; 103: 2394–2400.

37. A. Extra-intestinal manifestations are relatively common in chronic IBD, and affect the joints, skin, eyes, bile ducts, and various other organs. The most frequent manifestations are peripheral and axial arthropathies, erythema nodosum (EN), pyoderma gangrenosum (PG), episcleritis, iridocyclitis, and uveitis.

The aetiology of most of the manifestations remains obscure, and the diagnoses in such cases are based mainly on clinical manifestations. Inflammatory arthropathies are among the most common extra-intestinal manifestations in IBD, with a prevalence of 10–35%, and are found more commonly in patients with Crohn's disease. Erythema nodosum affects 2–20% of the IBD population. Women are more commonly affected than men.

Pyoderma gangrenosum affects 0.5–2% of the IBD population, and is characterized by the unpredictable development of chronic ulcerated skin lesions, up to 70% of which are distributed to the lower extremities. Another common lesion site is peristoma. Anterior uveitis (iridocyclitis) and episcleritis occur in up to 17% and 29% of the IBD population, respectively. Uveitis is often associated with coexisting joint and skin manifestations. Diagnosis is often based on clinical presentation, and treatment is usually symptomatic, along with treatment of underlying intestinal disease.

Sulfasalazine and methotrexate have been shown to be effective in peripheral and axial arthropathy, whereas anti-TNF drugs are reported to be successful treatment options in cases of ankylosing spondylitis, erythema nodosum and pyoderma gangrenosum.

Montilla Salas J, Muñoz Gomáriz E and Collantes E. Meta-analysis of efficacy of anti-TNF alpha therapy in ankylosing spondylitis patients. *Reumatologia Clínica* 2007; 3: 204–212.

Siemanowski B and Regueiro M. Efficacy of infliximab for extraintestinal manifestations of inflammatory bowel disease. *Current Treatment Options in Gastroenterology* 2007; 10: 178–184.

38. C. Crohn's disease is difficult to classify meaningfully, as it is such a heterogeneous disease. One system, known as the Vienna classification, was developed by the Working Party for the World Congress of Gastroenterology in Vienna in 1998 to assess the severity of Crohn's disease. The Vienna classification is designed to predict the changes in disease behaviour over the course of the disease. It does not assess the risk of colorectal cancer in IBD. Some have criticized it for having no consequence in the management of Crohn's disease.

Age at diagnosis (years)	Location	Behaviour
A1 < 40 years	L1 terminal ileal	B1 non-stricturing non-penetrating disease
A2 > 40 years	L2 colonic	B2 stricturing
	L3 ileocolonic	B3 penetrating; intra-abdominal or perianal fistula, perianal ulcer, inflammatory mass, and/or abscess
	L4 upper GI tract	

Reproduced from C. Gasche *et al.*, 'A simple classification of Crohn's disease: Report of the Working Party for the World Congress of Gastroenterology, Vienna 1998', *Inflammatory Bowel Disease*, 6, 1, pp. 8–15, 2000, with permission from Wiley.

Gasche C, Scholmerich J, Brynskov J *et al.* A simple classification of Crohn's disease: report of the Working Party for the World Congresses of Gastroenterology, Vienna 1998. *Inflammatory Bowel Disease* 2000; 6: 8–15.

39. D. This scenario raises the suspicion of acute severe colitis, but no diagnosis has been confirmed. Histology is the gold standard, but macroscopic features at endoscopy will allow urgent management. In acute severe colitis, bowel preparation and enemas carry a risk of perforation.

Both an unprepared rigid sigmoidoscopy and unprepared flexible sigmoidoscopy are reasonable options for the rapid diagnosis and assessment of the disease, and histological confirmation. Rigid sigmoidoscopy is readily available in most outpatient clinics and often on the ward; it offers an immediate endoscopic diagnosis of disease, allowing treatment to be started without further delay. Flexible or rigid sigmoidoscopy is the first choice for rapid diagnosis of IBD, and the choice is dependent on availability. Phosphate enema, barium enema, and colonoscopy are risky procedures in suspected severe acute colitis, due to the risk of bowel perforation.

Travis SPL, Strange EF, Lemann M *et al.* European evidence-based Consensus on the management of ulcerative colitis: current management. *Journal of Crohn's and Colitis* 2008; 2: 24–62.

Jakobovits SL and Travis SP. Management of acute severe colitis. *British Medical Bulletin* 2006; 75–76: 131–144.

40. B. Acute tachycardia with or without abdominal pain (often masked by steroids) is a worrying feature in acute severe ulcerative colitis. It warrants urgent assessment and investigation for complications that may require urgent surgery. CT scanning has become the gold standard for identifying perforation, and where available is preferable to a plain erect chest X-ray and abdominal film. *Clostridium difficile* is an important consideration, but should already have been tested for by day 5 of the presentation.

Indications for surgery in the acute setting include the following:

- Failure of medical management
- Perforation
- Toxic megacolon
- Severe haemorrhage
- Malignancy.

The mortality of acute severe colitis is associated with increasing age (> 50 years), male gender, and the presence of *C. difficile* diarrhoea. Short-term mortality is higher in emergency colectomies compared with elective colectomy, but nonetheless surgery can be life-saving.

The timing of surgery is often difficult, and should involve a comprehensive MDT approach, including surgeons, stoma nurses, IBD nurses, radiologists, dietitians, pharmacists, and pathologists where a diagnostic dilemma occurs. These people should be involved early in the admission. The latest BSG guidelines suggest that the operation of choice for acute severe colitis would be subtotal colectomy, end ileostomy, and preservation of a long rectal stump, which can be oversewn and remain in the peritoneal cavity or brought out as a mucous fistula. It is not recommended that an ileoanal pouch is created at the initial surgery. Completion of surgery should occur when the patient is fully recovered, to reduce complications.

Van Assche G, Vermeire S and Rutgeerts P. Management of acute severe ulcerative colitis. *Gut* 2011; 60: 130–133.

Carter M, Lobo A and Travis S. Guidelines for the management of inflammatory bowel disease in adults. *Gut* 2004; 53 (Suppl. V): v1–16.

41. C. Toxic dilatation is rapid widening of the colon in association with infection or inflammation; most cases are related to inflammatory bowel disease. Recently the incidence of this condition has increased due to the growing number of cases of pseudomembranous colitis. Symptoms include abdominal pain, shock, sepsis, and abdominal distension. Toxic dilatation is defined as a colon distended to more than 5.5 cm in the transverse colon or more than 9 cm at the caecum. Not all patients will need immediate surgery, and some can be managed with nasogastric tube, intravenous antibiotics, and intravenous fluids, but with close supervision and surgery should their condition worsen. Complications include perforation (around 35% of cases), sepsis, and shock.

NSAIDs, opiates, and anticholinergics should be avoided, as they may increase the incidence of colonic dilatation. The knee–elbow rolling manoeuvre has not been clinically proven to help with toxic megacolon, although there are isolated case reports which demonstrated that it was helpful.

Strong S. Management of acute colitis and toxic megacolon. *Clinics in Colon and Rectal Surgery* 2010; 23: 274–284.

Panos M, Wood M and Asquith P. Toxic megacolon: the knee-elbow position relieves bowel distension. *Gut* 1993; 34: 1726–1727.

42. D. Skin manifestations occur in up to 20% of IBD patients. This patient has peristomal pyoderma gangrenosum. Of the options provided, topical corticosteroids are the most appropriate first-line treatment, although all have a role.

Pyoderma gangrenosum (PG) presents in the ulcerative form as pain, and a pustule then rapidly develops into a painful ulcer with a serpiginous bluish edge, often on extensor surfaces, especially the legs. It can also be peristomal or perianal; 50% of patients have pathergy.

- PG occurs in up to 2% of IBD patients, with an equal gender distribution
- Treatment of PG includes moist wound management, topical steroids, topical tacrolimus, and intralesional steroids
- High-dose, prolonged courses of oral steroids and ciclosporin are the best-documented treatments. Azathioprine, sulphasalazine, tacrolimus, minocycline, and infliximab have also been used.

Mehta TA and Probert CSJ. Which extra-intestinal manifestations of IBD respond to biologics? In: Irving PM, Siegel CA, Rampton DS *et al.* (eds) *Clinical Dilemmas in Inflammatory Bowel Disease: new challenges*, 2nd edition. Oxford: Wiley-Blackwell; 2011. doi: 10.1002/9781444342574.ch28.

43. B. Facial erythema nodosum (EN) is unusual, and like all EN distributions tends to be associated with an IBD flare. Potassium iodide and NSAIDs can have a role; both are given orally, not topically. NSAID use is limited by the detrimental effect on colitis. Treatment of EN is best achieved by effective treatment of the IBD flare.

EN presents as multiple, bilateral, warm, tender violaceous nodules on the shins, but can occur on the calves, trunk, and face.

- EN has a female gender preponderance; systemic symptoms may occur
- A 3- to 6-week course is usually associated with an IBD flare
- Treatment of EN includes leg elevation, NSAIDs, and oral potassium iodide. The most important management of EN is the treatment of the IBD flare; corticosteroids are very effective in patients who need them for their active gut disease. EN can be treated with or be caused by infliximab.

Marshall JK and Irvine, EJ. Successful therapy of refractory erythema nodosum associated with Crohn's disease using potassium iodide. *Canadian Journal of Gastroenterology* 1997; 11: 501–502.

Mehta TA and Probert CSJ. Which extra-intestinal manifestations of IBD respond to biologics? In: Irving PM, Siegel CA, Rampton DS et al. (eds) Clinical Dilemmas in Inflammatory Bowel Disease: new challenges, 2nd edition. Oxford: Wiley-Blackwell; 2011. doi: 10.1002/9781444342574.ch28.

44. E. This patient described the onset of an acute febrile illness associated with a pathergy at the immunization site—this is Sweet's syndrome. Although infliximab may have a role, it is vital to rule out sepsis prior to immunosuppression, and alternative diagnoses have not been fully explored.

Sweet's syndrome is also known as 'acute febrile neutrophilic dermatosis', and this term outlines some of its features which are noted in this patient. Sweet's syndrome is associated with pathergy and can occur with inflammatory bowel disease.

Investigations:

- Patients commonly have raised inflammatory markers (WCC, ESR, and CRP)
- p-ANCA may be present
- Skin biopsy demonstrates diffuse polynuclear neutrophilic infiltration in the upper dermis.

Treatment:

- This most commonly involves the use of topical or oral steroids
- Potassium iodide, colchicine, metronidazole, and infliximab have a role.

Mehta TA and Probert CSJ. Which extra-intestinal manifestations of IBD respond to biologics? In: Irving PM, Siegel CA, Rampton DS et al. (eds) Clinical Dilemmas in Inflammatory Bowel Disease: new challenges, 2nd edition. Oxford: Wiley-Blackwell; 2011. doi: 10.1002/9781444342574.ch28.

45. C. Oral manifestations occur in up to 10% of IBD patients, and include:
- Aphthous ulcers
- Angular stomatitis
- Mucosal nodularity (cobblestoning)
- Pyostomatitis vegetans.

Angular stomatitis is less likely to be responsible for this man's deterioration and weight loss than painful aphthous ulcers and active IBD. Treatment of aphthous ulcers involves management of the underlying disease in conjunction with topical corticosteroids or NSAIDs. In severe cases, oral steroids may be warranted. This patient has significant weight loss, and oral corticosteroids may improve his underlying colitis, the aphthous ulcers, and his appetite. Iron supplementation may be indicated when angular stomatitis has resulted from iron deficiency.

Mehta TA and Probert CSJ. Which extra-intestinal manifestations of IBD respond to biologics? In: Irving PM, Siegel CA, Rampton DS et al. (eds) Clinical Dilemmas in Inflammatory Bowel Disease: new challenges, 2nd edition. Oxford: Wiley-Blackwell; 2011. doi: 10.1002/9781444342574.ch28.

46. B. The history does not mention pain or visual disturbance. Therefore episcleritis is most likely. Ocular complications of IBD occur in up to 6% of cases. Episcleritis and uveitis are more common than scleritis.

- Episcleritis is a painless hyperaemia of the sclera that occurs with flares of intestinal disease. It responds to topical corticosteroid treatment and causes no visual disturbance
- Scleritis is inflammation of deep scleral vessels, causing erythema, pain, and visual disturbance
- Uveitis runs a course independent of intestinal disease, and presents as an acute painful eye, with visual disturbance that can progress to blindness if it is not managed early with

corticosteroids, and, if refractory, with ciclosporin. It can be anterior, affecting the iris with or without the ciliary body, or posterior, affecting the choroid and the retina, or intermediate between the ciliary body and the retina.

Mehta TA and Probert CSJ. Which extra-intestinal manifestations of IBD respond to biologics? In: Irving PM, Siegel CA, Rampton DS et al. (eds) Clinical Dilemmas in Inflammatory Bowel Disease: new challenges, 2nd edition. Oxford: Wiley-Blackwell; 2011. doi: 10.1002/9781444342574.ch28.

47. D. Hepatobiliary complications of IBD include primary sclerosing cholangitis, autoimmune hepatitis, autoimmune pancreatitis, and gallstones. This patient is asymptomatic, with minimally abnormal liver function tests. Therefore non-alcoholic steatohepatitis (NASH) is the most likely diagnosis. Primary sclerosing cholangitis (PSC) is associated less frequently with Crohn's disease than with ulcerative colitis, where it occurs in 5% of cases. PSC has been identified in 3.4% of Crohn's patients with abnormal liver function tests. PSC would mandate annual colonoscopic surveillance for colonic Crohn's disease or ulcerative colitis.

Rasmussen HH, Fallingborg JF, Mortensen PB et al. Hepatobiliary dysfunction and primary sclerosing cholangitis in patients with Crohn's disease. Scandinavian Journal of Gastroenterology 1997; 32: 604–610.

Saich R and Chapman R. Primary sclerosing cholangitis, autoimmune hepatitis and overlap syndromes in inflammatory bowel disease. World Journal of Gastroenterology 2008; 14: 331–337.

48. A. Azathioprine use in thiopurine methyltransferase (TPMT) deficiency can result in higher levels of thioguanine nucleotide cytotoxic metabolites and myelosuppression. However, studies report that up to 75% of cases of azathioprine-induced myelosuppression have no TPMT mutation, and leucopenia most commonly occurs in individuals with a normal TPMT. TPMT does not predict clinical response or drug toxicity. The level of TPMT relates to genetic polymorphisms as follows:

Population percentage	Genetics	TPMT activity
90%	Homozygote wild-type	High/normal
10%	Heterozygote	Low
0.3% (1 in 300)	Homozygote variant type	None

Mowat C, Cole A, Windsor A et al. Guidelines for the management of inflammatory bowel disease in adults. Gut 2011; 60: 571–607.

49. C. This man is at risk of opportunistic infection, due to his age and comorbidities. Doses exceeding 20 mg daily for over 2 weeks of prednisolone treatment increase the risk of infection, as do all immunosuppressive agents. A trial of high-dose 5-ASA is the safest option in this case. Other treatment regimes could be considered, including surgery. However, this patient's respiratory disease might present a high anaesthetic risk.

Mowat C, Cole A, Windsor A et al. Guidelines for the management of inflammatory bowel disease in adults. Gut 2011; 60: 571–607.

1. **A 45-year-old premenopausal woman is referred to the gastroenterology outpatient department with abnormal blood tests. She is asymptomatic. Her mother had bowel cancer at the age of 62 years.**

    Investigations:
haemoglobin	105 g/L (115–165)
mean cell volume	78 fL (80–96)
serum ferritin	6 µg/L (15–300)

    What would be the most appropriate next step in her management plan?

    A. Colonoscopy

    B. FOB

    C. Monitor

    D. OGD

    E. TTG

2. **A 65-year-old man presented with several months' history of worsening diarrhoea. He also complained of increasing shortness of breath and wheeze. On examination his abdomen was soft and he had patches of dermatitis and peripheral oedema. He was mildly confused.**

    Investigations:
serum alanine aminotransferase	75 U/L (5–35)
serum alkaline phosphatase	190 U/L (45–105)
serum total bilirubin	50 µmol/L (1–22)

    What is the most appropriate treatment?

    A. Cobalamin

    B. Niacin

    C. Pyridoxine

    D. Riboflavin

    E. Thiamine

3. **A 37-year-old Caucasian woman attended clinic suffering from fatigue and increased bowel frequency. She had had a recent course of trimethoprim for a urinary tract infection, and she reported a heavy alcohol intake.**

Investigations:

haemoglobin	95 g/L (115 – 165)
mean cell volume	105 fL (80–96)
serum ferritin	276 µg/L (15–300)
serum folate	1.4 µg/L (2.0–11.0)
serum vitamin B_{12}	172 ng/L (160–760)

What is the most likely cause of her folate deficiency?

A. Coeliac disease

B. Poor dietary intake

C. Pregnancy

D. Small bowel Crohn's disease

E. Trimethoprim

4. **A 45-year-old woman was admitted on the medical take with cardiac-sounding chest pain. She had a body mass index of 34 kg/m². She suffered from osteoarthritis of both knees and had type 2 diabetes mellitus. She was keen to understand more about obesity and her potential treatment options.**

Which of the following is the best treatment option for her obesity at this stage?

A. Gastric banding

B. Lifestyle measures (dietary, exercise, and behavioural interventions)

C. Orlistat

D. Sibutramine

E. Surgical gastric bypass

5. **An 18-year-old girl is admitted to the gastroenterology ward for nutritional assessment. She has had profound weight loss of 2 kg per week for 4 weeks, has a BMI of 14 kg/m², and has a suspected underlying diagnosis of anorexia nervosa. She is frustrated about her admission, reporting no symptoms of ill health.**

Which of the following is most likely to be normal?

A. Albumin

B. Cortisol

C. Follicle-stimulating hormone

D. Growth hormone

E. Luteinizing hormone

6. **An otherwise fit and well 55-year-old man with a past medical history of type 2 diabetes mellitus and chronic lymphocytic leukaemia presented to clinic with abnormal blood tests. In the last 2 months he had developed reflux disease that resolved completely with ranitidine. He also took metformin for 10 years.**

   Investigations:
haemoglobin	98 g/L (115–165)
mean cell volume	103 fL (80–96)
serum ferritin	276 µg/L (15–300)
serum folate	2.4 µg/L (2.0–11.0)
serum vitamin B$_{12}$	123 ng/L (160–760)

   Which is the most likely underlying cause of his presentation?

   A. Age
   B. Chronic lymphocytic leukaemia
   C. Diet
   D. Metformin
   E. Ranitidine

7. **A 60-year-old man, diagnosed with oesophageal cancer, was admitted for an elective oesophagectomy. Six months ago his weight was 70 kg; on admission it was 66 kg with a body mass index of 20 kg/m^2. He was assessed for consideration of nutritional support prior to surgery.**

   Which of the following daily nutritional requirements is most accurate?

   A. Fibre requirements are 50 grams/day
   B. Nitrogen requirements are 0.13–0.24 g/kg/day
   C. Protein requirements are 1.5–2.5 g/kg/day
   D. Total energy requirements are 55–75 kcal/kg/day
   E. Water requirements are 50–80 mL/kg/day

8. **An 80-year-old woman with dementia was admitted with pneumonia. She was treated with antibiotics and improved over the course of a few days. She was then commenced on oral nutritional supplementation and a few days later had a seizure. Examination revealed a body mass index of 18 kg/m^2.**

   Investigations:
serum sodium	135 mmol/L (137–144)
serum potassium	2.1 mmol/L (3.5–4.9)
serum phosphate	0.3 mmol/L (0.8–1.4)
serum magnesium	0.4 mmol/L (0.75–1.05)

   Which of the following is the most appropriate immediate treatment?

   A. Intravenous magnesium
   B. Intravenous Pabrinex®
   C. Intravenous phosphate
   D. Intravenous potassium
   E. Parenteral nutrition

9. **A 36-year-old man with terminal ileal Crohn's disease attended clinic complaining of intermittent upper abdominal pain, constipation, and nausea. He has had Crohn's disease for 10 years; his maintenance therapy was azathioprine 2 mg/kg daily and 3-monthly vitamin B$_{12}$ injections. He has had one course of oral corticosteroids in the last year, and has also tried a low fibre diet. He has continued to smoke 20 cigarettes a day.**

Investigations:

haemoglobin	118 g/L (130–180)
white cell count	5.0 x 10^9/L (4–11)
platelet count	160 x 10^9/L (150–400)
MCV	80 fL (80–96)
serum vitamin B$_{12}$	913 ng/L (160–760)
red cell folate	420 µg/L (160–640)
serum C-reactive protein	6 mg/L (< 10)
faecal calprotectin	8 µg/g (< 50)
MRI small bowel	15 cm stricture in the terminal ileum causing obstruction; no evidence of active disease

What is the next most appropriate treatment option?

A. Anti-TNF therapy

B. Endoscopically dilate the stricture

C. Ileocaecal resection

D. Stop azathioprine and start methotrexate 15 mg once weekly

E. Stricturoplasty

10. **A 55-year-old woman with a 10-year history of type 2 diabetes mellitus was referred to the gastroenterology clinic. She complained of nausea, vomiting, and heartburn for the last year. Her symptoms had steadily worsened and she had lost 12 kg in weight over the last 4 months. She took regular metoclopramide and gliclazide, with Gaviscon as required.**

Investigations:

haemoglobin	114 g/L (115–165)
white cell count	5.7 x 10^9/L (4–11)
serum C-reactive protein	4 mg/L (< 10)
HbA1c	12.7% (< 6%)
OGD	normal, CLO negative

What is the most appropriate next investigation?

A. Abdominal ultrasound scan

B. Antroduodenal manometry

C. C-breath test

D. Gastric scintigraphy

E. Magnetic resonance imaging

11. **A 44-year-old woman was referred to the gastroenterology clinic with a 6-month history of diarrhoea, weight loss, and fatigue. She was diagnosed with scleroderma 10 years ago, but took no medications for this. She ate a varied diet, and no particular foods exacerbated her symptoms. On examination you noted skin bruising and a peripheral neuropathy in a glove-and-stocking distribution.**

Investigations:

haemoglobin	108 g/L (115–165)
mean cell volume	103 fL (80–96)
serum vitamin B_{12}	145 ng/L (160–760)
serum folate	10.5 µg/L (2.0–11.0)
anti-TTG antibodies	negative

Which would be the most appropriate investigation to make a diagnosis?

A. Faecal calprotectin

B. Flexible sigmoidoscopy

C. Gastroscopy with duodenal aspirate and D2 biopsies

D. Hydrogen breath test

E. SeHCAT scan

12. **A 65-year-old man who underwent a Billroth type I partial gastrectomy 20 years ago for recurrent gastric ulcers was seen in the gastroenterology clinic.**

Which of the following deficiencies is he most likely to suffer from?

A. Calcium

B. Folate

C. Iron

D. Vitamin B_{12}

E. Vitamin D

13. **A 35-year-old man was referred to you who underwent a Roux-en-Y gastric bypass in the USA 2 months ago for morbid obesity. Post-operatively he was diagnosed with dumping syndrome. He has tried dietary manipulation.**

Which of the following drugs would be the most appropriate to prescribe?

A. Acarbose

B. Methysergide maleate

C. Octreotide

D. Tolbutamide

E. Verapamil

14. **A 57-year-old woman was admitted with acute abdominal pain and a history of alcohol excess. She was sweaty, her heart rate was 115 beats/minute, and her blood pressure was 95/60 mmHg. Her amylase level was 1250 U/L (normal range 60–180 U/L), and she was diagnosed with acute severe pancreatitis. Her Apache II score was 9.**

    Which of the following would be the most appropriate for nutritional support?

    A. Elemental diet
    B. Nasogastric feeding
    C. Nasojejunal feeding
    D. Oral nutrition with nutritional supplements
    E. Parenteral nutrition

15. **A 65-year-old man was assessed in the pre-operative clinic for elective curative surgery for colorectal cancer. He had no significant past medical history. His weight was 50 kg, and his height was 1.63 cm. His pre-operative investigations were unremarkable.**

    His operation passed uneventfully and he returned to the surgical ward with intravenous fluids prescribed. On day 2 post-operatively his urine output was 25 mL/hour. He was managing sips of fluid only, but was starting to gain some appetite.

    Investigations:

serum sodium	143 mmol/L (137–144)
serum potassium	3.9 mmol/L (3.5–4.9)
serum phosphate	0.9 mmol/L (0.8–1.4)
serum magnesium	0.78 mmol/L (0.75–1.05)
serum corrected calcium	2.59 mmol/L (2.20–2.60)
urinary sodium	53 mmol/L

    Which of the following is the most appropriate fluid prescription for the next 24-hour period?

    A. 1000 mL compound sodium lactate (Hartmann's solution) with 20 mmol KCl
    B. 1000 mL 5% dextrose with 20 mmol KCl
    C. 1000 mL 5% dextrose with 40 mmol KCl and 500 mL 0.9% saline
    D. 1000 mL 0.9% saline with 20 mmol KCl
    E. 1000 mL 0.9% saline with 40 mmol KCl and 500 mL 5% dextrose

16. **A 54-year-old woman presented with intermittent epigastric pain that she had been experiencing for 10 years. She had lost 6 kg in weight, and noticed that her stools were pale and floating over the last month. She had Sjögren's syndrome, consumed 10 units of alcohol a week, and smoked 20 cigarettes a day.**

Investigations:

haemoglobin	124 g/L (115–165)
white cell count	7.5 x 10⁹/L (4.0–11.0)
serum C-reactive protein	2 mg/L (200)
CT abdomen	diffuse enlargemsent of the pancreas with loss of definition of pancreatic clefts

Which of the following factors is most important in determining the dose of pancreatic enzyme replacement?

A. Body weight
B. Faecal elastase
C. Serum amylase
D. Stool consistency
E. Weight loss

17. **A 59-year-old man with a long-standing history of ulcerative colitis underwent an elective panproctocolectomy and ileostomy formation. Two days post-operatively he developed increasing abdominal pain, fevers, and rigors. A CT abdomen was performed which showed a large intra-abdominal collection. He underwent a second laparotomy which revealed a small bowel perforation and necrosis. A small bowel resection and jejunostomy formation was performed.**

After a prolonged stay in the intensive care unit, the patient was transferred to the surgical ward and referred to the nutrition team. A small bowel contrast study was performed to assess the small bowel anatomy.

Investigations:

Gastrograffin small bowel enema	approximately 130 cm of small bowel extends from the duodenojejunal flexure that is of normal calibre with no evidence of stricturing or fistulation

Which of the following statements most accurately describes the patient's predicted long term requirements?

A. Enteral nutrition and oral glucose–saline solution
B. Enteral nutrition and parenteral saline
C. Modified diet and normal fluid intake
D. Normal diet and fluid intake
E. Parenteral nutrition and parenteral saline

18. **A 69-year-old woman with no significant past medical history underwent emergency surgery for acute abdominal pain. At laparotomy, she had evidence of extensive mesenteric infarction, and a small bowel resection with formation of a jejunostomy was performed. In the operation note the surgical team estimated that 60 cm of jejunum remained. After a short stay in the intensive care unit, the patient was transferred to a surgical ward. Her most recent fluid balance and blood investigations are shown below.**

Fluid balance chart (last 24 hours)

In			Total	Out			Total
Orally	IV Fluids	IV drugs		Urine	Stoma	Insensible	
2523	1000	200	3723	500	3556	500	4556

Investigations:
serum sodium	131 mmol/L (137–144)
serum potassium	3.2 mmol/L (3.5–4.9)
serum urea	16.2 mmol/L (2.5–7.0)
serum creatinine	119 µmol/L (60–110)
serum phosphate	1.9 mmol/L (0.8–1.4)
urinary sodium	<20 mmol/L (>20)

Which of the following interventions is the most important for reducing stoma output?

A. Loperamide 2 mg QDS
B. Low-residue diet
C. Omeprazole 40 mg OD
D. Oral glucose–saline solution 1L/24 hours to sip
A. Restrict intake of oral hypotonic fluid to 500 mL/24 hours

19. **A 65-year-old woman with a past medical history of atrial fibrillation underwent an emergency laparotomy and extensive small bowel resection for ischaemia. She made an uneventful post-operative recovery. Three years later, she presented to the Emergency Department with a 1-day history of severe right loin pain.**

Investigations:

haemoglobin	119 g/L (115–165)
white cell count	10.9 × 10⁹/L (4.0–11.0)
platelet count	373 × 10⁹/L (150–400)
serum sodium	135 mmol/L (137–144)
serum potassium	4.2 mmol/L (3.5–4.9)
serum urea	8.0 mmol/L (2.5–7.0)
serum creatinine	77 µmol/L (60–110)
spiral CT abdomen/pelvis	a large non-obstructing calculus is identified in the right renal pelvis

Which of the following is the most likely cause of her renal calculi?

A. Calcium bilirubinate

B. Calcium oxalate

C. Calcium phosphate

D. Cysteine

E. Uric acid

20. **A 45-year-old man with a long-standing history of small bowel Crohn's disease had undergone multiple ileal resections for stricturing disease. He was maintained on infliximab 5 mg/kg infusions at 8-weekly intervals. He presented with a 1-day history of severe left loin pain radiating into his groin with haematuria, but no change in his bowel habit.**

Investigations:

haemoglobin	131 g/L (11.5–16.5)
white cell count	14.4 × 10⁹/L (4.0–11.0)
platelets	373 × 10⁹/L (150–400)
serum sodium	137 mmol/L (137–144)
serum potassium	4.0 mmol/L (3.5–4.9)
serum urea	7.7 mmol/L (2.5–7.0)
serum creatinine	69 µmol/L (60–110)
KUB	large non-obstructing calculus seen at the left vesico-ureteric junction

Which of the following dietary measures would you recommend?

A. Increasing dietary beetroot

B. Increasing dietary fat

C. Increasing dietary wheat bran

D. Reducing dietary calcium

E. Reducing dietary spinach

21. **A 55-year-old woman with secondary progressive multiple sclerosis developed recurrent lower respiratory tract infections. She was assessed by a multidisciplinary team and was felt to be at high risk of aspiration. The patient successfully underwent insertion of a percutaneous endoscopic gastrostomy (PEG). Two years after the procedure, the patient presented with difficulty flushing the tube and leakage around the gastrostomy site.**

    An oesophagogastroduodenoscopy revealed a gastrostomy with a buried bumper.

    Which of the following statements about buried bumper syndrome is most accurate?

    A. It can be prevented by ensuring a 0.5 cm degree of 'play' between the external fixator and the skin site
    B. It can be prevented by rotating and pushing in the tube once a week
    C. It is diagnosed if the PEG can be pushed in easily
    D. It is less common in gastrostomies with a silicon internal disc
    E. The 'balloon push' technique is the standard method of removing a buried bumper endoscopically

22. **A 59-year-old man with extensive small bowel stricturing Crohn's disease underwent a large small bowel resection. It was complicated by an anastomotic breakdown which required a further resection and jejunostomy formation. He was referred to a local intestinal failure unit and, after a period of assessment, was discharged home on parenteral nutrition. He gained weight and made good progress, although an intermittently high-output stoma persisted.**

    When reviewed in clinic after a year on home parenteral nutrition, he complained of hair loss, a skin rash, and impairment of taste. Examination revealed a superficial scaling erythematous patchy rash that was most prominent in intertriginous areas and periorally.

    Which is the most likely nutrient deficiency?

    A. Niacin
    B. Selenium
    C. Vitamin A
    D. Vitamin E
    E. Zinc

23. **A 49-year-old woman with type 1 diabetes had associated diabetic retinopathy, and severe peripheral neuropathy with bilateral Charcot's joints at the ankles. Her blood glucose control had been suboptimal for many years. She presented with a 12-month history of persistent vomiting, which occurred within 30–60 minutes of eating. Her diabetologist had trialled her with a number of antiemetics, including maximal doses of metoclopramide and domperidone, without any significant effect. She had lost 12 kg in weight over a period of 6 months.**

Investigations:

haemoglobin A1c	11.3% (4.0–6.0)
gastric emptying scintigraphy	approximately 40% of the meal is still in the stomach at 4 hours

The decision was made to place an enteral feeding tube.

What type of enteral feeding tube would be most appropriate in the long term for this patient?

A. Laparoscopic placement of a jejunal feeding tube

B. Nasogastric tube

C. Nasojejunal tube

D. Percutaneous endoscopic gastrojejunostomy

E. Percutaneous endoscopic gastrostomy

24. **A 57-year-old man with severe Huntington's disease presented with aspiration pneumonia. He was treated with antibiotics and was assessed by the hospital speech and language therapists, the nutrition team, and the dietitian. He remained at continuing risk of aspiration and was kept nil by mouth. After 1 month of nasogastric feeding there was no improvement in his condition, and a percutaneous endoscopic gastrostomy was thought to be in his best interests.**

Since admission the patient had been confused, and a decline in his cognition due to Huntington's disease was diagnosed; his overall prognosis remained uncertain. The medical and psychiatric teams felt that he lacked capacity and would not regain this in the foreseeable future. There was no record of an advance directive, and no named next of kin or person assigned Lasting Power of Attorney. His only visitor was his elderly neighbour.

What is the most appropriate next step in the patient's management?

A. Appoint an Independent Mental Capacity Advocate (IMCA)

B. Insert a percutaneous endoscopic gastrostomy feeding tube

C. Involve the neighbour in a discussion with the responsible consultant

D. Seek advice from the Trust solicitor regarding Lasting Power of Attorney (LPA)

E. Seek a second opinion from another medical consultant

25. **A 20-year-old man presented to the dietitian with a new diagnosis of coeliac disease. He requested advice on what beverage he could drink at his 21st birthday celebration.**

    Which of the following beverages is most appropriate for a patient with coeliac disease?

    A. Ale
    B. Beer
    C. Cider
    D. Lager
    E. Stout

1. E. In the developing world, iron-deficiency anaemia (IDA) has a prevalence of 2–5% amongst adult men and post-menopausal women, the commonest cause being bleeding from the gastrointestinal tract. In pre-menopausal women, menstrual loss is the commonest cause. Other causes include occult GI blood loss (e.g. due to malignancy, gastric ulcers, oesophagitis, or angiodysplasia), malabsorption (e.g. due to coeliac disease, post bowel resection, or bacterial overgrowth) and non-GI blood loss (e.g. due to haematuria, blood donation, or epistaxis).

For IDA the BSG guidelines recommend that all men and all post-menopausal women undergo gastrointestinal investigations with OGD, colonoscopy, and coeliac serology. Pre-menopausal women under 50 years of age should have coeliac serology only checked; in this group, colonoscopy and/or OGD is reserved for symptomatic patients or those with a strong family history. As age is a strong predictor of pathology, guidelines suggest that all pre-menopausal women over the age of 50 years should have gastrointestinal investigations (as outlined above). Hypoferritinaemia (low ferritin without anaemia) is more common than IDA, but opinion is divided on the need for investigations; BSG guidelines suggest that only men over 50 years of age and post-menopausal women require investigation.

There is no role for FOB in the management of IDA. Small bowel imaging is only recommended if the patient becomes transfusion dependent.

Markers of IDA include low ferritin levels, low MCV, low red cell distribution width, and raised total iron-binding capacity. In chronic disease, ferritin levels can be raised and CRP should be checked (other causes of raised ferritin levels include infection/part of the acute phase reaction, malignancy, alcohol excess, haemochromatosis, and other causes of iron overload).

Goddard F, James MW, McIntyre AS et al. Guidelines for the management of iron deficiency anaemia. *Gut* 2011; 60: 1309–1316.

2. B. Pellagra is niacin (vitamin B_3) deficiency. It classically causes the 4 D's—dementia, dermatitis (often photosensitive), diarrhoea, and death. Other clinical features include dilated cardiomyopathy, aggression, headache, stupor, and seizures. Deficiency results from lack of dietary niacin, deficiency of tryptophan (due to poor dietary intake or increased usage), or excess leucine, although the exact mechanism is unclear. Carcinoid syndrome, resulting from increased serotonin production, typically presents with flushing and diarrhoea. It may cause niacin deficiency, as its precursor—tryptophan—is used to make serotonin and other similar metabolites, instead of niacin. Replacement is with nicotinamide.

Thiamine (vitamin B_1) deficiency causes dry or wet beriberi (the origin of this term is unclear, but it is the name given to thiamine deficiency, 'wet' being mainly heart failure symptoms and 'dry' being mainly neurological symptoms) and Wernicke–Korsakoff syndrome. Riboflavin (vitamin B_2) deficiency causes dermatitis, geographic tongue, and stomatitis. Pyridoxine (vitamin B_6) deficiency causes peripheral neuritis and seizures. Cobalamin (vitamin B$_{12}$) deficiency causes macrocytic anaemia, depression, and diarrhoea (for further information, see answer to Question 6).

Allen L. How common is vitamin B-12 deficiency? *American Journal of Clinical Nutrition* 2009; 89: 693S–696S.

Hudson B. Vitamin B-12 deficiency. *British Medical Journal* 2010; 340: c2305.

Wan P, Moat S and Anstey A. Pellagra: a review with emphasis on photosensitivity. *British Journal of Dermatology* 2011; 164: 1188–1200.

3. B. Folic acid (folate is the naturally occurring form) is a water-soluble member of the vitamin B$_9$ family that is not biologically active. It is found in animal products and leafy green vegetables in the polyglutamate form, and is cleaved to the monoglutamate form in the jejunum, where it is absorbed. Uptake occurs via specific receptors and it is then transformed into its active form, tetrahydrofolic acid. This is needed for DNA synthesis and repair in the same pathway as vitamin B$_{12}$, although deficiency does not appear to cause the same neurological defects.

The recommended daily intake is 400 mcg a day, increasing by 100–200 mcg if the patient is pregnant or lactating. Body stores are 5–10 mg and last 4 to 5 months. Causes of deficiency include inadequate diet, alcoholism, diseases of the small bowel that affect absorption (e.g. coeliac disease), and drugs that interfere with folate metabolism, namely trimethoprim, phenytoin, and methotrexate (which inhibits dihydrofolate reductase). Small bowel bacterial overgrowth tends to result in a high folate level due to production by bacteria.

Lucock M. Is folic acid the ultimate functional food component for disease prevention? *British Medical Journal* 2004; 328: 211–214.

4. B. Obesity and being overweight are defined as abnormal or excessive fat accumulation that may impair health.

Health risks include cardiovascular disease, hypertension, hypercholesterolaemia, diabetes, musculoskeletal problems, respiratory problems (obstructive sleep apnoea and asthma), fatty liver, gallstones, and increased risk of some cancers (colon, breast, and endometrial).

According to NICE guidelines, the first-line treatment is a combination of dietary, exercise, and behavioural interventions; pharmacological therapy is recommended if there is failure of first-line interventions. Orlistat should only be used when more than 3 months' use of dietary and lifestyle measures has failed. Orlistat prevents conversion of dietary fat into its absorbable form (via lipase inhibition), and consequently steatorrhoea is a significant side effect; this can be reduced by decreasing oral dietary fat intake. Meta-analyses show that the mean weight loss at 1 year is 2.9 kg. Sibutramine had its approval removed in 2010, as a European Medicines review found that an increased risk of cardiovascular events outweighed its benefits in weight reduction.

Surgery is recommended if:

- There is a failure of non-surgical measures (no clinically beneficial weight loss over 6 months)
- The patient has a BMI of 40 kg/m^2 or more, or a BMI of 35–40 kg/m^2 and other significant disease that could be improved if they lost weight
- The patient has a BMI greater than 50 kg/m^2
- The patient commits to long-term follow-up which needs to be done under the supervision of a specialist obesity team.

National Institute for Health and Clinical Excellence. *Obesity: guidance on the prevention, identification, assessment and management of overweight and obesity in adults and children.* NICE Clinical Guideline 43. London: NICE; 2006.

5. A. Anorexia nervosa is characterized by a refusal to maintain a normal weight and an intense fear of weight gain; the patient will have a distorted body image. The female:male ratio is 10:1, and the average age of onset is 15 years. It has the highest mortality of all the psychiatric disorders. Physical findings include lanugo hair, hypertrophy of salivary glands, loss of dental enamel, and abdominal distension. Biochemical abnormalities include thyroid dysfunction, raised amylase levels, pituitary–hypothalamic dysfunction (low follicle-stimulating hormone and luteinizing hormone levels, and raised growth hormone levels), and an increase in stress hormones such as cortisol. Albumin is a negative acute phase reactant but not a marker of nutritional status, and is therefore likely to be normal in this patient. Treatment is complex and involves inpatient and outpatient care, and the involvement of psychiatric services, family members, and primary care physicians. Recovery tends to follow the rule of thirds (a third will get better, a third will partially recover, and a third will have chronic problems). Recovery takes on average between 3 and 6 years.

Conversely, bulimia nervosa is an eating disorder that involves restricting food intake, followed by periods of binge eating, followed by bouts of vomiting or purging as a result of guilt and lack of self-esteem. Other methods of calorie loss include diuretic and laxative abuse, and excessive exercise. Patients with bulimia are more likely to be of normal weight and to suffer from affective disorders such as depression. They are more likely to be able to function in society without others being aware of their diagnosis. There is recognized overlap between bulimia nervosa and anorexia nervosa.

Morris J. Anorexia nervosa. *British Medical Journal* 2007; 334: 894.

Hay P. Bulimia nervosa. *British Medical Journal* 2001; 323: 33.

National Institute for Health and Clinical Excellence. *Eating Disorders: core interventions in the treatment and management of anorexia nervosa, bulimia nervosa and related eating disorders.* NICE Clinical Guideline 9. London: NICE; 2004.

6. D. Vitamin B_{12} (cobalamin) is a water-soluble vitamin. It is not made by the body, the only source being dietary (2–3 mcg a day). Total body stores are 2–5 mg, and 50% is stored in the liver. Excretion is mainly in the bile, but most is reabsorbed via the enterohepatic circulation. Deficiency can take up to 3 to 5 years to become apparent.

Blood abnormalities include raised MCV with or without anaemia, the presence of hypersegmented neutrophils, and pancytopenia (all as a result of inhibition of DNA synthesis). Symptoms include those related to anaemia, dementia, peripheral neuropathy, sensory ataxia, and signs of subacute combined degeneration of the cord.

Vitamin B_{12} absorption starts in the mouth in the mucous membranes. It is liberated from protein binding by acid and pepsin in the stomach, where it then binds to R factors (cobalamin-binding proteins). Pancreatic proteases cause it to be released from this complex in the duodenum, where it is bound to intrinsic factor (produced by gastric parietal cells). Its complex is then absorbed in the terminal ileum at specific intrinsic factor binding sites.

Causes of deficiency include the following:

- Poor dietary intake—vegans, alcoholics, and the elderly
- Gastric causes—autoimmune atrophic gastritis, pernicious anaemia (autoantibodies to parietal cells), atrophic gastritis from other causes (i.e. chronic *Helicobacter pylori* infection and achlorhydria, such as that due to PPI use, which is more common than with H2-receptor antagonists), and surgical gastrectomy
- Small bowel causes—coeliac disease, small bowel bacterial overgrowth, fish worm infection, surgical removal of the terminal ileum
- Medication—including metformin and nitrous oxide.

It has been shown that chronic leukaemias often cause a rise in the levels of vitamin B_{12}.

Allen L. How common is vitamin B-12 deficiency? *American Journal of Clinical Nutrition* 2009; 89: 693S–696S.

Annibale B, Lahner E and Fave GD. Diagnosis and management of pernicious anaemia. *Current Gastroenterology Reports* 2011; 13: 518–524.

7. B. NICE guidelines define those who are malnourished as having a BMI of less than 18.5 kg/m^2 or unintentional weight loss greater than 10% within the last 3–6 months, or a BMI of less than 20 kg/m^2 and unintentional weight loss greater than 5% within the last 3–6 months. Those at risk of malnutrition include individuals who have eaten little or nothing for more than 5 days and/or are likely to eat little or nothing for the next 5 days or longer, patients with poor absorptive capacity or high nutrient losses, and patients with increased nutritional requirements from causes such as sepsis or severe illness.

Nutritional support can be via oral supplementation, or enteral (into the gut) and parenteral (intravenous) nutrition. The choice of route is based on the extent of nutritional deficiency, the function of the gut and mucosal wall, the ability to gain and maintain intravenous access, and patient preference and compliance with treatment.

Nutritional support, under supervision of an expert nutrition team, should aim to provide protein, lipids, carbohydrates, and all minerals and vitamins. According to NICE guidelines, requirements for those who are severely unwell or at risk of refeeding syndrome are as follows:

- Total energy 25–35 kcal/kg/day
- Nitrogen 0.13–0.24 g/kg/day
- Protein 0.8–1.5 g/kg/day
- Water 30–35 mL fluid/kg/day.

National Institute for Health and Clinical Excellence. *Nutrition Support in Adults: oral nutrition support, enteral tube feeding and parenteral nutrition.* NICE Clinical Guideline 32. London: NICE; 2006.

8. C. Refeeding syndrome is a life-threatening condition of fluid and electrolyte shifts causing cardiac failure, pulmonary oedema, and dysrhythmias. It occurs in response to feeding after a period of relative starvation, and results from hypophosphataemia, hypokalaemia, hypomagnesaemia, and hyperglycaemia.

In starvation, intracellular minerals become depleted, although serum concentrations can remain normal. When feeding occurs, the relative glycaemia causes an increase in insulin production. Insulin stimulates protein, fat and glycogen synthesis, which requires electrolytes and cofactors such as thiamine. The shift of these electrolytes, especially phosphate, results in refeeding syndrome. Although mild hypophosphataemia is normally asymptomatic, severe hypophosphataemia can lead to seizures.

All patients at risk of refeeding syndrome should have electrolytes monitored daily and aggressive replacement therapy given, including IV vitamins (Pabrinex®). Patients at particular risk are those with poor intake for more than 5 days, existing electrolyte disturbance, low body mass index (BMI), significant recent unintentional weight loss, and a history of alcohol abuse. Recognition of patients at risk is the key to prevention of refeeding syndrome.

Nutritional assessment should be performed on all patients admitted to hospital, and includes the BMI (in kg/m^2) and the BAPEN Malnutrition Universal Screening Tool (MUST). A score is given for BMI, weight loss, and acute disease effect, which gives an overall score for risk of malnutrition that correlates with a score for management guidelines.

National Institute for Health and Clinical Excellence. *Nutrition Support in Adults: oral nutrition support, enteral tube feeding and parenteral nutrition.* NICE Clinical Guideline 32. London: NICE; 2006.

Skipper A. Refeeding syndrome or refeeding hypophosphatemia: a systematic review of cases. *Nutrition in Clinical Practice* 2012; 27: 34–40.

Mehanna H, Moledina J and Travis J. Refeeding syndrome: what it is, and how to prevent and treat it. *British Medical Journal* 2008; 336: 1495–1498.

9. C. Investigations suggest a mechanical stricture, with no active disease, causing obstructive symptoms; a change in medical therapy is not indicated. The stricture is 15 cm in length, and is therefore not amenable to endoscopic dilatation or stricturoplasty.

Endoscopic dilatation of strictures that develop post resection of ileocolonic Crohn's disease can delay further surgery by 3 years if they are more than 4 cm in length. It is beneficial in mild to moderate stricturing disease, and endoscopists should ensure that there is a 24-hour surgical service available on site. Conventional stricturoplasty (i.e. without bowel resection) is appropriate for strictures less than 10 cm in length. In patients with recurrent bowel resections, endoscopic dilatation and stricturoplasty are important alternatives when there is concern about remaining bowel length. Preservation is imperative to avoid short bowel syndrome.

Dignass A, Van Assche G, Lindsay J et al. The second European evidence-based Consensus on the diagnosis and management of Crohn's disease: current management. *Journal of Crohn's and Colitis* 2010; 4: 28–62.

10. D. This woman has poorly controlled diabetes, and her symptoms are most probably due to gastroparesis. This presents in patients with long-standing diabetes mellitus when there is evidence of end-organ damage. Systematic studies suggest that it occurs in 25–55% of type 1 diabetics and 30% of type 2 diabetics. Hyperglycaemia reversibly affects gastric motor function, so tighter control of blood sugar levels will improve symptoms.

All of the investigations listed can be used to assess gastric emptying, but gastric scintigraphy is the gold standard. The patient fasts overnight before eating an isotope-labelled solid test meal such as scrambled eggs or mashed potato. All drugs that delay gastric emptying should be discontinued. The most accurate measurement of gastric emptying is a residual content at 4 hours, with a value of more than 10% considered abnormal.

Transabdominal ultrasonography is best suited to liquid meals only, which is of little clinical use. It is also dependent on operator skill and patient habitus. The gastric emptying rate is calculated by measuring the sequential change in antral area following a test meal. MRI can be used to assess gastric emptying by allowing the calculation of gastric secretory rates. However this is just an estimate, and the technique has not been validated to the same degree as scintigraphy. In addition, it is more expensive to perform and less available for this indication.

Antroduodenal manometry provides important information about the mechanisms of gastroparesis, of which two have been identified—antral hypomotility and duodenal hypomobility causing resistance to emptying. It can also distinguish between neuropathic and myopathic diseases. C-breath testing is influenced by lung disease and small bowel maldigestion and malabsorption. Therefore, its use is limited in patients with lung, small bowel, pancreatic, and liver disease.

Patrick A and Epstein O. Review article: gastroparesis. *Alimentary Pharmacology and Therapeutics* 2008; 27: 724–740.

Szarka LA and Camilleri M. Clinical imaging: Gastric emptying. *Clinical Gastroenterology and Hepatology* 2009; 7: 823–827.

Abrahamsson H. Treatment options for patients with severe gastroparesis. *Gut* 2007; 56: 877–883.

11. D. When there is an increase in the bacterial colonization of the small bowel proximal to the distal ileum, it is referred to as small bowel bacterial overgrowth (SBBO). Patients can present with symptoms which include weight loss, abdominal pain, diarrhoea, and malnutrition. They may also exhibit neurological symptoms associated with vitamin B_{12} malabsorption and impaired absorption of fat-soluble vitamins (A, D, E, and K).

Causes of bacterial overgrowth

Reduced host defences	Hypogammaglobulinaemia
	Immunodeficiency (e.g. HIV)
	Old age
	Chronic pancreatitis
Excess bacterial entry to small bowel	Atrophic gastritis/gastric acid suppression (e.g. PPI)
	Gastrojejunostomy/Roux-en-Y anastomosis
	Gastrectomy
	Enteral fistulae
Delayed small bowel clearance	Small bowel/jejunal diverticula
	Scleroderma
	Strictures (e.g. Crohn's disease, post-surgical)
	Pseudo-obstruction
	Amyloidosis
	Autonomic neuropathy (e.g. diabetes mellitus, post-vagotomy)

Reproduced from Bloom S, Webster G, and Marks D, *Oxford Handbook of Gastroenterology and Hepatology*, second edition, Box 3.5, p. 227, 2012 with permission from Oxford University Press.

The most direct method of diagnosis of SBBO is microbiological culture of duodenal aspirate obtained at gastroscopy; bacteria levels of $> 10^5$ colonies/mL are diagnostic. However, hydrogen breath testing is less invasive, so is more commonly used as a first-line investigation. As this woman has symptoms suggestive of SBBO, this is the most appropriate investigation in this case.

The other options—faecal calprotectin, flexible sigmoidoscopy, and SeHCAT scan—may be useful to exclude other diagnoses, such as inflammatory bowel disease, microscopic colitis, and bile acid malabsorption, respectively. Treatment of SBBO includes surgical correction of the underlying abnormality, antibiotics (metronidazole is commonly used), and treatment of dysmotility.

Bloom S, Webster G and Marks D. *Oxford Handbook of Gastroenterology and Hepatology*, 2nd edition. Oxford: Oxford University Press; 2012. pp. 226–227.

12. C. Iron deficiency is the commonest vitamin deficiency post gastrectomy, and occurs approximately 10 years before the onset of vitamin B_{12} deficiency. Folate deficiency has also been documented, as has vitamin D deficiency with subsequent osteoporosis.

Following partial gastrectomy, 30–40% of patients experience long-term side effects; the risk of malignant change in the gastric remnant is 3% over 15 years. Dumping syndrome tends to present within 3 months of surgery, but can resolve within 1 year post-operatively. It occurs in 25–50% of patients, but causes significant symptoms in 5–10%.

A Billroth II gastrectomy is the surgical procedure of choice for a duodenal ulcer, whereas the Billroth I is used for a gastric ulcer.

Billroth I gastrectomy for gastric ulcer

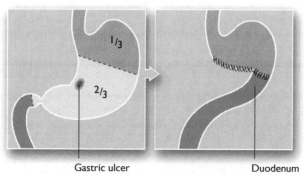

Gastric ulcer   Duodenum

Billroth II gastrectomy for duodenal ulcer

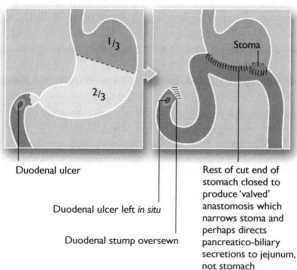

Duodenal ulcer

Duodenal ulcer left *in situ*

Duodenal stump oversewn

Rest of cut end of stomach closed to produce 'valved' anastomosis which narrows stoma and perhaps directs pancreatico-biliary secretions to jejunum, not stomach

Figure 4.1 Billroth I and Billroth II gastrectomy.

This figure was published in *Essential Surgery Problems, Diagnosis and Management*, 3rd edition, Burkitt HG and Quick CGR, Figure 14.11, p. 223. Copyright Elsevier 2001.

Burkitt HG and Quick CGR. *Essential Surgery: problems, diagnosis, and management*, 3rd edition. Philadelphia, PA: Churchill Livingstone; 2001. pp. 222–223.

Rogers C. Postgastrectomy nutrition. *Nutrition in Clinical Practice* 2011; 26: 126–136.

Tovey FI, Godfrey JE and Lewin MR. A gastrectomy population: 25–30 years on. *Postgraduate Medical Journal* 1990; 66: 450–456.

13. C. Dumping syndrome refers to the gastrointestinal and vasomotor symptoms experienced by patients after meals, following gastric surgery. The incidence and severity of symptoms depend on the type of surgery performed. Dumping syndrome occurs in 50–70% of patients during the early post-operative period following a Roux-en-Y gastric bypass. Symptoms often subside 15 to 18 months after surgery, but this is not always the case.

Symptomatic presentation can be divided into early and late dumping syndrome:

Early dumping syndrome	Late dumping syndrome
• 30–60 minutes after food	• 1–3 hours after food
• GI and vasomotor symptoms	• Vasomotor symptoms
• Abdominal pain, nausea, bloating, vomiting, diarrhoea	• Sweating, weakness, confusion, shakiness, hunger, hypoglycaemia
• Headache, flushing, fatigue, hypotension	• Due to reactive hypoglycaemia
• Due to a rapid influx of hyperosmolar contents into the duodenum, resulting in fluid shifts into the intestinal lumen and distension	• Diagnosed by an OGTT after an overnight fast

Data from Bloom S, Webster G, and Marks D, *Oxford Handbook of Gastroenterology and Hepatology*, second edition, 'Dumping syndrome', p. 290, 2012, Oxford University Press.

Dietary manipulation includes small, frequent meals (six times a day), eating a high-protein diet and complex carbohydrates, avoiding simple sugars, milk and dairy products, and avoiding drinking liquids for 30 minutes after eating food. Lying supine for 30 minutes after meals helps to delay gastric emptying for those with postprandial hypotension.

In 3–5% of patients, symptoms persist despite dietary modulation. Somatostatin analogues, such as octreotide, are the most effective medical therapy for dumping syndrome. Evidence supporting the use of acarbose is conflicting, although it may be most useful in late dumping syndrome. The other drugs listed have been used, but are not supported by significant evidence. If medical therapy fails, patients may be referred for surgery.

Ukleja A. Dumping syndrome: pathophysiology and treatment. *Nutrition in Clinical Practice* 2005; 20: 517–525.

Burkitt HG and Quick CGR. *Essential Surgery: problems, diagnosis, and management*, 3rd edition. Philadelphia, PA: Churchill Livingstone; 2001. p. 223.

Rogers C. Postgastrectomy nutrition. *Nutrition in Clinical Practice* 2011; 26: 126–136.

Tovey FI, Godfrey JE and Lewin MR. A gastrectomy population: 25–30 years on. *Postgraduate Medical Journal* 1990; 66: 450–456.

14. C. Early nutritional support plays a key role in recovery from acute pancreatitis, as the disease creates a catabolic stress response state, resulting in nutritional deterioration. Historically, management involved 'resting the pancreas' by limiting enteral intake and feeding parenterally; this concept is now thought to be incorrect. Early total parenteral nutrition may lead to a malfunction of the intestinal mucosal barrier, promoting sepsis from the gut.

Enteral nutrition maintains gut mucosal integrity and function. In severe pancreatitis, nutrition via a nasojejunal (NJ) tube results in fewer episodes of death, systemic infections, multiple organ failure, and operative interventions. The rationale is that food enters the small bowel distal to the ligament of Treitz and thus reduces pancreatic secretions. However, early studies of nasogastric (NG) feeding suggest that this may provide a suitable alternative, and further trials of NG feeding are being carried out. This would reduce the practical problems of inserting and maintaining an NJ tube. Patients with mild pancreatitis should be encouraged to eat and drink via the oral route as tolerated.

Al-Omran M, AlBalawi ZH, Tashkandi MF et al. Enteral versus parenteral nutrition for acute pancreatitis. *Cochrane Database of Systematic Reviews* 2010; Issue 1. Art. No.: CD002837.

UK Working Party on Acute Pancreatitis. UK guidelines for the management of acute pancreatitis. *Gut* 2005: 54 (Suppl. 3): iii1–9.

15. C. In practice, any of these fluid prescriptions is unlikely to cause harm, but the best answer is 1000 mL 5% dextrose with 40 mmol KCl and 500 mL 0.9% saline, to avoid excess sodium. In this case the urine output is in keeping with the patient's body weight (at 0.5 mL/kg/hour). A urinary sodium concentration higher than 20 mmol/L indicates adequate renal perfusion and hydration. This patient only requires maintenance fluids, especially as he is managing sips of fluid. Daily requirements are for 50–100 mmol/day of sodium, 40–80 mmol/day of potassium, and 1.5–2.5 litres of water.

	N saline 0.9%	Dextrose 5%	Hartmann's solution
Sodium (mmol/L)	154	0	131
Chloride (mmol/L)	154	0	111
Potassium (mmol/L)	0	0	5
Lactate (mmol/L)	0	0	29
Calcium (mmol/L)	0	0	2
Dextrose (g)	0	50	0

Surgical patients often have fluid deficits of 1–1.5 L pre-operatively due to a prolonged fast; guidelines suggest that clear non-particulate oral fluids should not be withheld for more than 2 hours prior to the induction of anaesthesia. The extracellular fluid compartment has a volume of more than 10 L. A deficit of more than 3 L in whole body fluid volume cannot be sustained, and intravascular volume becomes depleted.

Traditionally, bowel preparation was used to aggressively cleanse the bowel before colonic surgery, as it was thought to make it safer. However, it causes dehydration and electrolyte imbalances which, unless they are corrected pre-operatively, complicate intra-operative and post-operative fluid management. It can exacerbate hypovolaemia post-anaesthetic induction, resulting in over replacement and post-operative oedema. In addition, mechanical bowel preparation may increase anastomotic leak rates, and has failed to show a reduction in post-operative complication rates.

In recent years the length of time for pre-operative fasting has been reduced. Studies have shown that administration of a pre-operative carbohydrate load attenuates pre-operative thirst, anxiety, and post-operative nausea and vomiting. It also reduces post-operative insulin resistance, which improves the efficacy of post-operative nutritional support. This applies to patients who are undergoing elective surgery and who do not have disorders of gastric emptying or diabetes.

Powell-Tuck J, Gosling P, Lobo DN et al. *British Consensus Guidelines on Intravenous Fluid Therapy for Adult Surgical Patients*. GIFTASUP, on behalf of the British Association for Parenteral and Enteral Nutrition, March 2011.

16. D. The most likely diagnosis is autoimmune pancreatitis (AIP) as supported by the CT appearances and a raised immunoglobulin G4 level. There are also classical histopathological changes on pancreatic biopsies. It can clinically mimic pancreatic cancer, and causes chronic pancreatitis and pancreatic insufficiency. It is also associated with intrahepatic biliary strictures similar to PSC. AIP is characterized by:

- Diffuse pancreatic enlargement ('sausage pancreas')
- Pancreatic duct abnormality

- Low common bile duct stricture
- Lymphoplasmacytic infiltrate on biopsy
- Raised serum IgG4 levels
- Associated autoimmune disease (Sjögren's syndrome, Crohn's disease).

It is treated with steroids, and patients commonly have pancreatic insufficiency.

Pancreatin is a pancreatic enzyme replacement that is porcine in origin. Doses start at 40 000 IU with meals and 10 000 IU with snacks. The response to pancreatic enzyme therapy should be measured according to size, number, and consistency of stools. Treatment success is defined clinically by improved body weight and consistency of faeces. The high-strength pancreatin preparations Nutrizym 22® and Pancreatin HL® have been associated with the development of large bowel strictures (fibrosing colonopathy) in children with cystic fibrosis aged between 2 and 13 years. No such association was found with Creon®.

The most frequent side effects of pancreatic enzyme replacement are gastrointestinal, including nausea, vomiting, and abdominal discomfort. Hyperuricaemia and hyperuricosuria have been associated with very high doses.

The efficacy of pancreatin therapy is influenced by denaturation of lipase by gastric acid, improper timing of enzymes, coexisting small bowel mucosal disease, rapid intestinal transit, and effects of diabetes. Excessive heat should be avoided if mixing preparations with liquids or food, and the resulting mixture should not be kept for more than 1 hour.

Pain can be improved by smoking cessation, avoiding alcohol, a low-fat diet, and non-narcotic analgesics.

British Medical Association and the Royal Pharmaceutical Society of Great Britain. *British National Formulary. BNF 61*. London: BMJ Group and the Royal Pharmaceutical Society of Great Britain; 2011. pp. 79–80.

Hammer H. Pancreatic exocrine insufficiency: diagnostic evaluation and replacement therapy with pancreatic enzymes. *Digestive Diseases* 2010; 28: 339–343.

17. A. During the initial stages of recovery from surgery resulting in a short bowel, parenteral nutrition and fluid and electrolyte support are advised. After the initial post-operative period, it is helpful to establish the length of residual small bowel, as this can guide and predict future nutritional requirements.

Guide to bowel length and long-term fluid/nutritional support required by patients with a short bowel

Jejunal length (cm)	Jejunum–colon	Jejunostomy
0–50	PN	PN + PS
51–100	ON	PN + PS*
101–150	None	ON + OGS
151–200	None	OGS

PN, parenteral nutrition; PS, parenteral saline (with or without magnesium); ON, oral (or enteral) nutrition; OGS, oral (or enteral) glucose/saline solution.

*At 85–100 cm, may require PS only.

Reproduced from *Gut*, J Nightingale and J M Woodward, 'Guidelines for The Management of Patients with a Short Bowel', 55 (Supplement IV), pp. iv1–iv12. Copyright 2006, with permission from BMJ Publishing Group Ltd.

18. E. The patient described has a jejunostomy with less than 100 cm of small bowel remaining, which will have an impact on the absorption of sodium and water. The capacity to absorb nutrients is higher in the proximal small bowel than in the distal small bowel, so patients with less than 100 cm of jejunum (or less than 50 cm of jejunum with an intact colon) will be overall net secretors of fluid and electrolytes. Net absorbers are patients with more than 100 cm of jejunum remaining. This patient has 60 cm of jejunum remaining, and will be an overall net secretor, so increasing fluid intake will cause a higher stoma output.

Jejunal output and resulting fluid and electrolyte depletion may be managed in a number of different ways. BSG guidelines suggest a number of different therapeutic interventions that can be used to reduce stoma output. Restricting the intake of hypotonic and most hypertonic fluid can help to reduce stomal output. Oral glucose–saline solutions, ideally with a sodium concentration of 90–120 mmol/L (e.g. WHO solution made up at 1.5 x strength, St Mark's solution), can increase the absorption of sodium and water from the jejunal lumen. Adjuncts can include salt tablets or adding salt to food.

Antimotility drugs (e.g. loperamide, codeine) reduce intestinal motility, thus decreasing stomal output. Antisecretory drugs such as omeprazole, cimetidine, and ranitidine help to reduce gastric acid secretion, particularly in patients with a stomal output of more than 2000 mL/24 hours. Octreotide can also reduce diarrhoea and stomal output.

Nightingale J and Woodward JM on behalf of the Small Bowel and Nutrition Committee of the British Society of Gastroenterology. Guidelines for the management of patients with a short bowel. *Gut* 2006; 55 (Suppl. IV): iv1–12.

19. B. Calcium oxalate stone formation results from increased absorption of oxalate unbound from calcium (which is instead bound to free fatty acids) from the colon. This leads to hyperoxaluria, and calcium oxalate precipitates in the renal tract as renal calculi or diffuse nephrocalcinosis. Chronic renal failure can develop. This process is exacerbated by malabsorption of fats, increasing the amount of free fatty acid available in the jejunal lumen. Other contributing factors include increased levels of bile acids in the lumen, which increase the colonic permeability to oxalate and other compounds (and hence absorption), reduced oxalate degradation by intestinal bacteria, and hypocitraturia. Jejunum–colon patients have a 25% chance of developing symptomatic calcium oxalate renal stones.

Earnest DL, Johnson G, Williams HE *et al.* Hyperoxaluria in patients with ileal resection: an abnormality in dietary oxalate absorption. *Gastroenterology* 1974; 66: 1114–1122.

Rudman D, Dedonis JL, Fountain MT *et al.* Hypocitraturia in patients with gastrointestinal malabsorption. *New England Journal of Medicine* 1980; 303: 657–661.

Nightingale JMD, Lennard-Jones JE, Gertner DJ *et al.* Colonic preservation reduces the need for parenteral therapy, increases the incidence of renal stones but does not change the high prevalence of gallstones in patients with a short bowel. *Gut* 1992; 33: 1493–1497.

Nightingale J and Woodward JM on behalf of the Small Bowel and Nutrition Committee of the British Society of Gastroenterology. Guidelines for the management of patients with a short bowel. *Gut* 2006; 55 (Suppl. IV): iv1–12.

20. E. Patients with short bowel syndrome, particularly jejunum–colon patients, are thought to be at risk of forming calcium oxalate renal stones. BSG guidelines advise a number of dietary measures, including maintaining a low-oxalate diet, avoiding dehydration, reducing fat intake, and increasing the amount of dietary calcium.

Foods high in oxalate are listed in the following table:

Food type	Examples
Fruit	Blackberries, blueberries, raspberries, strawberries, grapes, plums, currants, kiwis, tangerines, figs, citrus peel
Vegetables	Spinach, parsley, green pepper, leeks, olives, celery, swiss chard, beet greens, okra, green beans, swede
	Non-green vegetables: carrots, beets, beans (baked, dried, and kidney beans), summer squash, sweet potatoes
Nuts and seeds	Almonds, cashews, peanuts
Legumes	Tofu, other soy products
Grains	Wheat bran, wheat germ, quinoa (a vegetable often used like a grain)
Other	Black tea, hot chocolate, coffee, dark or robust beers
	Black pepper

Nightingale J and Woodward JM on behalf of the Small Bowel and Nutrition Committee of the British Society of Gastroenterology. Guidelines for the management of patients with a short bowel. *Gut* 2006; 55 (Suppl. IV): iv1–12.

21. B. A gastrostomy provides nutrition for those who need enteral feeding, and can either be placed endoscopically (PEG) or radiologically inserted (RIG). A RIG may be considered in patients with oesophageal stricturing or head and neck malignancy where there is a perceived risk of tumour seeding. Complications can be immediate (e.g. respiratory failure, bleeding, perforation of a viscus, peritonitis), early (e.g. pneumonia, infection, early tube displacement), or late (e.g. aspiration pneumonia, infection, hypergranulation, leakage, fistula formation, small bowel ischaemia and obstruction, tumour seeding, and tube malfunction and displacement). Around 40% of patients who undergo percutaneous feeding tube placement may show pneumoperitoneum on X-rays, which is often asymptomatic and may last for several days.

A buried bumper occurs when the gastrostomy tube is pulled tightly up against the gastric mucosa, and over the course of time erosion of the gastric mucosa occurs. Eventually the mucosa grows over the bumper and buries it. One of the first signs of a buried bumper is when the PEG becomes difficult to push in or rotate easily. Eventually it may be hard to flush as it becomes slowly obstructed and leakage around the site occurs. A silicon internal disc increases the likelihood of a buried bumper.

A buried bumper may be prevented during the procedure by ensuring a 1 cm degree of play between the external fixator and the skin, which avoids excess tension. Patients and carers should be taught to ensure that they can push in and rotate the PEG on a weekly basis, as this helps to prevent a buried bumper from developing.

BSG guidelines describe a number of endoscopic techniques which have been used to remove a buried bumper. These include the 'balloon push technique', the 'balloon pull technique', the 'snare technique' and use of a 'needle knife.' Surgery may be required to remove a deeply buried bumper in some patients. In certain patients, who may be considered high risk for surgery or further endoscopic procedures, the PEG tube may be left *in situ* and a jejunal extension passed to allow feeding to continue.

Westaby D, Young A, O'Toole P *et al*. The provision of a percutaneously placed enteral tube feeding service. *Gut* 2010; 59: 1592–1605.

22. E. Zinc deficiency causes a characteristic skin rash (mainly affecting the intertriginous and perioral areas), alopecia, taste impairment, glucose intolerance, and diarrhoea. In children, acrodermatitis enteropathica is an autosomal-recessive disorder of zinc uptake, and features include the characteristic periorificial rash with nail changes, secondary skin infections, alopecia, and diarrhoea.

Zinc is considered to be an essential trace element for human nutrition, and has an important role in many enzyme systems, including that of DNA polymerase. In addition to the above symptoms, deficiency also causes acne, visual problems, impaired ability to smell, subtle cognitive and memory changes, and increased susceptibility to respiratory infections. Secondary skin infections may develop with extensive skin rashes. Nail changes, including white spots, bands, lines, or leuconychia, may also be evident.

Similar symptoms and signs have been seen in patients on total parenteral nutrition who do not receive zinc supplementation. Diarrhoea, stomal and fistula losses increase the loss of zinc, and hypercatabolism also causes increased urinary losses of zinc.

Jeejeebhoy (2009) made a number of recommendations, one of which was that zinc should be added to all parenteral nutrition mixtures. The recommended amounts are 3–4 mg per day for adult patients. Those patients who have higher gastrointestinal losses were felt to need additional supplementation—around 12 mg per litre of loss. It was also felt that patients on long-term parenteral nutrition may require zinc infusions, but more research was deemed necessary.

Vitamin A deficiency causes night blindness and eventually xerophthalmia. It can also lead to impaired immune function, cancer, and birth defects. Vitamin E deficiency can lead to neuromuscular problems such as spinocerebellar ataxia and myopathies, and anaemia, due to oxidative damage to red blood cells. The presence of vitamin deficiency should be evaluated in patients with malabsorption.

Selenium deficiency has been seen in patients with malabsorption and in those on total parenteral nutrition. The effects include myocardial necrosis leading to congestive cardiomyopathy, and degeneration and necrosis of cartilage tissue. There is also increased susceptibility to infection. Selenium is also necessary for the conversion of the thyroid hormone thyroxine (T_4) into its more active counterpart, triiodothyronine (T_3), and as such a deficiency can cause symptoms of hypothyroidism.

Niacin deficiency causes pellagra. Symptoms and signs are wide-ranging and include skin changes such as sensitivity to sunlight, dermatitis, alopecia, oedema, and glossitis. Psychological changes include emotional problems, aggression, insomnia, confusion, and dementia. Neurological signs include weakness, ataxia, paralysis, and peripheral neuritis. Diarrhoea and a dilated cardiomyopathy may also occur. Pellagra is due to either chronic dietary vitamin B_3 deficiency or alterations in protein metabolism, such as carcinoid syndrome, where tryptophan deficiency may occur.

Wolman SL, Anderson GH, Marliss GB et al. Zinc in total parenteral nutrition: requirements and metabolic effects. *Gastroenterology* 1979; 76: 458–467.

Jeejeebhoy K. Zinc: an essential trace element for parenteral nutrition. *Gastroenterology* 2009; 137: S7–12.

23. A. Gastric emptying scintigraphy of a radiolabelled solid meal (99-m technetium-labelled egg white) is used in the diagnosis of gastroparesis. Retention of over 10% of the solid meal after 4 hours is abnormal. In research studies, an attempt to grade the severity of the delay in gastric emptying has been made, and it has been suggested that it might be used clinically.

Grading for severity of delayed gastric emptying based on 4-hour values is as follows:

Grade 1 (mild)	11–20% retention at 4 hours
Grade 2 (moderate)	21–35% retention at 4 hours
Grade 3 (severe)	36–50% retention at 4 hours
Grade 4 (very severe)	> 50% retention at 4 hours

Post-pyloric feeding is indicated in the presence of severe gastroparesis. Other indications would include situations where enteral feeding is required but intra-gastric feeding is either difficult (e.g. gastric outlet obstruction) or poorly tolerated (e.g. gastro-oesophageal reflux, recurrent pulmonary aspiration).

A short-term trial of nasojejunal (NJ) feeding acutely would be recommended to ensure that feeding can be safely tolerated. Long-term nasoenteric (NG or NJ) feeding is prone to failure due to tube occlusion or dislodgement, which in turn interrupts feeding and medication. Therefore it is not recommended for more than 1 month, and this patient is likely to need enteral feeding indefinitely.

A PEGJ (percutaneous endoscopic gastrojejunostomy) describes a jejunal extension tube passed via the PEG tube, which can either be done at the same time as the PEG insertion or added at a later date. It is useful when enteral feeding is required at the same time as gastric decompression. Displacement remains the major limitation, with 30–40% migrating back into the stomach within 2 months despite adequate placement beyond the ligament of Treitz using a guidewire.

Direct percutaneous endoscopic jejunostomy (DPEJ) is an evolving technique that is used to establish jejunal feeding. It involves direct placement of the feeding tube into the jejunum using either a paediatric colonoscope or an enteroscope. Its success is dependent on the expertise of the endoscopist and assistant.

Arts J, Caenepeel P, Verbeke K et al. Influence of erythromycin on gastric emptying and meal-related symptoms in functional dyspepsia with delayed gastric emptying. *Gut* 2005; 54: 455–460.

Shike M, Berner YH, Gerdes H et al. Percutaneous endoscopic gastrostomy and jejunostomy for long-term feeding in patients with cancer of the head and neck. *Otolaryngology – Head and Neck Surgery* 1989; 101: 549–554.

Westaby D, Young A, O'Toole P et al. The provision of a percutaneously placed enteral tube feeding service. *Gut* 2010; 59: 1592–1605.

24. A. The multidisciplinary team (MDT) is not responsible for making decisions but for determining the most appropriate and agreed course of action from the medical perspective. A second opinion may be useful, but will have no legal bearing on the situation. Similarly, although a collateral history from a neighbour may be helpful, the neighbour has no legal responsibility or requirement to make decisions on behalf of the patient.

The Mental Capacity Act 2005 outlines the steps involved in creating a Lasting Power of Attorney. It states that the party involved must have reached the age of 18 years and have the capacity to execute such a decision, which is not applicable in this case.

The Mental Capacity Act 2005 recommends that the appropriate authority should make arrangements to enable an Independent Mental Capacity Advocate (IMCA) to be available to represent and support individuals who lack capacity to make decisions about the provision of serious medical treatment by an NHS body. Before the treatment is provided, the NHS body must instruct an IMCA to represent the individual. In addition, the NHS body must, in providing or securing the provision of treatment for the patient, take into account any information given or submissions made by the IMCA. Inserting a PEG feeding tube without the assessment and advice of an IMCA would be going against the Mental Incapacity Act 2005.

'Serious medical treatment' refers to that which involves providing, withholding, or withdrawing treatment of a kind prescribed by regulations made by the appropriate authority.

The National Archives. *Mental Capacity Act 2005*. www.legislation.gov.uk/ukpga/2005/9/contents (accessed 20 June 2011).

25. C. Safe beverages include cider, wine, sherry, champagne, spirits, port, and liquor. Distillation of spirits removes gluten, so all spirits—including malt whisky—are suitable. Stout, beer, ale, and lager all contain gluten.

Non-alcoholic beverages that contain gluten include malted drinks, barley squash, and some colas. Tea, coffee, fruit drinks, cordials, and flavoured water are all gluten free.

Coeliac UK. *Alcohol*. www.coeliac.org.uk/gluten-free-diet-lifestyle/keeping-healthy/alcohol (accessed 20 October 2011).

1. **A 46-year-old man with chronic liver disease secondary to alcohol misuse was seen in the outpatient clinic.**

   Which of the following factors is most important for variceal development?

   A. Child–Pugh grade C cirrhosis
   B. Concomitant diagnosis of non-alcoholic steatohepatitis (NASH)
   C. Continued alcohol intake
   D. Haemophilia A
   E. Hepatic venous pressure gradient (HVPG) greater than 10 mmHg

2. **A 40-year-old man with cirrhosis and known oesophageal varices presented to hospital with haematemesis. He was encephalopathic.**

   Initial observations:

blood pressure	87/55 mmHg
pulse	120 beats/minute
temperature	36.1°C
oxygen saturations	91% on room air
respiratory rate	21 breaths/minute

   Investigations:

haemoglobin on venous gas	902 g/L (130–180)
platelet count	15 × 10⁹/L (150–400)
ABO blood group	A negative

   Which of the following statements about the resuscitation of patients with variceal haemorrhage is most accurate?

   A. Blood loss can be estimated to be 750–1500 mL
   B. Fresh frozen plasma (FFP) contains only clotting factors II, VII, IX, and X
   C. Give Group-O-negative platelets if no ABO-matched platelets are available
   D. Resuscitation is needed with packed red cell transfusions to a haemoglobin concentration of more than 100 g/L
   E. Terlipressin and broad-spectrum antibiotics should be given pre-endoscopy

3. **A variceal screening gastroscopy was performed on a 42-year-old woman with recently diagnosed chronic liver disease secondary to non-alcoholic fatty liver disease (NAFLD). She had not had a variceal bleed before. She was intolerant of propranolol and had Child–Pugh grade C cirrhosis. Her endoscopy revealed grade II/medium oesophageal varices with no visible 'red signs.'**

    Which of the following is the best treatment plan?

    A. Endoscopic sclerotherapy and referral for transplantation
    B. Oral nitrate therapy and repeat surveillance endoscopy in 1 year's time
    C. Referral for transjugular intrahepatic portosystemic shunt (TIPSS)
    D. Trial of a selective beta-blocker and repeat surveillance endoscopy in 1 year's time
    E. Variceal band ligation and repeat surveillance endoscopy in 1 year's time

4. **A 52-year-old man with advanced alcoholic liver cirrhosis was admitted with a fall. He was not known to have chronic renal impairment. He was taking spironolactone, which was stopped on admission, and he had moderate volume ascites.**

    Investigations on admission:

sodium	124 mmol/L (137–144)
potassium	5.8 mmol/L (3.5–4.9)
urea	10.4 mmol/L (2.5–7.0)
creatinine	180 µmol/L (60–110)
urine dipstick	protein: trace
USS renal tract	normal sized kidneys with no hydronephrosis
septic screen	negative

    After 48 hours of fluid resuscitation, including human albumin solution, his bloods results were as follows:

sodium	127 mmol/L (137–144)
potassium	5.7 mmol/L (3.5–4.9)
urea	7.2 mmol/L (2.5–7.0)
creatinine	150 µmol/L (60–110)

    What is the next best option for management?

    A. Administer 2 L of IV colloid
    B. Commence haemofiltration
    C. Commence terlipressin
    D. Drainage of ascites
    E. Renal biopsy

5. **A 61-year-old woman was diagnosed with hepatorenal syndrome.**

    Which of the following findings best describes the earliest manifestation of hepatorenal syndrome (HRS)?

    A. Activation of the renin–angiotensin–aldosterone system
    B. Increased creatinine levels
    C. Peripheral vasodilation
    D. Renal vasoconstriction
    E. Retention of sodium

6. **A 54-year-old man was diagnosed with type 1 hepatorenal syndrome. He had no past medical history of ischaemic heart disease and was euvolaemic. He weighed 70 kg.**

    What is the most appropriate initial treatment?

    A. Human albumin solution 70 g on day 1, and 20–40 g of human albumin solution on subsequent days
    B. Human albumin solution 100 g for 5 days
    C. Terlipressin 0.5 mg to 2 mg IV QDS
    D. Terlipressin 0.5 mg to 2 mg IV QDS plus 70 g of human albumin solution on day 1 and 20–40 g of human albumin solution on subsequent days
    E. Terlipressin 0.5 mg to 2 mg IV QDS plus 70 g of human albumin solution per day

7. **A 43-year-old man with alcoholic liver disease and portal hypertension was admitted with confusion. He was taking propranolol, spironolactone, vitamin B$_{12}$, and thiamine; these medications were continued over the next 3 days. He was initially treated with intravenous fluids and lactulose.**

    Investigations on admission:

urea	4.0 mmol/L (2.5–7.0)
creatinine	70 µmol/L (60–110)

    Investigations 3 days later

urea	8.0 mmol/L (2.5–7.0)
creatinine	150 µmol/L (60–110)

    Which of the following investigations favours a diagnosis of acute tubular necrosis over hepatorenal syndrome?

    A. Granular casts and renal epithelial cells seen on urine microscopy
    B. High urinary osmolarity
    C. Low urinary sodium
    D. Normal renal USS
    E. Urinary protein of 250 mg in 24 hours

8. **A 59-year-old man with cirrhosis and moderate ascites was admitted
    to the medical assessment unit with encephalopathy and deteriorating
    renal function. On examination his abdomen was mildly tender, without
    peritonism, and his chest was clear to auscultation.**

    **His observations were temperature 38.2°C, blood pressure 99/59 mmHg,
    pulse 97 beats/minute, and oxygen saturations 98% on room air. He was
    commenced on empirical intravenous antibiotics, after sending ascitic
    fluid and blood cultures.**

    Investigations:
        acitic polymorphonuclear leucocytes (PMNs)   178 (< 250 cells/mm^3)
        serum-ascites albumin gradient (SAAG)   15 g/dL

    What is the subsequent best course of action?

    A. Continue antibiotics and await cultures
    B. Continue antibiotics and CT abdomen
    C. Continue antibiotics and portal vein Doppler
    D. Stop antibiotics and erect chest X-ray
    E. Stop antibiotics and await cultures

9. **A 59-year-old man with cirrhosis and moderate ascites was admitted
    with encephalopathy and deteriorating renal function. On examination
    his abdomen was mildly tender, without peritonism, and his chest was
    clear on auscultation.**

    Investigations:
        ascitic polymorphonuclear leucocytes (PMNs)   178 (< 250 cells/mm^3)
        serum-ascites albumin gradient (SAAG)   15 g/dL

    **He was treated empirically with ceftriaxone, and after 48 hours his
    ascitic culture grew Gram-negative rods.**

    **Observations after 48 hours were temperature 37.6°C, blood pressure
    100/59 mmHg, pulse 82 beats/minute, and oxygen saturations 98%
    on room air. His abdomen was mildly tender to palpation, but
    not peritonitic.**

    What is the next best course of action?

    A. Continue antibiotics and add metronidazole
    B. Continue antibiotics and repeat ascitic tap
    C. Continue antibiotics and treat for SBP
    D. Request CT abdomen
    E. Stop antibiotics, and repeat ascitic tap and cultures

10. **A 44-year-old woman from Pakistan with chronic liver disease presented with jaundice and abdominal distension. She was found to have ascites, and an ascitic tap was performed.**

    Investigations:

serum white cell count	9.6×10^9/L (4.0–11.0)
serum total albumin	30 g/L (37–49)
serum CA-125	200 U/mL (< 35)
ascitic white cell count	100 cells/mm³ with 75 PMNs
	(WCC < 500 cells/mm³ and PMNs < 250 cells/mm³)
ascitic albumin	15 g/L
ascitic Gram stain	no organisms seen

    Which of the following is the most likely diagnosis?

    A. Cirrhosis

    B. Gynaecological malignancy

    C. Hepatocellular carcinoma

    D. Nephrotic syndrome

    E. Tuberculosis

11. **A 35-year-old woman visited the UK from Malaysia when she was 30 weeks pregnant. She was referred by the Emergency Department with malaise, nausea, vomiting, headache, pruritus, and abnormal blood results. On examination she had a gravid uterus, no stigmata of chronic liver disease, and no dependent oedema. Her blood pressure was 162/66 mmHg, her pulse was 87 beats/minute, her oxygen saturations was 98% on room air, and her temperature was 36.3°C.**

Investigations:

haemoglobin	117 g/L (115–165)
white cell count	16.3 x 10⁹/L (4.0–11.0)
platelets	190 x 10⁹/L (150–400)
prothrombin time	21 seconds (15–19)
activated partial thromboplastin time	45 seconds (30–40)
serum lactate dehydrogenase	236 U/L (10–250)
serum bilirubin	76 µmol/L (1–22)
serum alkaline phosphatase	115 U/L (45–105)
serum alanine aminotransferase	402 U/L (5–35)
serum bile acid	6 µmol/L (< 10)
uric acid	11.0 mg/dL (2.0–6.5)
urine dipstick	protein: positive
	glucose: negative
	blood: negative
	ketones: negative
	leucocytes: negative
liver biopsy	microvesicular steatosis, foamy hepatocytes, and hepatic necrosis

What is the most likely diagnosis?

A. Acute fatty liver of pregnancy

B. HELLP syndrome

C. Hepatitis E

D. Intrahepatic cholestasis of pregnancy (ICP)

E. Pre-eclampsia

12. **A 26-year-old woman who was 20 weeks pregnant presented to the gastroenterology outpatients clinic for a routine follow-up appointment. She had irritable bowel syndrome and had recently had some blood tests.**

Which one of the following results is usually unchanged in pregnancy?

A. Alkaline phosphatase

B. Aminotransferases

C. Cholesterol

D. Globulin

E. Haemoglobin

13. **A 36-year-old man with a history of alcohol excess presented to the Emergency Department following a haematemesis. A previous abdominal ultrasound scan had revealed radiological evidence of cirrhosis.**

On examination, he had moderate ascites and grade 3 encephalopathy. His abdomen was soft and non-tender. He had a gastroscopy which revealed three grade 4 oesophageal varices; these were banded. His oral intake remained inadequate on the ward for 48 hours after endoscopy.

Investigations:

haemoglobin	97 g/L (130–180)
white cell count	11.5 x 10⁹/L (4.0–11.0)
platelet count	89 x 10⁹/L (150–400)
serum bilirubin	163 µmol/L (1–22)
serum alkaline phosphatase	213 U/L (45–105)
serum alanine aminotransferase	79 U/L (5–35)
serum amylase	204 U/L (60–180)
prothrombin time	21 s (11.5–15.5)

What is the most appropriate nutritional management?

A. Nasogastric feeding
B. Nasojejunal feeding
C. Oral nutrition
D. Parenteral nutrition
E. Supplemented oral nutrition

14. **A 56-year-old man who was drinking 34 units of alcohol per week presented to the Emergency Department with jaundice.**

Investigations:

haemoglobin	117 g/L (130–180)
white cell count	12.5 x 10⁹/L (4.0–11.0)
platelet count	89 x 10⁹/L (150–400)
serum bilirubin	187 µmol/L (1–22)
serum alkaline phosphatase	149 U/L (45–105)
serum alanine aminotransferase	86 U/L (5–35)
prothrombin time	18 (lab PT = 12.5)

What is his Maddrey's Discriminant Function score?

A. 30
B. 32
C. 34
D. 36
E. 38

15. **A 45-year-old man with chronic hepatitis B was found to have three liver nodules, all of which were less than 3 cm in size. He had no other comorbidities. On examination, he had no ascites and was not encephalopathic. He was on no regular medications.**

    Investigations:

haemoglobin	12.7 g/dL (130–180)
white cell count	10.5 x 10⁹/L (4.0–11.0)
platelet count	89 x 10⁹/L (150–400)
serum bilirubin	107 µmol/L (1–22)
serum alkaline phosphatase	149 U/L (45–105)
serum alanine aminotransferase	86 U/L (5–35)
serum albumin	30 g/L (37–49)
serum α-fetoprotein	500 kU/L (< 10)
prothrombin time	21 seconds (11.5–15.5)

    Which of the following will best determine appropriate referral for liver transplant assessment?

    A. Barcelona Clinic Liver Cancer (BCLC) staging classification
    B. Child–Turcotte–Pugh (CTP) score
    C. Maddrey's Discriminant Function (MDF) score
    D. Model for End-Stage Liver Disease (MELD) score
    E. United Kingdom End-Stage Liver Disease (UKELD) score

16. **A 49-year-old woman presented to clinic with a history of alcohol excess.**

    Investigations:

haemoglobin	10.7 g/dL (130–180)
mean cell volume	104.3 fL (80–96)
white cell count	4.2 x 10⁹/L (4.0–11.0)
platelet count	89 x 10⁹/L (150–400)
serum bilirubin	44 µmol/L (1–22)
serum alkaline phosphatase	230 U/L (45–105)
serum alanine aminotransferase	53 U/L (5–35)
serum albumin	30 g/L (37–49)
prothrombin time	21 seconds (11.5–15.5)

    Which of the following markers is most suggestive of a diagnosis of chronic liver disease complicated by portal hypertension?

    A. Elevated alanine aminotransferase
    B. Hyperbilirubinaemia
    C. Hypoalbuminaemia
    D. Macrocytosis
    E. Thrombocytopenia

17. **A 58-year-old man who admitted to consuming 20 units of alcohol per day presented to the Emergency Department febrile and icteric. Abdominal examination revealed a 6 cm tender hepatomegaly with moderate ascites.**

    Investigations:

haemoglobin	137 g/L (130–180)
white cell count	15.5 x 10⁹/L (4.0–11.0)
platelet count	109 x 10⁹/L (150–400)
serum bilirubin	187 µmol/L (1–22)
serum alkaline phosphatase	149 U/L (45–105)
serum alanine aminotransferase	86 U/L (5–35)
prothrombin time	21 seconds (11.5–15.5)

    His Maddrey's Discriminant Function score was 36, and he was considered for corticosteroid therapy.

    Which one of the following is least likely to be of benefit in the management of his alcoholic hepatitis?

    A. Corticosteroids
    B. Enteral nutrition
    C. N-acetylcysteine
    D. Non-steroidal anti-inflammatory drugs (NSAIDs)
    E. Pentoxifylline

18. **A 45-year-old woman, who consumed more than 60 units of alcohol per week, presented to the Emergency Department with a fractured tibia. She had no evidence of chronic liver disease on examination. She was seen by the orthopaedic team, who requested a gastroenterology opinion.**

    Which of the following would be first-line therapy to treat delirium tremens if it occurs in this patient?

    A. Oral chlordiazepoxide
    B. Oral haloperidol
    C. Oral lorazepam
    D. Oral oxazepam
    E. Oral risperidone

19. **A 33-year-old man presented to the Emergency Department with a 4-week history of rigors, weight loss, and right sided abdominal pain which radiated to his right shoulder. He had returned from a business trip to China 9 months ago. He reported two episodes of fresh rectal bleeding on return to the UK following his trip.**

On examination, he had a temperature of 39°C, blood pressure of 100/60 mmHg, heart rate of 90 beats/minute, and hepatomegaly.

Investigations:

haemoglobin	140 g/dL (130–180)
white cell count	22 × 10⁹/L (4.0–11.0)
platelet count	220 × 10⁹/L (150–400)
prothrombin time	14 seconds (11.5–15.5)
serum albumin	30 g/L (37–49)
serum total bilirubin	22 μmol/L (1–22)
serum alanine aminotransferase	50 U/L (5–35)
serum alkaline phosphatase	350 U/L (45–105)
serum C-reactive protein	356 mg/L (< 10)

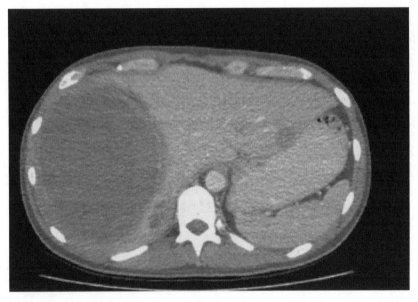

Figure 5.1 CT abdomen.

What is the most likely diagnosis?

A. Cavernous haemangioma

B. Hepatocellular carcinoma

C. Hydatid cyst

D. Liver abscess

E. Metastases to the liver

20. **A 22-year-old bodybuilder presented to the Emergency Department with a 6-week history of jaundice, pruritus, and right upper abdomen pain. He drank 4 units of alcohol per day. There was no family history of liver disease. Examination of the abdomen showed 6 cm hepatomegaly, with no splenomegaly or ascites.**

Investigations:

haemoglobin	140 g/L (130–180)
white cell count	10 x 10⁹/L (4.0–11.0)
platelet count	475 x 10⁹/L (150–400)
prothrombin time	17 seconds (11.5–15.5)
serum albumin	30 g/L (37–49)
serum total bilirubin	552 μmol/L (1–22)
serum alanine aminotransferase	250 U/L (5–35)
serum alkaline phosphatase	650 U/L (45–105)
serum ferritin	810 μg/L (15–300)
hepatitis virus serology	B and C negative
autoimmune profile	negative
liver ultrasound	hepatomegaly with normal calibre of both extrahepatic and intrahepatic bile ducts
MRI liver	normal bile duct and hepatomegaly with normal pancreas

His liver function tests improved slowly.

What is the most likely diagnosis?

A. Alcoholic hepatitis
B. Drug-induced cholestatic jaundice
C. Gallstone in the common bile duct
D. Haemochromatosis
E. Hepatitis A

21. **A 55-year-old man with no symptoms had a routine blood check, and was found to have abnormal liver function tests. He was overweight, with a BMI of 38 kg/m², and drank 2 units of alcohol per week. There were no risk factors for viral hepatitis.**

    Investigations:

serum cholesterol	9 mmol/L (< 5.2)
serum total bilirubin	89 µmol/L (1–22)
serum alanine aminotransferase	235 U/L (5–35)
serum alkaline phosphatase	229 U/L (45–105)
prothrombin time	14 seconds (11.5–15.5)
antinuclear antibodies	1:80 (negative at 1:20 dilution)
antimitochondrial antibodies	1:20 (negative at 1:20 dilution)
serum immunoglobulin G	25 g/L (6.0–13.0)
serum immunoglobulin A	5 g/L (0.8–3.0)
serum immunoglobulin M	12 g/L (0.4–2.5)
hepatitis virus serology	negative
US abdomen	mild hepatomegaly with fatty infiltration and normal biliary tree

    Which is the best investigation to explain the abnormal liver function tests?

    A. Computed tomography abdomen
    B. Endoscopic retrograde cholangiopancreatography
    C. Liver biopsy
    D. Magnetic resonance cholangiopancreatography
    E. Transient elastography

22. **A 25-year-old woman, who was 30 weeks pregnant, presented to the Emergency Department with jaundice. She had flown in on holiday from her country of origin in south-east Asia. Over the last month her family had noticed a yellow discoloration of her eyes. During the flight she became disorientated.**

    Investigations:

haemoglobin	118 g/L (130–180)
white cell count	3.8 x 10⁹/L (4.0–11.0)
platelet count	324 x 10⁹/L (150–400)
serum total protein	68 g/L (61–76)
serum albumin	32 g/L (37–49)
serum total bilirubin	361 µmol/L (1–22)
serum alanine aminotransferase	92 U/L (5–35)
serum aspartate aminotransferase	76 U/L (1–31)
serum alkaline phosphatase	178 U/L (45–105)
prothrombin time	46 seconds (11.5–15.5)

    Which of the following is the most likely aetiology?

    A. Acute hepatitis B
    B. Black cohosh
    C. Hepatitis A
    D. Hepatitis E
    E Leptospirosis

23. **A 19-year-old woman presented to the Emergency Department with jaundice, lethargy, and vomiting. Her mother reported that she had been unwell for several weeks.**

Investigations:

haemoglobin	134 g/L (130–180)
white cell count	12.3 x 10⁹/L (4.0–11.0)
platelet count	365 x 10⁹/L (150–400)
serum total protein	72 g/L (61–76)
serum albumin	34 g/L (37–49)
serum total bilirubin	213 µmol/L (1–22)
serum alanine aminotransferase	123 U/L (5–35)
serum aspartate aminotransferase	87 U/L (1–31)
serum alkaline phosphatase	191 U/L (45–105)
prothrombin time	18.9 seconds (11.5–15.5)

In this scenario, which of the following most accurately reflects the percentage of patients with no discernible cause?

A. 6%

B. 17%

C. 33%

D. 41%

E. 50%

24. **A 42-year-old woman presented with a 2-day history of jaundice. She had developed easy bruising, and her partner noticed that she was sleepy during the daytime.**

Investigations:

haemoglobin	167 g/L (130–180)
white cell count	14.5 x 10⁹/L (4.0–11.0)
platelet count	402 x 10⁹/L (150–400)
serum albumin	34 g/L (37–49)
serum total bilirubin	178 µmol/L (1–22)
serum alanine aminotransferase	98 U/L (5–35)
serum aspartate aminotransferase	75 U/L (1–31)
serum alkaline phosphatase	245 U/L (45–105)
prothrombin time	19.1 seconds (11.5–15.5)

Which of the following treatments is most likely to be effective?

A. Corticosteroids for autoimmune hepatitis

B. Lamivudine for hepatitis B

C. Milk thistle (silibinin) for mushroom poisoning

D. N-acetylcysteine for paracetamol overdose

E. Penicillamine for Wilson's disease

25. **A 27-year-old man with no past medical history presented with acute liver failure. He denied paracetamol use and was haemodynamically stable.**

    Investigations:

haemoglobin	154 g/L (130–180)
white cell count	13.0 x 10⁹/L (4.0–11.0)
platelet count	369 x 10⁹/L (150–400)
serum albumin	39 g/L (37–49)
serum total bilirubin	464 μmol/L (1–22)
serum alanine aminotransferase	109 U/L (5–35)
serum aspartate aminotransferase	100 U/L (1–31)
serum alkaline phosphatase	179 U/L (45–105)
prothrombin time	53 seconds (11.5–15.5)
paracetamol	< 10 (< 10)

    Which one of the following is a poor prognostic indicator, without a liver transplant, in the setting of non-paracetamol-induced acute liver failure?

    A. Age > 50 years
    B. Bilirubin > 200 μmol/L
    C. INR > 3.0
    D. Serum creatinine > 300 mmol/L
    C. Viral aetiology

26. **A 46-year-old woman was prescribed clarithromycin for a community acquired pneumonia.**

    Which of the following is not a cytochrome P450 enzyme inhibitor?

    A. Carbamazepine
    B. Clarithromycin
    C. Fluconazole
    D. Omeprazole
    E. Ritonavir

27. **A 66-year-old woman was found to have cholestatic derangement in her liver function tests, most probably due to recently prescribed antibiotics. Which of the following is not an example of an idiosyncratic reaction in the context of drug-induced liver injury?**

    A. Co-amoxiclav
    B. Co-trimoxazole
    C. Halothane
    D. Paracetamol
    E. Phenytoin

28. **A 57-year-old man was referred to hospital with cholestatic jaundice, and had recently started new medications.**

    Which of the following causes a predominantly cholestatic type of liver injury?

    A. Baclofen
    B. Irbesartan
    C. Lisinopril
    D. Omeprazole
    E. Sodium valproate

29. **A 37-year-old man presented with a paracetamol overdose. Regarding the metabolism of paracetamol, which one of the following does not increase the amount of toxic metabolite?**

    A. Alcohol excess
    B. Concomitant use of isoniazid
    C. Concomitant use of phenytoin
    D. Fasting
    E. Presentation to a hospital within less than 10 hours after ingestion

30. **A 27-year-old Chinese woman presented with deranged liver function tests.**

    Which one of the following is not known to cause hepatotoxicity?

    A. Black cohosh
    B. Chinese green tea extract
    C. Usnic acid
    D. Vitamin A supplement
    E. Vitamin D supplement

31. **A 57-year-old man is about to be discharged following an orthotopic liver transplant for hepatitis C. He is concerned about potential complications.**

    Which of the following is a recognized early complication following orthotopic liver transplantation?

    A. Cytomegalovirus infection
    B. Diabetes mellitus
    C. Lymphoproliferative disorders
    D. Neutropenia
    E. Recurrence of hepatitis C

32. **A Vietnamese man was diagnosed with hepatitis B as a child. He moved to the UK 10 years ago. He is married with two children; his wife is positive (ETC). His wife is positive for anti-HBsAg and anti-HBcAg. He was well apart from some intermittent vague right upper quadrant pain. He drank no alcohol, and had a family history of hepatocellular carcinoma.**

    Investigations:
    HBeAg   positive
    HBV DNA   230 000 IU/mL (< 250 IU/mL)
    serum alanine aminotransferase   99 U/L (5–35)
    liver ultrasound   normal
    Fibroscan®   8.2 kPa (< 7 kPa)

    What is the most appropriate primary treatment end point in order to prevent long-term negative clinical outcomes such as cirrhosis, hepatocellular carcinoma, and death?

    A. Decrease or normalize serum ALT
    B. Improve liver histology
    C. Induce HBeAg loss or seroconversion
    D. Induce HBsAg loss or seroconversion
    E. Sustained decrease in serum HBV DNA level to low or undetectable

33. **A 30-year-old woman was receiving treatment for hepatitis B with 0.5 mg entecavir daily. After 12 months, the viral load dropped to 100 000 IU/mL (pre-treatment value was 230 000 IU/mL) and the ALT normalized.**

    What would be the next best management step?

    A. Check for resistant mutations
    B. Continue the same dose of entecavir until the viral load is undetectable
    C. Increase the dose of entecavir to 1 mg
    D. Stop the entecavir treatment
    E. Switch to tenofovir

34. **A 36-year-old woman with chronic hepatitis C was referred to clinic for consideration of treatment. There was no relevant past medical history and she had no signs of chronic liver disease.**

    Investigations:

haemoglobin	130 g/dL (115–165)
white cell count	7 x 10⁹/L (4–11)
platelets	230 x 10⁹/L (150–400)
international normalized ratio	1.0 (< 1.4)
serum alkaline phosphatase	47 U/L (45–105)
serum gamma glutamyl transferase	43 U/L (4–35)
serum alanine aminotransferase	110 U/L (5–35)
serum aspartate aminotransferase	67 U/L (1–31)
serum bilirubin	12 µmol/L (1–22)
serum albumin	38 g/L (37–49)
HCV genotype	2
HCV RNA	740 000 IU/mL (lower detection limit 15)
Fibroscan®	5.6 kPa (< 7 kPa)

    ### What would you advise in terms of management?

    A. Hepatocellular carcinoma surveillance with 6-monthly ultrasound and alpha fetoprotein

    B. Liver biopsy

    C. No treatment

    D. Pegylated interferon and ribavirin for 24 weeks

    E. Pegylated interferon and ribavirin for 48 weeks

35. **A 30-year-old woman was referred to the outpatient clinic with epigastric pain and a 6 cm right liver lobe mass on ultrasonography. She had no comorbidities and was on the oral contraceptive pill.**

    Investigations:

serum alkaline phosphatase	52 U/L (45–105)
serum gamma glutamyl transferase	34 U/L (4–35)
serum alanine aminotransferase	21 U/L (5–35)
serum aspartate aminotransferase	26 U/L (1–31)
serum bilirubin	15 µmol/L (1–22)
serum albumin	39 g/L (37–49)
multiphase CT	well-demarcated mass with early enhancement in the arterial phase before iso-attenuation in the delayed phase
magnetic resonance imaging of liver	hyperintense lesion on T1 and T2 weighted imaging, with early enhancement with gadolinium

    ### Following discussion at the multidisciplinary meeting, what would be the most appropriate recommendation?

    A. Chemoembolization

    B. Liver biopsy

    C. Referral for liver transplantation

    D. Referral for surgical resection

    E. Stopping the oral contraceptive pill and monitoring

36. **A 52-year-old woman was referred to the outpatient clinic with asymptomatic jaundice. She had a BMI of 24 kg/m² and drank 22 units of alcohol per week. She had a past medical history of hypothyroidism, for which she was prescribed levothyroxine.**

    Investigations:

haemoglobin	133 g/L (130–180)
MCV	89 fL (80–96)
platelet count	360 x 10⁹/L (150–400)
serum total bilirubin	92 µmol/L (1–22)
serum alanine transaminase	162 U/L (5–35)
serum alkaline phosphatase	197 U/L (45–105)
serum albumin	39 g/L (37–49)
international normalized ratio	0.9 (< 1.4)
antinuclear antibody	negative at 1:20 dilution
antimitochondrial antibody	positive at 1:160 dilution
anti-smooth muscle antibody	negative at 1:20 dilution
anti-liver/kidney microsome type 1 antibodies	negative
serum immunoglobulin G	32 g/L (6.0–13.0)
serum immunoglobulin A	6 g/L (0.8–3.0)
serum immunoglobulin M	8 g/L (0.4–2.5)
liver ultrasound	normal

    Which of the following is the most likely diagnosis?

    A. Autoimmune hepatitis

    B. Non-alcoholic steatohepatitis

    C. Primary biliary cirrhosis

    D. Primary biliary cirrhosis–autoimmune hepatitis overlap syndrome

    E. Primary sclerosing cholangitis

37. **A 46-year-old woman was seen in your gastroenterology outpatient clinic and diagnosed with primary biliary cirrhosis.**

    Investigations:

serum total bilirubin	60 µmol/L (1–22)
serum alanine transaminase	120 U/L (5–35)
serum aspartate transaminase	120 U/L (1–31)
serum alkaline phosphatase	1000 U/L (45–105)
serum gamma glutamyl transpeptidase	300 U/L (4–35)
serum albumin	40 g/L (37–49)
liver ultrasound	normal liver echotexture

    Which of the following best defines response to treatment in this patient?

    A. Serum alanine transaminase 72 U/L

    B. Serum alkaline phosphatase 600 U/L

    C. Serum aspartate transaminase 72 U/L

    D. Serum gamma glutamyl transferase 180 U/L

    E. Serum total bilirubin 30 µmol/L

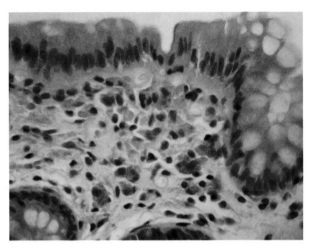

Plate 1 See also Figure 2.2a. Permission granted by Dr N. Ryley, Torbay Hospital; slides from his personal collection.

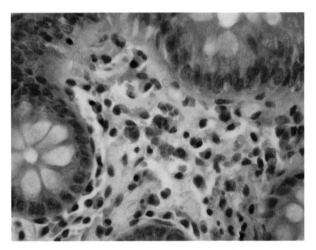

Plate 2 See also Figure 2.2b. Permission granted by Dr N. Ryley, Torbay Hospital; slides from his personal collection.

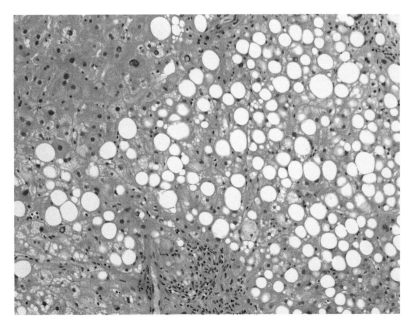

Plate 3 Liver biopsy, haematoxylin and eosin stain. See also Figure 5.3. Reproduced with permission from Dr Michael L Texler, PathWest, Australia.

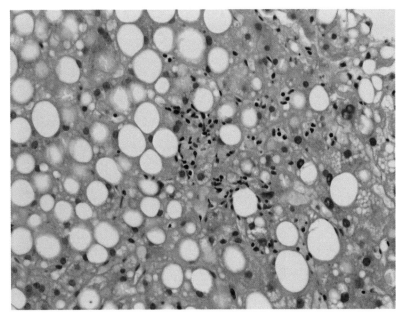

Plate 4 Haematoxylin and eosin staining. See also Figure 5.9. Reproduced with permission from Dr Michael L Texler, PathWest, Australia.

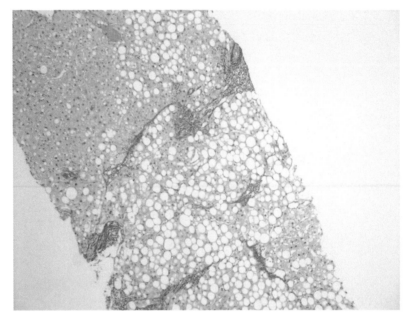

Plate 5 Van Gieson stain; red = fibrous tissue. See also Figure 5.10. Reproduced with permission from Dr Michael L Texler, PathWest, Australia.

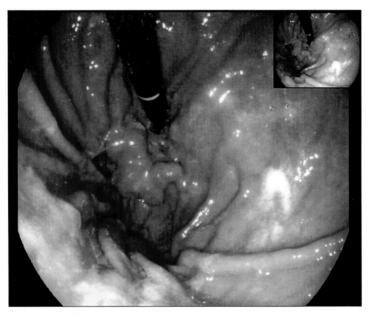

Plate 6 See also Figure 7.1.

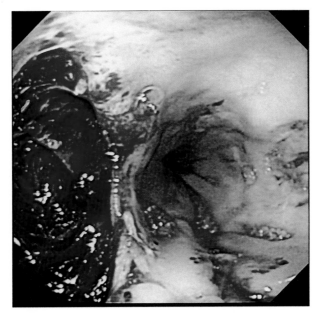

Plate 7 See also Figure 7.2. Reprinted from *Journal of Gastrointestinal Endoscopy*, 68, 4 Matull WR, Cross TJ, Yu D et al. pp. 767–768. Copyright 2008, with permission from Elsevier.

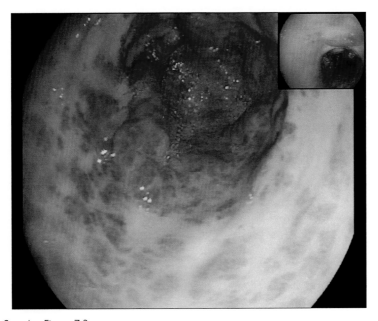

Plate 8 See also Figure 7.3.

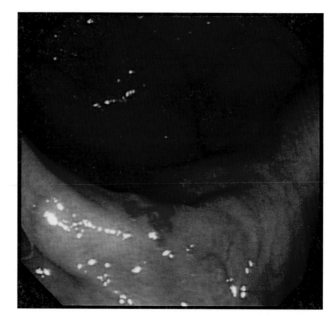

Plate 9 See also Figure 7.4.

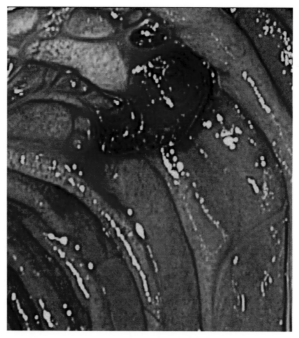

Plate 10 Endoscopic image of the second part of the duodenum. See also Figure 7.6.

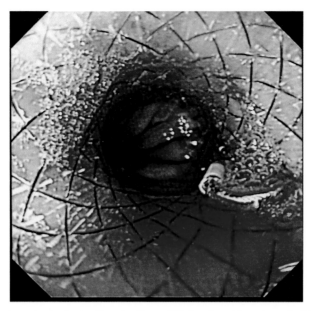

Plate 11 Oesophageal stent *in situ*. See also Figure 7.8. Reprinted from *Journal of Gastrointestinal Endoscopy*, 68, 4, Matull WR, Cross TJ, Yu D et al., 'A removable covered self-expanding metal stent for the management of Sengstaken–Blakemore tube-induced oesophageal tear and variceal hemorrhage', pp. 767–768. Copyright 2008, with permission from Elsevier.

38. **A 22-year-old man was seen in your IBD clinic for follow-up of his Crohn's colitis. His bowel symptoms were stable, but he complained of recurrent right upper quadrant pain over the past few months, with associated fever and chills.**

Investigations:

serum bilirubin	21 μmol/L (1–22)
serum alanine transaminase	35 U/L (5–35)
serum alkaline phosphatase	186 U/L (45–105)
serum albumin	39 g/L (37–49)
antinuclear antibody	positive at 1:640 dilution
antimitochondrial antibody	negative at 1:20 dilution
anti-smooth muscle antibody	positive at 1:320 dilution
serum immunoglobulin M	12.7 g/L (0.4–2.5)

Which of the following investigations is most likely to establish the diagnosis?

A. Abdominal computerized tomography

B. Abdominal ultrasound

C. Endoscopic retrograde cholangiopancreatography

D. Liver biopsy

E. Magnetic resonance cholangiopancreatography

39. **A 41-year-old man with primary sclerosing cholangitis was seen in the hepatology clinic 1 year previously with unremarkable blood tests. He now complains of worsening fatigue and pruritus.**

Investigations:

serum total bilirubin	134 μmol/L (1–22)
serum alanine transaminase	54 U/L (5–35)
serum alkaline phosphatase	410 U/L (45–105)
serum albumin	34 g/L (37–49)
magnetic resonance cholangiopancreatography	1 mm stricture of the distal common bile duct with extrahepatic and left hepatic duct dilatation and irregularity

Which of the following is the most appropriate next intervention?

A. Endoscopic retrograde cholangiopancreatography and dilatation

B. Endoscopic retrograde cholangiopancreatography and sphincterotomy

C. Endoscopic retrograde cholangiopancreatography and stenting

D. Pancreaticoduodenectomy

E. Referral for liver transplantation

40. **A 23-year-old man with primary sclerosing cholangitis was seen in the hepatology clinic as a routine follow-up. His general practitioner had organized an ultrasound scan, as he had complained of episodes of right upper quadrant pain.**

Investigations:

liver ultrasound   there is a 6 mm soft tissue mass of homogenous echotexture in the gallbladder, consistent with a polyp. The CBD and the biliary tree are normal. The liver is of normal size and echotexture

What is the most appropriate next step in his management?

A. Cholecystectomy

B. Endoscopic retrograde cholangiopancreatography

C. Liver transplantation

D. Monitoring with serial ultrasound imaging at 12-monthly intervals

E. Pylorus-sparing pancreaticoduodenectomy

41. **A 60-year-old woman was referred to clinic following 3 weeks of jaundice, lethargy, and itching. She consumed 20 units of alcohol a week and smoked 20 cigarettes a day. She had taken simvastatin 20 mg for the past 5 years for hypercholesterolaemia, and levothyroxine for hypothyroidism. On clinical examination she was icteric, had palmar erythema, and had a palpable liver edge.**

Investigations:

serum total bilirubin	223 µmol/L (1–22)
serum alkaline phosphatase	213 U/L (45–105)
serum alanine transaminase	701 U/L (5–35)
serum aspartate transaminase	900 U/L (1–31)
serum gamma glutamyl transferase	1201 U/L (4–35)
serum albumin	34 g/L (37–49)
international normalized ratio	1.6 (< 1.4)
antinuclear antibody	positive at 1:40 dilution
antimitochondrial antibody	negative at 1:20 dilution
anti-liver/kidney microsome type 1 antibody	negative
immunoglobulin M	2.4 g/L (0.4–2.5)
immunoglobulin A	4.0 g/L (0.5–4.0)
immunoglobulin G	28 g/L (5.0–13.0)
liver ultrasound	hepatomegaly with normal portal vein flow and a normal-sized spleen
liver biopsy	interface hepatitis of moderate activity with lobular hepatitis. There is no central portal bridging necrosis or biliary lesions

What would be the most appropriate next step?

A. Azathioprine and prednisolone

B. Azathioprine and tacrolimus

C. Cessation of alcohol and repeat the liver function tests in a week

D. Cessation of simvastatin and repeat the liver function tests in a week

E. Pentoxifylline and repeat the liver function tests in a week

42. **A 52-year-old woman with abnormal liver function tests was seen in clinic. Blood tests and the autoimmune profile suggested a diagnosis of autoimmune hepatitis. A liver biopsy was performed.**

    Which of the following is most consistent with this diagnosis?

    A. Blue staining of hepatocytes with Perl's Prussian stain
    B. Florid duct lesions with granulomas
    C. Interface hepatitis with portal branching fibrosis
    D. Non-caseating granulomas and perigranulomatous mononuclear cell inflammation with hepatic necrosis
    E. Steatosis with hepatocyte balloon degeneration and pericellular fibrosis

43. **A patient with newly diagnosed autoimmune hepatitis was started on prednisolone 30 mg and azathioprine 60 mg. She contacted her GP 3 months later as she noticed that she had become jaundiced and she found it difficult to sleep at night due to excessive itching.**

    Investigation:
    liver ultrasound   normal

    What would be the most appropriate change to her treatment?

    A. Azathioprine 120 mg and prednisolone 60 mg
    B. Azathioprine 60 mg and prednisolone 60 mg
    C. Azathioprine 120 mg and tacrolimus 3.5 mg twice daily
    D. Budesonide 9 mg once daily
    E. Mycophenolate mofetil 1.5 g twice daily

44. **A 63-year-old woman was referred to the outpatient gastroenterology clinic with abnormal liver function tests. She was asymptomatic. She had a history of hypothyroidism, type 1 diabetes, and bipolar disorder.**

Investigations:

serum total bilirubin	32 µmol/L (1–22)
serum alanine aminotransferase	42 U/L (5–35)
serum gamma glutamyl transferase	48 U/L (4–35)
serum alkaline phosphatase	112 U/L (45–105)
serum albumin	41 g/L (37–49)
international normalized ratio	1.0 (< 1.4)
antinuclear antibody	1:80 dilution (negative at 1:20 dilution)
antimitochondrial antibody	1:20 dilution (negative at 1:20 dilution)
anti-liver/kidney microsomal type 1 antibody	negative
serum immunoglobulin G	17 g/L (6.0–13.0)
serum immunoglobulin A	4.0 g/L (0.8–3.0)
serum immunoglobulin M	2.4 g/L (0.4–2.5)
liver ultrasound	normal
liver biopsy	mild activity interface hepatitis

What is the most appropriate option?

A. Azathioprine and low dose prednisolone

B. Methotrexate

C. Monitor liver function tests 3-monthly

D. Mycophenolate mofetil

E. Prednisolone

45. **A 64-year-old man was referred to the outpatient clinic with abdominal pain and abnormal liver function tests. He drank 36 units of alcohol per week.**

Investigations:

liver ultrasound	2 cm lesion in segment III, in an otherwise normal appearing liver
serum α-fetoprotein	453 kU/L (< 10)
quadruple-phase CT of the liver	hypervascular lesion in the arterial phase, followed by washout in the portal venous phase

Which is the most appropriate treatment?

A. Doxorubicin chemotherapy

B. Liver transplantation

C. Radiofrequency ablation

D. Resection

E. Transarterial chemoembolization

46. **A 54-year-old man with Child–Pugh grade B cirrhosis secondary to alcoholic liver disease was under surveillance for hepatocellular carcinoma. He had been abstinent for 4 years and had no other comorbidities.**

Investigations:

serum α-fetoprotein	753 kU/L (< 10)
liver ultrasound	possible liver lesion
magnetic resonance imaging of the liver with gadolinium	two separate 3 cm lesions in segment II and segment III which are hypervascular in the arterial phase, followed by washout in the portal venous phase

What is the most appropriate management for this patient?

A. Doxorubicin chemotherapy

B. Liver transplantation

C. Radiofrequency ablation

D. Resection

E. Transarterial chemoembolization

47. **A 64-year-old man with a BMI of 36 kg/m² presented with jaundice, nausea, and abdominal pain and distension that had developed over 6 weeks. He consumed 4 units of alcohol a week. Clinical examination revealed hepatomegaly, splenomegaly, and ascites.**

Investigations:

haemoglobin	173 g/L (130–180)
haematocrit	0.58 (0.4–0.52)
white cell count	14.2 x 10⁹/L (4.0–11.0)
platelet count	690 x 10⁹/L (150–400)
serum sodium	136 mmol/L (137–144)
serum potassium	4.3 mmol/L (3.5–4.9)
serum urea	6.2 mmol/L (2.5–7.0)
serum creatinine	78 μmol/L (60–110)
serum total bilirubin	63 μmol/L (1–22)
serum alanine aminotransferase	85 U/L (5–35)
serum aspartate aminotransferase	102 U/L (1–31)
serum alkaline phosphatase	500 U/L (45–105)
serum albumin	32 g/L (37–49)
ascitic fluid albumin	22 g/L

What is the most likely cause of his presentation?

A. Alcoholic liver disease

B. Hepatic vein thrombosis

C. Non-alcoholic fatty liver disease

D. Portal vein thrombosis

E. Right-sided heart failure

48. A 65-year-old man with known alcoholic liver disease was admitted with acute decompensation of his liver disease.

Investigations:

liver ultrasound   6 x 7 cm mass in the right lobe of the liver

He was referred for transarterial chemoembolization (TACE), which involved gaining access to the arterial supply to the liver.

From which artery does the common hepatic artery arise directly?

A. Aorta

B. Coeliac artery

C. Left gastric artery

D. Right gastric artery

E. Superior mesenteric artery

49. A 23-year-old Kenyan healthcare worker attended her GP concerned that she might have hepatitis B, as her husband was recently diagnosed with the disease. On further questioning, she reported that her mother and sister both had hepatitis B. She was asymptomatic.

Investigations:

serum total bilirubin	18 μmol/L (1–22)
serum alanine aminotransferase	34 U/L (5–35)
serum aspartate aminotransferase	23 U/L (1–31)
serum alkaline phosphatase	85 U/L (45–105)
serum albumin	39 g/L (37–49)
HBsAg	negative
HBeAg	negative
anti-HBs	positive
anti-HBc IgG	positive
anti-HBe	negative

What is the most likely cause of the above hepatitis B serology?

A. Chronic hepatitis with pre-core mutant

B. Chronic infection with low replication

C. Resolved infection

D. Susceptible individual

E. Vaccinated

50. A 68-year-old man from Libya was referred by his GP with a new diagnosis of hepatitis B. On history and examination he appeared well. The patient asked about the likelihood of successful treatment.

Investigations:

serum bilirubin	13 μmol/L (1–22)
serum alkaline phosphatase	153 U/L (45–105)
serum alanine aminotransferase	278 U/L (5–35)
serum albumin	39 g/L (37–49)
HBsAg	positive
HBcAb	positive
HBeAg	positive
anti-HBe	negative
anti-HBc IgM	negative
anti-HBc IgG	positive
anti-HBs	negative
viral load	6×10^7 IU/mL (lower detection 250 IU/mL)
genotype	A
liver biopsy	METAVIR activity score A2(A0–A3) and fibrosis score 1(1–4).

With regard to nucleoside analogue treatment of hepatitis B, which of the following factors is least useful for predicting the response to therapy?

A. Age

B. Genotype A

C. High activity scores in the liver biopsy pre-treatment

D. High ALT (above three times the upper limit of normal) pre-treatment

E. Low viral load (below 10^8 IU/mL) pre-treatment

51. A 43-year-old man presented with a 5-month history of lethargy, abdominal discomfort, and a non-productive cough, associated with mild shortness of breath. He had been working in Yemen and had returned to the UK to visit. His wife reported weight loss of 5 kg in the last 2 months.

Investigations:

haemoglobin	134 g/L (130–180)
MCV	86 fL (80–96)
white cell count	8.7 × 10⁹/L (4.0–11.0)
neutrophil count	5.1 × 10⁹/L (1.5–7.0)
lymphocyte count	2.9 × 10⁹/L (1.5–4.0)
monocyte count	0.3 × 10⁹/L (< 0.8)
eosinophil count	0.4 × 10⁹/L (0.04–0.40)
basophil count	< 0.1 × 10⁹/L (< 0.1)
platelet count	453 × 10⁹/L (150–400)
serum sodium	135 mmol/L (137–144)
serum potassium	4.5 mmol/L (3.5–4.9)
serum urea	6.7 mmol/L (2.5–7.0)
serum creatinine	78 μmol/L (60–110)
serum total bilirubin	47 μmol/L (1–22)
serum alanine aminotransferase	23 U/L (5–35)
serum aspartate aminotransferase	26 U/L (1–31)
serum alkaline phosphatase	160 U/L (45–105)
serum albumin	37 g/L (37–49)

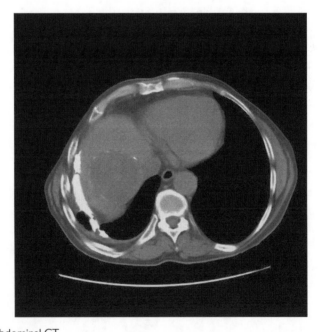

Figure 5.2 Abdominal CT.

Reproduced with kind permission from Dr Paul Burn, Consultant Radiologist.

What is the most likely diagnosis?

A. Caroli's syndrome

B. Hepatocellular carcinoma

C. Hydatid cysts

D. Liver abscesses

E. Polycystic liver disease

52. A 65-year-old man was referred to the liver clinic with abnormal liver function tests. He had a BMI of 32 kg/m^2, a history of hypertension, and type 2 diabetes. He reported drinking 2 units of alcohol per week.

Investigations:

serum total bilirubin	12 μmol/L (1–22)
serum alanine aminotransferase	123 U/L (5–35)
serum aspartate aminotransferase	112 U/L (1–31)
serum alkaline phosphatase	103 U/L (45–105)
serum albumin	38 g/L (37–49)
serum ferritin	554 μg/L (15–300)
transferrin saturations	17% (20–50)
liver ultrasound	normal sized liver with increased echogenicity consistent with steatosis

Which pharmacotherapy is least likely to be effective for his hepatitis?

A. Beta-carotene

B. Metformin

C. Orlistat

D. Pioglitazone

E. Vitamin E

53. **A 34-year-old woman, who was abstinent from alcohol, had a background of hyperlipidaemia, hypertension, type 2 diabetes, and hypothyroidism. She presented to the gastroenterology outpatient clinic. Her medication history included metformin and ramipril. She had had a recent course of trimethoprim for a urinary tract infection.**

Investigations:

serum total bilirubin	24 µmol/L (1–22)
serum alanine aminotransferase	87 U/L (5–35)
serum alkaline phosphatase	132 U/L (45–105)
serum albumin	42 g/L (37–49)
serum ferritin	545 µg/L (15–300)
anti-smooth muscle antibody	positive

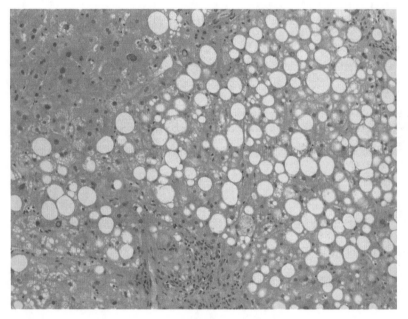

Figure 5.3 Liver biopsy, haematoxylin and eosin stain. See also Plate 3.

Reproduced with permission from Dr Michael L Texler, PathWest, Australia.

What is the most likely cause of her abnormal liver function tests?

A. Autoimmune hepatitis

B. Drug-induced cholestasis

C. Haemochromatosis

D. Non-alcoholic steatohepatitis

E. Wilson's disease

54. A 16-year-old girl, who was struggling with school and not socializing, attended her GP regarding depression.

Investigations:

serum total bilirubin	46 µmol/L (1–22)
serum alanine aminotransferase	53 U/L (5–35)
serum alkaline phosphatase	115 U/L (45–105)
serum albumin	42 g/L (37–49)
serum copper	8 µmol/L (12–26)
serum caeruloplasmin	145 mg/L (200–350)
24-hour urinary copper	> 3 µmol (0.2–0.6)

Which of the following foods is least harmful for this patient?

A. Chocolate

B. Mushrooms

C. Nuts

D. Salmon

E. Shellfish

55. A 33-year-old Caucasian man was referred with a history of tiredness. The general practitioner was concerned that the patient had haemochromatosis. In clinic genotyping was arranged.

Investigations:

serum ferritin	> 2000 µg/L (15–300)

What is the most likely finding on genotyping?

A. C282Y/H63D

B. C282Y heterozygote

C. C282Y/S65C

D. Hepcidin gene (HAMP)

E. Transferrin receptor 2 gene

56. A 26-year-old man was referred to the hepatology clinic with malaise, lethargy, and joint pain.

Investigations:

serum total bilirubin	24 µmol/L (1–22)
serum alanine aminotransferase	31 U/L (5–35)
serum alkaline phosphatase	92 U/L (45–105)
serum albumin	42 g/L (37–49)
transferrin saturations	54% (20–50)
serum ferritin	839 µg/L (15–300)
HFE genotype	C282Y homozygote

What is the most appropriate next step in his management?

A. Echocardiogram

B. Liver biopsy

C. Repeat liver function tests and ferritin 3 monthly

D. Serum glucose

E. Therapeutic venesection

57. **A 56-year-old woman was referred to the liver clinic with a ferritin level of 453 µg/L with concerns that the patient had haemochromatosis. She had an extensive past medical history.**

    Which of the following conditions is least likely to cause raised serum ferritin levels?

    A. Diabetes mellitus
    B. Hyperthyroidism
    C. Inflammation
    D. Neoplasm
    E. Non-alcoholic fatty liver disease

58. **A 63-year-old woman was referred by the GP with abnormal liver function tests after the GP had performed some routine blood tests. She was diagnosed with autoimmune hepatitis and commenced on azathioprine for immunosuppression.**

    Which of the following adverse effects is least likely to occur with azathioprine?

    A. Arthralgia
    B. Fever
    C. Leucopenia
    D. Lymphoproliferative disorder
    E. Pancreatitis

1. E. Development of varices

The strongest predictor of the development of varices in cirrhotic patients without varices at the time of initial endoscopic screening is an HVPG of more than 10 mmHg. HVPG is an indirect measure of sinusoidal pressure, and is raised in intrahepatic causes of portal hypertension but not in prehepatic causes. The normal HVPG is in the range 3–5 mmHg, with portal hypertension at pressures greater than 5 mmHg.

Continued hepatic injury—for example, with ongoing alcohol misuse—is another strong predictor of the development of varices. Haemophilia A is a risk factor for bleeding, but is unrelated to variceal development. All of the other factors relate to the development of varices, but HVPG is the most important.

Risk factors for variceal bleeding

The factors that predict variceal haemorrhage are (1) pressure within the varix, (2) variceal size, (3) tension on the variceal wall, and (4) severity of the liver disease. The two most important risk factors for variceal haemorrhage are the size of the varices and the severity of the liver disease.

Portal pressure, size of varices, and variceal wall tension

All three of these factors are interrelated. Large varices and those with a higher wall tension have an increased risk of bleeding. The pressure within the varix is directly related to the HVPG. Interestingly, there is no linear relationship between HVPG and the risk of variceal haemorrhage. Variceal bleeding is significantly reduced when the HVPG is reduced to less than 12 mmHg, and this pressure is often the target for pharmacological therapy.

Endoscopic visible warning signs called 'red signs' reflect changes in the variceal wall structure and tension due to the formation of microtelangiectasias.

The following 'red signs' have been described:

- *Red wale marks* are longitudinal red streaks on varices
- *Cherry red spots* are discrete red cherry-coloured spots that are flat and overlie varices
- *Haematocystic spots* are raised discrete red spots overlying varices that resemble 'blood blisters'
- *Diffuse erythema* denotes a diffuse red colour of the varix.

Severity of liver disease

The North Italian Endoscopy Club found that the risk of variceal bleeding correlated with the severity of liver disease (in addition to variceal size and red wale markings) as measured by the Child–Pugh classification. In their study, 321 patients with cirrhosis and varices were followed up for between 1 and 38 months (median 23 months). In total, 85 patients had a variceal haemorrhage, and of those that bled, 17% had Child–Pugh class A, 31% had Child–Pugh class B, and 39% had Child–Pugh class C disease.

Epidemiology of varices

- Varices are present in almost half of patients with cirrhosis at the time of diagnosis
- Approximately 7% of patients with varices have a variceal bleed per year (5% for small varices and 15% for large varices)
- The 6-week mortality with each variceal bleed ranges from almost 0% in patients with Child–Pugh class A disease to approximately 30% among patients with class C disease.

Garcia-Tsao G, Sanyal AJ, Grace ND et al. Prevention and management of gastroesophageal varices and variceal hemorrhage in cirrhosis. *Hepatology* 2007; 46: 922–938.

Jalan R and Hayes PC. UK guidelines on the management of variceal haemorrhage in cirrhotic patients. *Gut* 2000; 46 (Suppl. 3): iii1–15.

Bacon B and O'Grady J. *Comprehensive Clinical Hepatology*. Oxford: Elsevier Mosby; 2006.

The North Italian Endoscopic Club for the Study and Treatment of Esophageal Varices. Prediction of the first variceal hemorrhage in patients with cirrhosis of the liver and esophageal varices. A prospective multi-center study. *New England Journal of Medicine* 1988; 319: 983–989.

Garcia-Tsao G and Bosch J. Management of varices and variceal hemorrhage in cirrhosis. *New England Journal of Medicine* 2010; 362: 823–832.

2. E. Recommendations for treatment of active variceal bleeding in cirrhosis

- Aggressive restoration of intravascular volume with large-bore venous access
- Cross-match 6 units of blood; blood loss should be replaced by packed red cells and clotting factors
- Correction of coagulopathy with FFP which contains all of the clotting factors found in whole blood (the role of recombinant factor VIIa awaits further clarification)
- Careful monitoring to avoid over-transfusion with volume overload resulting in rebound portal hypertension and induction of rebleeding
- Consensus guidelines recommend a target haemoglobin concentration of approximately 70–80 g/L, depending on other factors such as patient comorbidities, age, haemodynamic status, and the presence of ongoing bleeding clinically
- Consider airway protection with elective intubation if there is:
  - severe uncontrolled variceal bleeding
  - severe encephalopathy
  - inability to maintain oxygen saturations above 90%
  - aspiration pneumonia.
- Oesophageal variceal haemorrhage should undergo variceal band ligation; aim for early endoscopic examination within 12 hours of initial presentation
- Gastric variceal haemorrhage should be managed endoscopically, preferably with cyanoacrylate injection. If this is unavailable, transjugular intrahepatic portosystemic stent (TIPSS) is very effective in controlling bleeding. If bleeding is not controlled after the first endoscopy, consider TIPSS rather than a second endoscopy
- Prior to endoscopic diagnosis, terlipressin should be given to patients with suspected variceal haemorrhage

- Antibiotic therapy should be commenced in patients with chronic liver disease who present with acute upper gastrointestinal haemorrhage
- TIPSS shunting is recommended as the treatment of choice for uncontrolled variceal haemorrhage
- Balloon tamponade should be considered as a temporary (< 24 hours) salvage treatment for uncontrolled variceal haemorrhage
- After endoscopic treatment of acute oesophageal variceal haemorrhage, patients should receive vasoactive drug treatment (terlipressin, somatostatin, vapreotide, or octreotide) for up to 5 days.

Platelet transfusion

The most important risk associated with giving group-mismatched platelets is no longer thought to be due to ABO proteins but to plasma antibody incompatibility—in particular, high-titre anti-A antibodies in Group O platelets which have caused acute haemolytic reactions.

Platelets do not need to be matched from the point of view of efficacy, although this is desirable. Some of the early studies suggested that platelet increments were lower in mismatched transfusions, but more recent data are conflicting, and haemostatic effectiveness is not thought to be compromised in a clinically significant way. The recommendation is that recipients should receive ABO-matched platelets as first choice. Group A platelets are now the first choice for 'emergency group-unknown' transfusions, and the second choice if group-matched platelets are unavailable. Group O platelets should not be given to non-group O patients unless they have been screened for high-titre antibodies.

Quantifying blood loss

It is difficult to estimate the total volume of blood loss in patients with chronic liver disease using traditional surgical trauma guidelines, as such patients frequently have a lower mean arterial pressure compared with people without liver disease. A bleed is deemed clinically significant if a patient requires 2 units of packed red cells or more within 24 hours, together with any of the following features: systolic blood pressure < 100 mmHg, a postural change of > 20 mmHg or pulse rate > 100 beats/minute. Be aware that the use of beta-blockers may mask a tachycardia.

Serious Hazards of Transfusion (SHOT). *Report and Summary 2008.*

British Committee for Standards in Haematology (BCSH). Guidelines for the use of platelet transfusions. *British Journal of Haematology* 2003; 122: 10–23.

de Franchis R. Revising consensus in portal hypertension: report of the Baveno V consensus workshop on methodology of diagnosis and therapy in portal hypertension. *Journal of Hepatology* 2010; 53: 762–768.

Scottish Intercollegiate Guidelines Network (SIGN). *Management of Acute Upper and Lower Gastrointestinal Bleeding.* Edinburgh: SIGN; 2008.

Garcia-Tsao G and Bosch J. Management of varices and variceal hemorrhage in cirrhosis. *New England Journal of Medicine* 2010; 362: 823–832.

Garcia-Tsao G, Sanyal AJ, Grace ND *et al.* Prevention and management of gastroesophageal varices and variceal hemorrhage in cirrhosis. *Hepatology* 2007; 46: 922–938.

3. E. Therapies that should not be used as primary prophylaxis include nitrates alone, endoscopic variceal sclerotherapy, shunt therapy (either transjugular intrahepatic portosystemic shunt or surgical shunt), non-selective beta-blockers (NSBBs) in combination with endoscopic band ligation (EBL), and NSBBs in combination with nitrates. As this patient is intolerant of beta-blockers and yet has grade II/medium varices with Child–Pugh grade C cirrhosis, one should consider EBL. NSBBs reduce portal pressure by decreasing cardiac output and producing splanchnic bed vasodilation. Selective beta-blockers are suboptimal and are not recommended. Recent trials of carvedilol, an NSBB with mild anti-α_1-adrenergic effects, have shown a possible advantage over propranolol in terms of a reduction in HVPG, although it may possibly cause higher rates of systemic hypotension.

Size of varices

Some guidelines refer to varices as small, medium, or large, whereas others refer to them as grade I, II, or III.

- Small = grade I: varices that collapse to inflation of the oesophagus with air
- Medium = grade II: varices between grades I and III
- Large = grade III: varices that are large enough to occlude the lumen of the endoscope.

Recommendations for the prevention of a first variceal haemorrhage (primary prophylaxis)

- All patients should be endoscoped at the time of diagnosis
- Patients without varices should not be started on pharmacological treatment. Beta-blockers are associated with side effects and do not prevent the development of varices
- Patients with small/grade I varices who are Child–Pugh class C or have red wale signs at endoscopy should receive an NSBB. Such patients have a similar risk of variceal haemorrhage to those patients with medium and large varices with Child–Pugh class A disease, and should be considered as high risk. Patients with small/grade I varices without high-risk features can be considered for pharmacotherapy
- Patients with medium/grade II and large/grade III varices should receive primary prophylaxis with either an NSBB or EBL. Practice is determined by local resources and expertise, patient preference and characteristics, side effects, and contraindications. Where neither beta-blockers nor EBL can be used, consider treatment with nitrates.

Advantages and disadvantages of NSBBs

- *Advantages*: low cost, expertise not required for use, and may prevent other complications such as ascites, bleeding from portal hypertensive gastropathy, and spontaneous bacterial peritonitis
- *Disadvantages*: frequent side effects lead to discontinuation in 15–20% of cases, and between half and a third of patients with cirrhosis who are taking NSBBs fail to achieve a therapeutic reduction in HVPG < 12 mmHg (further exacerbated by non-compliance and under-dosing)
- Propranolol can be started at 40 mg twice daily and increased to 80 mg twice daily if necessary. Long-acting propranolol (80 mg or 160 mg) can be used to improve compliance.

Advantages and disadvantages of EBL

- *Advantages*: performed at the time of endoscopy, and not dependent on long-term patient compliance
- *Disadvantages*: potential haemorrhage from ulcers post treatment, and the need for expertise.

Recommendations for secondary prophylaxis after variceal haemorrhage

- Patients with cirrhosis who have not received primary prophylaxis should be treated with NSBBs, EBL, or both
- Patients with cirrhosis who were on beta-blockers for primary prevention and have a variceal bleed should have EBL.

Recommendations for patients who rebleed after endoscopic therapy and pharmacotherapy for secondary prophylaxis

- TIPSS or surgical shunts are effective for those with Child–Pugh class A and B disease
- Transplantation provides good long-term outcomes in Child–Pugh class B and C cirrhosis, and should be considered.

Classification of gastric varices

- *Type 1 gastro-oesophageal varices (GOV-1)*: continuous with oesophageal varices and extend for 2–5 cm below the gastro-oesophageal junction (GOJ) along the lesser curve
- *Type 2 gastro-oesophageal varices (GOV-2)*: as above, but extend beyond the GOJ into the fundus of the stomach
- *Type 1 isolated gastric varices (IGV-1)*: occur in the fundus of the stomach
- *Type 2 isolated gastric varices (IGV-2)*: occur in any other part of the stomach or duodenum.

Recommendations for secondary prophylaxis after gastric variceal haemorrhage

- IGV and GOV-2 should be treated with cyanoacrylate, TIPSS, or NSBBs
- GOV-1 should be treated with cyanoacrylate, EBL, or NSBBs.

de Franchis R. Revising consensus in portal hypertension: report of the Baveno V consensus workshop on methodology of diagnosis and therapy in portal hypertension. *Journal of Hepatology* 2010; 53: 762–768.

Garcia-Tsao G and Bosch J. Management of varices and variceal hemorrhage in cirrhosis. *New England Journal of Medicine* 2010; 362: 823–832.

Garcia-Tsao G, Sanyal AJ, Grace ND *et al*. Prevention and management of gastroesophageal varices and variceal hemorrhage in cirrhosis. *Hepatology* 2007; 46: 922–938.

Jalan R and Hayes PC. UK guidelines on the management of variceal haemorrhage in cirrhotic patients. *Gut* 2000; 46 (Suppl. 3): iii1–15.

4. C. One should ensure that the patient is adequately filled and that there is an absence of hypovolaemia prior to diagnosing hepatorenal syndrome and commencing terlipressin. This patient has been fluid resuscitated, yet this has not reduced his creatinine level to < 133 mmol/L. A central line is not essential in the management of fluid balance, although it may be useful.

The European Association for the Study of the Liver (EASL) has defined hepatorenal syndrome (HRS) as 'The occurrence of renal failure in a patient with advanced liver disease in the absence of an identifiable cause of renal failure. Thus, the diagnosis is essentially one of exclusion of other causes of renal failure.'

International Ascites Club (IAC) guidelines: criteria for the diagnosis of hepatorenal syndrome (2005)

- Cirrhosis with ascites
- Serum creatinine > 133 mmol/L
- Absence of hypovolaemia—no improvement in serum creatinine levels (decreased to < 133 mmol/L) after at least 2 days with diuretic withdrawal (if on diuretics) and volume expansion with albumin. The recommended dose of albumin is 1 g/kg/day up to a maximum of 100 g/day
- Absence of shock—renal failure in the setting of ongoing bacterial infection, but in the absence of septic shock, can now be regarded as HRS
- No current or recent treatment with nephrotoxic drugs
- Absence of parenchymal kidney disease as indicated by proteinuria > 500 mg/day, microhaematuria (> 50 red blood cells per high power field), and/or abnormal renal USS.

Differences between type 1 and type 2 hepatorenal syndrome

Type 1	Type 2
• Rapidly progressive	• Moderate renal failure with a slowly progressive course
• Commonly precipitated by bacterial infections such as SBP	• Occurs in patients with refractory ascites
• Not a terminal event of hepatic failure, but potentially reversible	• Survival better than with type 1 HRS

Data from International Ascites Club (IAC) Guidelines. Criteria for the diagnosis of hepatorenal syndrome criteria (2005). http://www.icascites.org/about/guidelines

The IAC HRS criteria apply a rigid cut-off with regard to diagnostic creatinine levels. More recent collaborations of these experts have suggested that patients with milder degrees of renal dysfunction, which do not meet the 2005 IAC criteria, may also experience adverse outcomes. Adaptations of the acute and chronic kidney injury classifications to include renal dysfunction in liver disease have yet to be validated.

European Association for the Study of the Liver. EASL clinical practice guidelines on the management of ascites, spontaneous bacterial peritonitis, and hepatorenal syndrome in cirrhosis. *Journal of Hepatology* 2010; 53: 397–417.

Arroyo V, Gines P, Gerbes AL *et al*. Definition and diagnostic criteria of refractory ascites and hepatorenal syndrome in cirrhosis. *Hepatology* 1996; 23: 164–176.

Runyon BA. Management of adult patients with ascites due to cirrhosis: an update. *Hepatology* 2009; 49: 2087–2107.

Moore KP and Aithal GP. Guidelines on the management of ascites in cirrhosis. *Gut* 2006; 55: 1–12.

Salerno F, Gerbes A, Gines P *et al*. Diagnosis, prevention and treatment of hepatorenal syndrome in cirrhosis. *Gut* 2007; 56: 1310–1318.

Wong F, Nadim MK, Kellum JA *et al*. Working Party proposal for a revised classification system of renal dysfunction in patients with cirrhosis. *Gut* 2011; 60: 702–709.

5. C. Pathogenesis of HRS

- Splanchnic arterial vasodilation is mainly due to nitrous oxide (NO) release
- Vasodilators also cause a reduction in the peripheral vascular resistance
- NO and other vasodilators result in the splanchnic bed being resistant to endogenous vasocontrictors such as angiotensin II, norepinephrine, vasopressin, and endothelin
- Elsewhere in the body these endogenous vasoconstrictors have an effect and lead to renal, hepatic, and cerebral vasoconstriction
- Renal vasoconstriction secondary to effects of the renin–angiotensin–aldosterone (R-A-A) system and sympathetic nervous system result in a shift in the renal autoregulatory curve which makes renal perfusion more sensitive to changes in mean arterial pressure
- A compensatory hyperdynamic circulation is often present in order to meet tissue demands in the face of a reduced peripheral resistance, which would otherwise result in an effective hypovolaemic state
- Over time, cardiac function declines secondary to cirrhotic cardiomyopathy, and this results in hypoperfusion of the kidneys—another key element of HRS pathogenesis.

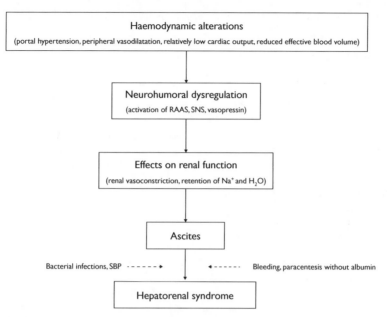

Figure 5.4 Pathogenetic mechanisms of hepatorenal syndrome in cirrhosis. Dotted arrows indicate that precipitating factors are frequent but not necessary. RAAS, renin–angiotensin–aldosterone system; SBP, spontaneous bacterial peritonitis; SNS, sympathetic nervous system.

Reproduced from *Gut*, Salerno F, Gerbes A, Gines P et al., 'Diagnosis, prevention and treatment of hepatorenal syndrome in cirrhosis', 56, 9, pp. 1310–1318. Copyright 2007, with permission from BMJ Publishing Group Ltd.

Salerno F, Gerbes A, Gines P et al. Diagnosis, prevention and treatment of hepatorenal syndrome in cirrhosis. *Gut* 2007; 56: 1310–1318.

European Association for the Study of the Liver. EASL clinical practice guidelines on the management of ascites, spontaneous bacterial peritonitis, and hepatorenal syndrome in cirrhosis. *Journal of Hepatology* 2010; 53: 397–417.

Runyon BA. Management of adult patients with ascites due to cirrhosis: an update. *Hepatology* 2009; 49: 2087–2107.

Moore KP and Aithal GP. Guidelines on the management of ascites in cirrhosis. *Gut* 2006; 55: 1–12.

Arroyo V, Gines P, Gerbes AL et al. Definition and diagnostic criteria of refractory ascites and hepatorenal syndrome in cirrhosis. *Hepatology* 1996; 23: 164–176.

6. D. Terlipressin

- Initial dose of 0.5–1 mg every 4–6 hours
- If there is no early response (defined as less than a 25% decrease in creatinine after 3 days of treatment), the dose can be increased in a stepwise manner up to a maximum of 2 mg/4-hourly (12 mg in 24 hours)
- If, after 14 days of treatment, the creatinine level does not fall below 133 μmol/L, stop terlipressin
- Use with caution in patients with ischaemic cardiovascular disease, hypertension, cardiac dysrhythmias, or atherosclerosis
- Contraindicated in pregnancy.

Albumin

- The recommended albumin dose is 1 g/kg of body weight on the first day, up to a maximum of 100 g, followed by 20–40 g/day.

A combination of albumin and terlipressin has been shown to reverse hepatorenal syndrome in about 60% of cases of type 1 HRS. The use of terlipressin and albumin in type 2 HRS has not been widely studied. The few studies that have been conducted show a temporary improvement in renal function which later deteriorates after stopping treatment.

Terlipressin leads to a rise in blood pressure, decreases plasma renin levels, and increases GFR. It may do this by causing splanchnic bed vasoconstriction, redistributing circulatory volume, and correcting renal hypoperfusion. Whether treatment of type 1 HRS with terlipressin confers a long-term survival advantage has yet to be seen, but it is an important support measure for improving renal function in patients who are awaiting liver transplantation.

Albumin leads to an expansion of the central blood volume, which reduces stimulation of the R-A-A system and may also bind vasodilators.

Response to treatment is usually quicker in patients with a lower baseline creatinine level. After withdrawal of successful treatment for HRS, approximately 20% of patients relapse, but renal function often improves again on commencing treatment.

Liver transplantation remains the best treatment for type 1 and type 2 HRS, although many patients still require dialysis afterwards. HRS should be treated before transplantation, as it may improve post-transplant outcome. Some patients who require prolonged (> 12 weeks) renal support before transplantation should be considered for combined renal and liver transplant.

TIPSS has been shown in several trials to improve renal function and improve survival in type 1 HRS. However, as the trials excluded almost all patients with a history of severe encephalopathy, high bilirubin levels, and high Child–Pugh scores, the relevance of these findings to everyday practice is unclear. Nevertheless, there is some support for its use in selected patients with no or only a partial response to albumin and vasopressor therapy as a bridge to liver transplantation in type 1 HRS.

Renal replacement therapy with haemofiltration and haemodialysis may be useful in patients who fail to respond to vasoconstrictor therapy and who fulfil the criteria for renal support. Severe hyperkalaemia, metabolic acidosis, and volume overload are rare in type 1 HRS.

Salerno F, Gerbes A, Gines P et al. Diagnosis, prevention and treatment of hepatorenal syndrome in cirrhosis. *Gut* 2007; 56: 1310–1318.

European Association for the Study of the Liver. EASL clinical practice guidelines on the management of ascites, spontaneous bacterial peritonitis, and hepatorenal syndrome in cirrhosis. *Journal of Hepatology* 2010; 53: 397–417.

Nazar A, Pereira GH, Guevara M et al. Predictors of response to therapy with terlipressin and albumin in patients with cirrhosis and type 1 hepatorenal syndrome. *Hepatology* 2010; 51: 219–226.

7. A. Granular casts can be found in both acute tubular necrosis (ATN) and HRS, but renal epithelial cells are more suggestive of ATN. A normal USS is useful for excluding an obstructed urinary system and parenchymal disease, but could be seen in both ATN and HRS. A low urinary sodium concentration and high urinary osmolarity are consistent with HRS, as renal tubular integrity is usually maintained, in contrast to ATN, although these findings are not a criterion for the diagnosis of HRS. Importantly, this patient remained on diuretics and therefore the urinary electrolyte measurements are uninterpretable. Diuretics should be stopped for at least 2 days before a diagnosis of HRS is made. Hypovolaemia or septic shock often precede ATN, whereas

HRS commonly occurs with severe alcoholic hepatitis or in patients with advanced cirrhosis following a septic insult, such as SBP.

Urinalysis in renal dysfunction in cirrhosis

Cause	Osmolality (mOsm/kg)	Urinary sodium (mmol/L)	Sediment	Protein (mg/day)
Pre-renal hypovolaemia	> 500	< 20	Normal	< 500
Hepatorenal syndrome	> 500	< 20	Nil/few granular casts	< 500
Acute tubular necrosis	< 350	> 40	Granular casts, renal epithelial cells	500–1500
Acute interstitial nephritis	< 350	> 40	White blood cells	500–1500
Acute glomerulonephritis	Variable	Variable	Red cell casts	> 2000

Main causes of renal dysfunction in cirrhosis

- Hepatorenal syndrome:
  - Type 1
  - Type 2
- Nephrotoxic drugs:
  - Aminoglycosides
  - NSAIDs
  - Contrast agents
- Hypovolaemia induced:
  - Gastrointestinal bleeding
  - Diuretics
  - Diarrhoea, including lactulose induced
- Parenchymal renal disease:
  - Acute tubular necrosis
  - Glomerulonephritis (hepatitis B, hepatitis C)
  - IgA nephropathy.

Arroyo V, Gines P, Gerbes AL et al. Definition and diagnostic criteria of refractory ascites and hepatorenal syndrome in cirrhosis. *Hepatology* 1996; 23: 164–176.

European Association for the Study of the Liver. EASL clinical practice guidelines on the management of ascites, spontaneous bacterial peritonitis, and hepatorenal syndrome in cirrhosis. *Journal of Hepatology* 2010; 53: 397–417.

Gines P and Schrier R. Renal failure in cirrhosis. *New England Journal of Medicine* 2009; 361: 1279–1290.

Runyon BA. Management of adult patients with ascites due to cirrhosis: an update. *Hepatology* 2009; 49: 2087–2107.

Salerno F, Gerbes A, Gines P et al. Diagnosis, prevention and treatment of hepatorenal syndrome in cirrhosis. *Gut* 2007; 56: 1310–1318.

8. A. Patients with cirrhosis and ascites who have convincing signs and symptoms of SBP at the time of tapping their ascites, but who are found to have a PMN count of < 250 cells/mm³, often do not clear the infection spontaneously and develop SBP. Therefore empirical antibiotics should be continued and cultures awaited. Ascitic culture is negative in up to 60% of patients with clinical signs suggestive of SBP and a PMN count of > 250 cells/mm^3.

A diagnostic paracentesis should be performed in any cirrhotic patients with ascites and gastrointestinal bleeding, shock, fever, or other signs of systemic inflammation, local signs of peritonitis, gastrointestinal symptoms (vomiting, diarrhoea, ileus), worsening liver and/or renal function, or hepatic encephalopathy. SBP can also be asymptomatic, particularly in outpatients.

Secondary bacterial peritonitis, due to viscous perforation or loculated abscess, can mimic SBP with similar signs and symptoms which fail to differentiate between the two diagnoses.

Although characteristic ascitic fluid findings have been described as being suggestive of a secondary peritonitis, these are not reliable, and both the BSG and EASL guidelines urge caution when using them. Instead, abdominal CT and an erect chest X-ray should be used to investigate patients in whom such a diagnosis is suspected.

Characteristic findings in secondary peritonitis
- PMN count > 250 cells/mm^3 (usually > 1000 cells/mm^3)
- Multiple organisms (frequently fungi and enterococcus)
- At least two of the following:
  - Total protein > 1 g/dL
  - LDH greater than the upper limit of normal for serum
  - Glucose < 50 mg/dL
- Failure of response to therapy for SBP.

CEA (> 5 ng/mL) and ascitic ALP (> 240 U/L) have also been used to help to detect secondary peritonitis.

If a patient is diagnosed with SBP and is treated with an appropriate antibiotic, after 48 hours the PMN count should fall by at least 25% of its pre-treatment value. In secondary peritonitis the PMN count will continue to rise despite treatment. If there is a failure to respond to antibiotics, consider broadening antibiotics to cover for secondary peritonitis, and further imaging such as an erect chest X-ray and abdominal CT.

Runyon BA. Management of adult patients with ascites due to cirrhosis: an update. *Hepatology* 2009; 49: 2087–2107.

European Association for the Study of the Liver. EASL clinical practice guidelines on the management of ascites, spontaneous bacterial peritonitis, and hepatorenal syndrome in cirrhosis. *Journal of Hepatology* 2010; 53: 397–417.

Moore KP and Aithal GP. Guidelines on the management of ascites in cirrhosis. *Gut* 2006; 55: 1–12.

9. C. Continuing antibiotics and repeating the ascitic tap is reasonable, but given the abdominal tenderness and low-grade pyrexia, treating as for SBP is the best course of action.

Bacterascites is defined as a PMN count of < 250 cells/mm^3 with a positive culture. These infections can represent a spontaneous colonization of ascites, and such patients can either be clinically asymptomatic or have abdominal pain and fever. In other cases bacterascites develops as a result of secondary bacterial colonization of ascites from an extraperitoneal infection. Bacterascites is sometimes cleared spontaneously—yet in other instances, often when the patient is symptomatic, it is the precursor to SBP.

EASL and BSG guidelines suggest that any symptomatic patients with bacterascites should be treated according to SBP treatment protocols. However, if the patient is asymptomatic, the ascitic tap can be repeated while continuing antibiotics. If the second tap reveals a PMN count of > 250 cells/mm³, treatment according to SBP treatment protocols is recommended. If the second ascitic tap reveals a PMN count of < 250 cells/mm³, the antibiotics can be stopped, while awaiting the second culture results with careful follow-up.

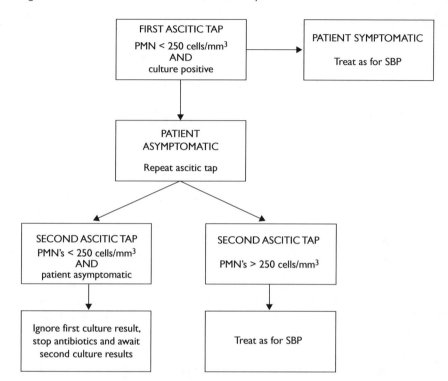

Figure 5.5 Algorithm for managing monomicrobial bacterascites.

Culture-negative neutrocytic ascites

This describes the patient with an ascitic tap showing a PMN count of > 250 cells/mm³ and a negative ascitic culture. These patients present similarly to those with SBP, and should be treated in the same way, as both groups of patients have similar morbidity and mortality.

Spontaneous bacterial peritonitis

An ascitic fluid neutrophil count of > 250 cells/mm³ is diagnostic of SBP, and patients should be commenced on empirical antibiotic therapy. The percentage of PMNs in the fluid is usually greater than 50%. Antibiotics should not be started prior to ascitic cultures being taken, as even a single dose of an effective broad-spectrum drug causes the culture to produce no growth in up to 86% of cases.

Third-generation cephalosporins such as cefotaxime (2 g for 5 days) can be commenced empirically. When the ascitic culture is positive (around 40% of cases), the most common pathogens include Gram-negative bacteria, usually *E. coli* and Gram-positive cocci (mainly *Streptococcus* species and enterococci). Anaerobic bacteria are not associated with SBP. Piperacillin and tazobactam (Tazocin) are frequently used in the UK.

Use of IV albumin in SBP

Up to 30% of patients with SBP treated with antibiotics alone develop type 1 HRS. The administration of IV albumin at 1.5 g albumin/kg in the first 6 hours on day 1, followed by

1 g/kg on day 3, reduces the frequency of HRS and improves survival. It is unclear whether albumin is beneficial in patients with normal bilirubin and creatinine levels, and until further evidence is available the guidelines suggest that albumin should be given to all patients with SBP.

Primary and secondary prophylaxis of SBP with antibiotics

Patients with both severe liver disease and low protein ascites (< 15 g/L) may benefit from norfloxacin antibiotic prophylaxis, which has been shown to reduce the risk of SBP and improve survival. In patients who have recovered from SBP, secondary prophylaxis with norfloxacin reduces the risk of recurrent SBP. Other antibiotics are also used. Patients should also be considered for transplantation, as those who have recovered from SBP have a poor long-term prognosis.

European Association for the Study of the Liver. EASL clinical practice guidelines on the management of ascites, spontaneous bacterial peritonitis, and hepatorenal syndrome in cirrhosis. *Journal of Hepatology* 2010; 53: 397–417.

Moore KP and Aithal GP. Guidelines on the management of ascites in cirrhosis. *Gut* 2006; 55: 1–12.

Runyon BA. Management of adult patients with ascites due to cirrhosis: an update. *Hepatology* 2009; 49: 2087–2107.

Sort P, Navasa M, Arroyo V *et al.* Effect of intravenous albumin on renal impairment and mortality in patients with cirrhosis and spontaneous bacterial peritonitis. *New England Journal of Medicine* 1999; 341: 403–409.

10. A. This patient has a serum-ascites albumin gradient (SAAG) of 15 g/L; a SAAG of ≥ 11 g/L is suggestive of portal hypertension. The cause of ascites can be ascertained by calculating the SAAG, as it correlates directly with portal pressure (> 97% cases). Around 5% of patients with ascites have a mixed ascites with two or more causes present.

- SAAG ≥ 11 g/L suggests portal hypertension
- SAAG < 11 g/L suggests non-portal hypertensive causes.

Analysis of ascitic fluid

	White cell count > 500/μL Neutrophil count > 250/μL	White cell count 250/μL	Lymphocyte count > 250/μL
SAAG ≥ 11 g/L	• Cirrhosis • Acute liver failure • Portal vein thrombosis • Right heart failure	• SBP in portal hypertension	• Tuberculosis or malignancy in portal hypertension • Partially treated SBP
SAAG < 11 g/L	• Malnutrition • Protein-losing enteropathy • Nephrotic syndrome	• Peritonitis • Pancreatitis • SBP in hypoalbuminaemia	• Malignancy • Tuberculosis • Connective tissue disease

Data from Bloom S, Webster G, and Marks D, *Oxford Handbook of Gastroenterology and Hepatology*, second edition, Figure 1.1, p. 23, 2012, Oxford University Press.

Serum CA-125 is frequently elevated in female and male patients with ascites or pleural fluid of any cause, and levels fall when the ascites is controlled. Raised levels of CA-125 in female patients with ascites can often lead to unnecessary investigation for gynaecological malignancy.

The concentration of red cells in ascites is usually less than 1000 cells/mm³, and bloody ascites (> 50 000 cells/mm³) occurs in about 2% of cirrhotics. About a third of patients with cirrhosis and bloody ascites have a hepatocellular carcinoma. To calculate the estimated true neutrophil count in a patient with an ascitic RBC count of > 1000 cells/mm³, subtract one neutrophil for every 250 RBCs.

Bloom S, Webster G and Marks D. *Oxford Handbook of Gastroenterology and Hepatology*, 2nd edition. Oxford: Oxford University Press; 2012. p. 23.

Runyon BA. Management of adult patients with ascites due to cirrhosis: an update. *Hepatology* 2009; 49: 2087–2107.

Moore KP and Aithal GP. Guidelines on the management of ascites in cirrhosis. *Gut* 2006; 55: 1–12.

11. A. This woman has pre-eclampsia, there is no evidence of haemolysis or thrombocytopenia, and her LFTs and uric acid levels are elevated. These features in combination with her liver biopsy are suggestive of acute fatty liver of pregnancy. Often a liver biopsy would not be performed, in order to avoid treatment delay.

Liver dysfunction in pregnancy is mostly related to one of the following:

- Pre-eclampsia (hypertension and proteinuria, with or without oedema)
- Haemolysis, elevated liver enzymes, and low platelets (HELLP)
- Acute fatty liver of pregnancy
- Cholestasis of pregnancy
- Hyperemesis gravidarum.

These can be separated into those that can occur with pre-eclampsia (pre-eclampsia, HELLP, and acute fatty liver of pregnancy) and those that have no relationship to pre-eclampsia (cholestasis of pregnancy and hyperemesis gravidarum).

Acute fatty liver of pregnancy

- Onset occurs in late pregnancy (30–38 weeks), mostly in the third trimester, and can start with a prodromal illness of malaise, nausea, vomiting, right upper quadrant pain, fever, headache, and pruritus
- Aminotransferase and bilirubin levels may be moderately high
- Serum creatinine and uric acid levels are commonly high
- Clinical severity varies from very mild to a fulminant hepatic failure with disseminated intravascular coagulation
- Around 50% of cases have pre-eclampsia, and there is an overlap with HELLP; it can be difficult to distinguish between them
- There is an association between the condition and patients with a maternal BMI of < 20 kg/m² and twin pregnancies
- Liver biopsy demonstrates microvesicular steatosis (zone 1 sparing), foamy hepatocytes and hepatic necrosis, but is rarely performed, due to the need for prompt treatment and coagulopathy
- Treatment is to deliver the foetus
- With good supportive treatment, maternal mortality is now rare
- Liver transplantation is rarely required except in cases of massive hepatic haemorrhage, rupture, or fulminant liver failure
- It rarely recurs in subsequent pregnancies.

Pre-eclampsia

- Pre-eclampsia and HELLP are probably different manifestations of the same pathology
- Pre-eclampsia occurs in about 5 in 100 pregnancies
- Pathogenesis is thought to be related to uteroplacental ischaemia, which leads to endothelial dysfunction and the release of cytotoxic factors
- It presents with a triad of hypertension, proteinuria, and non-dependant oedema after 20 weeks gestation
- Approximately 20–30% of cases of pre-eclampsia have abnormal LFTs
- The fetus must be delivered urgently in order to avoid eclampsia, hepatic rupture, and necrosis.

HELLP (haemolysis, elevated liver enzymes, and low platelets)

- Occurs in approximately 1 to 6 in 1000 pregnancies, and between 16 weeks' gestation and 3 days postpartum (70% occur between 27 and 37 weeks, mostly in the third trimester)
- Up to 65% of pre-eclamptics will demonstrate features of HELLP
- Mortality is rare in HELLP, but when maternal death does occur it is often a consequence of hepatic rupture
- Hypertension and proteinuria may be absent in HELLP
- Warning signs include a high LDH, ALT > 100 U/L, high uric acid levels, and a platelet count of < 50
- Jaundice is uncommon; fibrinogen and prothrombin time are usually normal
- Treatment includes urgent hospitalization, magnesium, antihypertensives, and antiplatelet drugs
- Delivery is the only definitive treatment for prepartum cases
- About 25% of cases occur in the postpartum period.

Differences between HELLP, intrahepatic cholestasis of pregnancy (ICP), and acute fatty liver of pregnancy

	HELLP	ICP	Acute fatty liver of pregnancy
Onset	Third trimester or postpartum	25–32 weeks	Third trimester or postpartum
Presence of pre-eclampsia	Yes	No	50% of cases
Features	Haemolysis, thrombocytopaenia	Pruritus, mild jaundice, elevated bile acids	Liver failure and coagulopathy, encephalopathy, hypoglycaemia, disseminated intravascular coagulation
Aminotransferases	Mild to 10- to 20-fold elevation	Mild to 10- to 20-fold elevation	300- to 500-fold elevation typical, but variable
Bilirubin	< 5 mg/dL unless massive necrosis	< 5 mg/dL	Often < 5 mg/dL, higher if severe

Reproduced from Hay JE, 'Liver disease in pregnancy', *Hepatology*, 47, 3, pp. 1067–1076, 2008, with permission from Wiley and the American Association for the Study of Liver Diseases.

Intrahepatic cholestasis of pregnancy (ICP)/obstetric cholestasis

- A common familial condition that occurs in 0.1–1.5% of European pregnancies
- It presents in the second and third trimester with intense pruritus, possibly a mild jaundice, and infrequently with a rash
- The disease usually follows a benign course with a mild elevation of ALT and raised serum bile acids, which are the most specific and sensitive marker (bile acid levels > 10 μmol/L, and up to 100-fold elevation)

- The main risk is to the foetus. There is an increased risk of premature labour, intrauterine death, and placental insufficiency, and therefore the patient should be referred to an obstetrician
- Treatment with ursodeoxycholic acid provides symptomatic relief from pruritus, and reduces ALT and serum bile acids, but it is not certain whether it improves foetus outcome
- An adverse foetus outcome can be avoided by delivery when the foetus lungs are mature.

Hyperemesis gravidarum

- Intractable vomiting in the first trimester of pregnancy; around 50% of patients with this condition have abnormal liver tests (AST raised by up to 20-fold, occasional jaundice)
- Viral hepatitis should be excluded
- Treatment is with IV fluids, nutritional support, anti-emetics and (rarely) corticosteroids.

Hay JE. Liver disease in pregnancy. *Hepatology* 2008; 47: 1067–1076.

European Association for the Study of the Liver. EASL Clinical Practice Guidelines: management of cholestatic liver diseases. *Journal of Hepatology* 2009; 51: 237–267.

12. B. The following alterations to normal ranges of serological tests can be found in pregnancy:

Unchanged

- Bilirubin, aminotransferases, prothrombin time.

Increased

- White blood cells, caeruloplasmin, triglycerides, and α- and β-globulins
- α-fetoprotein, especially in twins
- Cholesterol levels increase by twofold
- Alkaline phosphatase levels increase by two- to fourfold
- Fibrinogen levels increase by 50%.

Decreased

- Gamma globulin
- Haemoglobin, in later pregnancy.

Hay JE. Liver disease in pregnancy. *Hepatology* 2008; 47: 1067–1076.

13. A. The role of nutrition in the management of decompensated chronic liver disease is important. In this encephalopathic patient, his oral intake will be inadequate to meet his energy requirements. His oesophageal varices have been banded, so a nasogastric tube can be placed safely.

Nasojejunal feeding is not indicated. Parenteral nutrition can be considered if the patient cannot be fed via the enteral route. It is rarely indicated in the care of patients with decompensated chronic liver disease.

Enteral nutrition (EN) improves nutritional status and survival in severely malnourished patients with alcoholic hepatitis. It is as effective as corticosteroids in patients with severe alcoholic hepatitis. Patients treated with EN who survive have a better outcome in the following year.

Parenteral nutrition (PN) should be considered in patients with alcoholic steatohepatitis who are moderately or severely malnourished, and who are unable to be fed adequately orally or enterally.

Plautha M, Cabre E, Riggio O *et al.* ESPEN Guidelines on Enteral Nutrition: liver disease. *Clinical Nutrition* 2006; 25: 285–294.

Plauth M, Cabre E, Campillo B *et al.* ESPEN Guidelines on Parenteral Nutrition: hepatology. *Clinical Nutrition* 2009; 28: 436–444.

14. D. Severe alcoholic hepatitis has a high mortality, and there are several prognostic models available to determine patients at high risk of death who may benefit from corticosteroid or other pharmacological treatments.

Maddrey's Discriminant Function (MDF) score

$$MDF = (4.6 \times PT \text{ prolongation}) + \frac{\text{total serum bilirubin in } \mu mol/L}{17}$$

An MDF score of > 32 identifies patients with severe alcoholic hepatitis. This score correlates with a mortality of greater than 50% at 1 month, compared with 17% mortality if the MDF is < 32.

Glasgow Alcoholic Hepatitis Score (GAHS)

A GAHS score of ≥ 9 is associated with a poorer outcome.

The score is calculated as follows:

Score	1	2	3
Age (years)	< 50	> 50	–
WCC (x 10^9/L)	< 15	> 15	–
Urea (mmol/L)	< 5	> 5	–
PT ratio or INR	1.5	1.5–2.0	> 2.0
Bilirubin (μmol/L)	< 125	125–250	> 250

Reproduced from *Gut*, EH Forrest et al., 'Analysis of factors predictive of mortality in alcoholic hepatitis and derivation and validation of the Glasgow alcoholic hepatitis score', 54, 8, pp. 1174–1179. Copyright 2005, with permission from BMJ Publishing Group Ltd.

Patients with a GAHS score of ≥ 9 have a 28-day survival of 52% in untreated patients, compared with 78% in corticosteroid-treated patients. The 84-day survival is 38% in untreated patients, compared with 59% in corticosteroid-treated patients.

National Institute for Health and Clinical Excellence. *Alcohol-Use Disorders: diagnosis and clinical management of alcohol-related physical complications*. NICE Clinical Guideline 100. London: NICE; 2010.

Forrest EH, Morris AJ, Stewart S et al. The Glasgow alcoholic hepatitis score identifies patients who may benefit from corticosteroids. Gut 2007; 56: 1743–1746.

15. A. In this patient, who has a Child–Turtcotte–Pugh (CTP) score of B, with three nodules less than 3 cm and no other comorbidities, the BCLC staging classification is most appropriate for liver transplant referral.

The BCLC staging classification is based on cohort studies and randomized controlled trials by the Barcelona Liver Clinic Group. It is not a scoring system but a staging system which aids selection of patients who will benefit from curative therapies, as described in Figure 5.6.

The CTP score was originally designed to assess the prognosis of cirrhotic patients undergoing surgical treatment for portal hypertension. It can be used to select the most appropriate management of hepatocellular carcinoma (HCC).

The MELD score was originally introduced to measure the mortality risk in patients with end-stage liver disease undergoing transjugular intrahepatic portosystemic shunts. It was subsequently modified for use as a disease severity index to determine referral to transplant programmes and organ allocation priorities. Patients with the highest scores are prioritized for organ allocation.

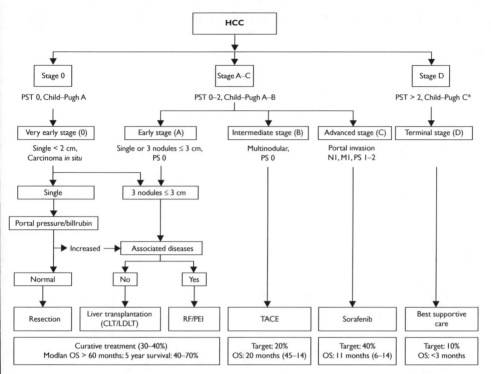

Figure 5.6 The BCLC staging classification.

Reprinted from *Journal of Hepatology*, 56, 4, European Association for the Study of the Liver, European Organisation for Research and Treatment of Cancer, 'EASL–EORTC Clinical Practice Guidelines: Management of hepatocellular carcinoma', pp. 908–943. Copyright 2012, with permission from European Association for the Study of the Liver, published by Elsevier.

The UKELD score is the UK version of the established MELD score. It is intended for use in stratifying patients for liver transplant assessment. The UKELD score is derived from the patient's serum sodium, creatinine, and bilirubin levels and the international normalized ratio (INR) of the prothrombin time. A score of > 49 predicts a 1-year mortality of > 9%, and is the minimum criterion for entry to the waiting list.

Liver transplantation is the most effective therapeutic option in many patients with acute or chronic liver failure. Most are performed using the whole organ from a deceased donor. The term 'orthotopic' is derived from the position in which the donor liver is placed. Donor organs can be split and used in two adults or a child and an adult. Surgically, the same technique is used if a living donor organ is used. The most common surgical technique is an end-to-end anastomosis of the proximal donor bile duct to the distal recipient duct. If the ducts are diseased in the recipient (e.g. in cases of primary sclerosing cholangitis), the donor duct is anastomosed to the jejunum of the recipient using a Roux-en-Y loop.

HCC and hepatopulmonary syndrome are two indications for transplant in which the MELD does not reflect the mortality. The criteria for transplantation in cases of HCC are:

- One single nodule less than 5 cm in size, *or*
- Three nodules, none of which is larger than 3 cm.

Hepatopulmonary syndrome is defined as arterial deoxygenation and widespread intrapulmonary vasodilatation in the context of chronic liver disease. Portopulmonary hypertension, on the other hand, is not in itself an indication for a liver transplant.

Other indications for liver transplantation are a number of metabolic diseases with hepatic manifestations, such as hereditary amyloidosis and hyperoxaluria.

European Association for the Study of the Liver. EASL–EORTC clinical practice guidelines: management of hepatocellular carcinoma. *Journal of Hepatology* 2012; 56: 908–943.

Kamath PS and Kim WR. The model for end-stage liver disease (MELD). *Hepatology* 2007; 45: 797–805.

Neuberger J, Gimson A, Davies M *et al*. Selection of patients for liver transplantation and allocation of donated livers in the UK. *Gut* 2008; 57: 252–257.

Bloom S, Webster G and Marks D. *Oxford Handbook of Gastroenterology and Hepatology*, 2nd edition. Oxford: Oxford University Press; 2012.

Hauser S, Pardi D and Poterucha J. *Mayo Clinic Gastroenterology and Hepatology Board Review*, 3rd edition. New York: Mayo Clinic Scientific Press; 2008.

NHS Blood and Transplant and the Liver Advisory Group. *Protocols and Guidelines for Adults Undergoing Deceased Donor Liver Transplantation in the UK*. Watford: NHS Blood and Transplant; 2009.

Murray KF and Carithers RL Jr. AASLD practice guidelines: evaluation of the patient for liver transplantation. *Hepatology* 2005; 41: 1407–1432.

Said A, Einstein M and Lucey MR. Liver transplantation: an update 2007. *Current Opinion in Gastroenterology* 2007; 23: 292–298.

16. E. Thrombocytopenia is found in 76% of patients with cirrhosis. The pathophysiology is thought to be multifactorial, and includes splenic sequestration when complicated by portal hypertension, bone-marrow suppression secondary to toxicity, reduced thrombopoietin levels, and autoantibody platelet destruction.

Macrocytosis is associated with alcohol excess, and has a number of other causes, including vitamin B_{12} deficiency, folate deficiency, and hypothyroidism. Hypoalbuminaemia may occur due to an acute or chronic inflammatory process, malnutrition, malabsorption, or renal losses. Hyperbilirubinaemia and raised alanine aminotransferase (ALT) levels are not predictors of portal hypertension.

Afdhal N, McHutchison J, Brown R *et al*. Thrombocytopenia associated with chronic liver disease. *Journal of Hepatology* 2008; 48: 1000–1007.

Goulis J, Chau TN, Jordan S *et al*. Thrombopoietin concentrations are low in patients with cirrhosis and thrombocytopenia and are restored after orthotopic liver transplantation. *Gut* 1999; 44: 754–758.

Kajihara M, Okazaki Y, Kato S *et al*. Evaluation of platelet kinetics in patients with liver cirrhosis: similarity to idiopathic thrombocytopenic purpura. *Journal of Gastroenterology and Hepatology* 2007; 22: 112–118.

17. D. National Institute for Health and Clinical Excellence (NICE) guidelines state that corticosteroids (prednisolone 40 mg once daily for 4 weeks) are associated with a significant reduction in both all-cause mortality and liver-related mortality at 1 month and 6 months. No significant differences were found between corticosteroids and a control for gastrointestinal bleeding and infection.

Pentoxyfylline is a non-selective phosphodiesterase inhibitor (400 mg orally 3 times daily for 4 weeks) which can also be considered in patients with severe disease (Maddrey's Discriminant Function score > 32) in whom corticosteroid therapy is contraindicated. Those with severe disease should be treated aggressively with enteral nutritional therapy, which is as effective as corticosteroids in the management of alcoholic hepatitis.

NSAIDs can precipitate hepatorenal syndrome, due to their effects on prostaglandin-modulated renal blood flow, and are therefore contraindicated. One trial of N-acetylcysteine and corticosteroid therapy suggested that there is an improvement in mortality at 1 month, but 6-month mortality is not improved.

National Institute for Health and Clinical Excellence. *Alcohol-Use Disorders: diagnosis and clinical management of alcohol-related physical complications.* NICE Clinical Guideline 100. London: NICE; 2010.

O'Shea RS, Dasarathy S and McCullough AJ. Alcoholic liver disease. *American Journal of Gastroenterology* 2010; 105: 14–32.

Nguyen-Khac E, Thevenot T, Piquet M *et al.* Glucocorticoids plus N-acetylcysteine in severe alcoholic hepatitis. *New England Journal of Medicine* 2011; 365: 1781–1789.

18. A. Alcohol withdrawal syndromes develop when alcohol intake is abruptly stopped or reduced. It can occur as early as 6–8 hours after stopping alcohol consumption, it peaks at between 10–30 hours, and it subsides after 40–50 hours. Alcohol withdrawal seizures may occur within the first 12–48 hours.

Delirium tremens occurs in less than 5% of individuals who withdraw from alcohol. It usually starts 48–72 hours after abstinence, and is characterized by coarse tremor, agitation, fever, tachycardia, profound confusion, delusions, and hallucinations. It may lead to hyperpyrexia, ketoacidosis, and profound circulatory collapse.

The NICE guidelines for delirium tremens recommend offering short-acting benzodiazepines as first-line treatment. If symptoms persist or oral medication is declined, parenteral lorazepam, haloperidol, or olanzapine should be considered. Oxazepam is a short-acting benzodiazepine which is sometimes used in hepatic impairment, but would not be a first-line medication.

Dosing regimens in use include fixed dosing of benzodiazepines, front-loading dosing, or symptom-triggered dosing (the reader should refer to the NICE guidelines for examples of dosing regimens).

Prophylactic oral or parenteral thiamine should be used in patients at risk of developing Wernicke's encephalopathy. Parenteral followed by oral thiamine should be offered to dependent alcohol users who are at risk of malnourishment, have decompensated liver disease, are acutely withdrawing, are admitted for detoxification, or have an acute illness. Patients with signs of Wernicke's encephalopathy should have 5 days of treatment with parenteral thiamine.

National Institute for Health and Clinical Excellence. *Alcohol-Use Disorders: diagnosis and clinical management of alcohol-related physical complications.* NICE Clinical Guideline 100. London: NICE; 2010.

National Institute for Health and Clinical Excellence. *Alcohol Use Disorders: diagnosis, assessment and management of harmful drinking and alcohol dependence.* NICE Clinical Guideline 115. London: NICE; 2011.

19. D. The CT scan demonstrates multiple liver lesions in both the right and left lobe of the liver, consistent with multiple liver abscesses. Radiologically, the typical findings for an abscess are a low-density mass with smooth margins, and a contrast-enhancing peripheral rim. This patient had symptoms suggestive of dysentery, but did not seek medical advice at the time.

More than 90% of patients with amoebic liver abscesses have a leucocytosis and positive anti-amoebic serum antibodies. Serology may be negative in the first week, and antibody titres reach a peak by the second or third month. They then fall, but are still detectable at 9 months. Around 85–90% of patients are positive for indirect haemagglutination, which is the most sensitive and specific test. *Entamoeba histolytica* Gal/GalNAc lectin antigen is positive in almost all patients. The role of microscopic stool examination is limited.

Hepatic adenomas are radiologically well-demarcated lesions that enhance early in the arterial phase due to blood supply from the hepatic artery. They are benign liver tumours which are at risk of malignant transformation or rupture and intra-abdominal bleeding. They are strongly associated with the oral contraceptive pill, anabolic steroid use, and glycogen storage disease.

Hepatocellular carcinomas are hypervascular in the arterial phase, followed by washout in the portal venous phase in multiphase imaging such as CT or MRI.

Hydatid disease occurs mainly in the liver. The cysts have a thick wall on imaging, with focal or circumferential calcification, and daughter cysts may also be present.

Torre A and Kershenobich D. Amebic liver abscess. *Annals of Hepatology* 2002; 1: 45–47.

Rodes J, Benhamou J and Mizzetto M. *The Textbook of Hepatology: from basic science to clinical practice,* 3rd edition. Malden, MA: Blackwell Publishing Ltd; 2007.

20. B. Alcoholic hepatitis would be very unlikely with an alcohol intake of 28 units per week, and an ALT of > 200 U/L would also argue against this. Hepatitis A might fit this scenario, but drug-induced cholestasis is most likely. Liver function tests usually improve spontaneously and slowly. Bodybuilders may use supplements containing anabolic steroids or prohormones that can lead to the development of jaundice. A negative autoimmune screen, viral hepatitis screen, and normal imaging exclude the other causes of jaundice.

Bloom S and Webster G. *Oxford Handbook of Gastroenterology and Hepatology,* 2nd edition. Oxford: Oxford University Press; 2012.

21. C. Liver biopsy is a useful investigation for patients with atypical clinical features, and can help to distinguish between autoimmune hepatitis (AIH) and non-alcoholic fatty liver disease (NAFLD) in an obese patient with raised immunoglobulin G (IgG) levels and a positive antinuclear antibody (ANA) titre. It can be helpful in identifying patients with coexisting liver disease, such as overlap syndrome of primary biliary cirrhosis with autoimmune hepatitis. The use of liver biopsy in the evaluation of focal liver disease is highly variable, and can be complicated by the nature of the lesions, which may be cystic, solid, or vascular.

Contraindications to liver biopsy include extrahepatic biliary obstruction, bacterial cholangitis, abnormal coagulation, thrombocytopenia, ascites, cystic lesions, and a diagnosis of amyloidosis.

BSG guidelines are as follows:
- If the platelet count is > 60 x 10^9/L, the biopsy can be safely performed
- If the platelet count is 40–60 x 10^9/L, platelet transfusion may increase the count sufficiently for the percutaneous biopsy to be performed safely
- If platelet transfusion does not increase the platelet count, or the count is < 40 x 10^9/L, alternative biopsy methods should be considered

- Drugs that affect platelet function (e.g. aspirin, clopidogrel) should be discontinued at least 2 days before biopsy
- If the prothrombin time is prolonged by less than 4 seconds, percutaneous biopsy can be safely performed
- If the prothrombin time is prolonged by 4–6 seconds, a fresh frozen plasma transfusion is required
- If the prothrombin time is prolonged by more than 6 seconds, an alternative route of biopsy should be considered.

Neuberger J, Grant A, Day C et al. Guidelines on the Use of Liver Biopsy in Clinical Practice. London: British Society of Gastroenterology; 2004.

Rockey D, Caldwell SH, Goodman ZD et al. Liver biopsy. Hepatology 2009; 49: 1017–1044.

22. D. Acute liver failure (ALF) is a rare condition that involves the development of hepatic encephalopathy and coagulopathy in a non-cirrhotic person with no prior history of liver disease (splenomegaly is rare). It is an illness of less than 26 weeks' duration. The American Association for the Study of Liver Diseases guidelines state that further divisions of time of onset of encephalopathy or coagulopathy from jaundice do not have helpful prognostic significance. Transplant-free survival can be greater than 50% if acute liver failure is due to paracetamol, ischaemia or pregnancy related causes.

Hepatitis E is a significant cause of ALF in south-east Asia, India, Pakistan, and China, and tends to be more severe in pregnant women. In western Europe and the USA, acute liver failure is more commonly caused by drugs than by viral hepatitis. Hepatitis E is transmitted by the faecal–oral route, and is often caused by a contaminated water supply. In pregnancy, infection is more frequent, and the third trimester carries the highest risk, although outcomes are not affected by pregnancy.

Acute hepatitis B causes acute liver failure in 8% of patients in the USA, and antiviral therapy such as tenofovir or entecavir may be considered in patients with acute hepatitis B.

Black cohosh extract is sometimes used as a herbal remedy to treat symptoms of the menopause. There are conflicting views as to whether it works, and there have also been questions raised about its safety, with some reports of liver failure.

Hepatitis A-related acute liver failure may occur a few weeks after exposure, but may be prevented by vaccination prior to travel to areas of high endemicity.

Leptospirosis occurs after the organism directly enters the human body via the skin. It has an incubation period of 7–14 days, and is diagnosed by checking the Leptospira IgM.

Other causes of acute liver failure worldwide include the following:

- Paracetamol overdose
- Drug-induced liver disease
- Infection (viral/bacterial):
  + Hepatitis B (anti-HB core IgM positive)
  + Hepatitis C (rare)
  + Epstein–Barr virus (EBV)
  + Cytomegalovirus (CMV)
- Ischaemia—the history may elicit recent episodes of hypotension
- Autoimmune liver disease
- Pregnancy related (acute fatty liver of pregnancy, HELLP)
- Wilson's disease

- Budd–Chiari syndrome—history of venous thromboembolism
- Toxins (*Amanita phalloides* mushrooms).

Bernal W, Auzinger E, Dhawan A *et al*. Acute liver failure. *Lancet* 2010; 376: 190–201.

Lee WM, Larson AM and Stravitz RT. *AASLD Position Paper: the management of acute liver failure: update 2011*. Baltimore, MD: American Association for the Study of Liver Diseases; 2011.

23. B. The history and investigations are suggestive of acute liver failure. Around 17% of patients have no discernible cause; this is often called seronegative hepatitis.

Other causes in the USA include the following:

- Paracetamol (40%)
- Drug induced (13%)
- Hepatitis B (6%)
- Hepatitis A (4%)
- Ischaemic hepatitis (6%)
- Other (autoimmune, Wilson's disease, Budd–Chiari syndrome, pregnancy associated) (14%)
- Idiopathic (17%).

Bernal W, Auzinger E, Dhawan A *et al*. Acute liver failure. *Lancet* 2010; 376: 190–201.

24. D. The management of acute liver failure can be divided into general measures, which include screening for all causes, and disease-specific measures.

General management

Cerebral oedema

- This can lead to uncal herniation and hypoxic brain injury
- It can be predicted by the degree of encephalopathy
- Patients with grade 1 or 2 encephalopathy should be transferred to a transplant facility for consideration of transplantation
- Grade 2 encephalopathy warrants ITU care. Grade 3 encephalopathy warrants intubation and ventilation
- CT is advised, to exclude other causes of depressed consciousness
- Consider lactulose. Studies show a small increase in survival time, but there is no evidence that it reduces the severity of encephalopathy or improves overall outcome
- Minimize intravenous fluids, avoid sedation, and nurse the patient at 30 degrees prone
- Intracranial pressure (ICP) monitoring is not routinely used. However, when it is used, cerebral perfusion pressure should be maintained in the range 60–100 mmHg and intracranial pressure at less than 40 mmHg
- A clinical diagnosis of raised ICP should be treated with boluses of 20% mannitol (0.5g/kg IV bolus, but not if the serum osmolality is > 320 mOsm/L). Hyperventilation to a $PaCO_2$ of 25 mmHg may also be beneficial
- Phenytoin is indicated for seizures.

Kidney injury

- Avoid nephrotoxic agents (e.g. aminoglycosides, ACE inhibitors, NSAIDs)
- Maintain adequate haemodynamics with inotropes if necessary
- Continuous (rather than intermittent) venovenous haemodialysis is indicated when potassium is > 6 mmol/L, bicarbonate is < 15 mmol/L, or creatinine is > 400 umol/L.

Infection

- Prophylactic antibiotics and antifungal agents are routinely administered, but there is no evidence of a survival benefit. They may prevent worsening encephalopathy and subsequent cerebral oedema.

Coagulopathy

- Routine correction of abnormal clotting with blood products is not advised, due to the volume load and masking progression of ALF, unless bleeding or invasive procedures are planned.
- Vitamin K, 5–10 mg intravenously or subcutaneously, is routine.

Hypoglycaemia

- This occurs due to inadequate degradation of insulin and diminished production of glucose by the liver
- Monitor blood sugar levels regularly
- Treat with intravenous dextrose.

Gastric protection

- Routine use of proton pump inhibitors or H2-receptor antagonists is advised, to prevent haemorrhagic gastritis.

Nutrition

- Early nasogastric feeding is advised.

Disease-specific management

Paracetamol toxicity

- This is the most common cause of acute liver failure in the UK
- N-acetylcysteine (NAC) can be administered empirically when there is doubt about the aetiology of the liver failure
- The King's College criteria for poor prognostic indicators in acute liver failure (without a transplant) are an arterial pH < 7.3 OR a prothrombin time > 100 seconds (INR 6.5) AND a creatinine > 300 umol/L AND Grade 3 or 4 encephalopathy.

Drug-induced liver failure

- This is mostly idiosyncratic, unlike paracetamol toxicity
- No antidotes are available
- Common drugs include antibiotics, NSAIDS, and anticonvulsants
- Remember to consider herbal remedies and dietary supplements.

Infection

- Consider lamivudine if due to hepatitis B
- Acute liver failure due to reactivation of hepatitis B may occur if the patient is immunocompromised, or during chemotherapy. Give prophylactic treatment with nucleoside analogue (lamivudine) if HBsAg positive during immunocompromised state, and for 6 months afterwards
- Give doxycycline or intravenous penicillin treatment for leptospirosis.

Autoimmune disorders

- Autoantibodies may be negative; liver biopsy may be required
- While awaiting transplant, consider a therapeutic trial of corticosteroids.

Pregnancy related

- Early recognition and prompt delivery are needed, with supportive treatment thereafter.

Wilson's disease

- This disease is fatal without transplant
- Haemolytic anaemia with serum bilirubin level > 20 µmol/L; unconjugated and total bilirubin levels are high
- Low serum caeruloplasmin (not specific in ALF), low (or normal) serum copper and high urinary copper levels
- Note that raised urinary copper levels are not exclusive to Wilson's disease; elevated levels may be found in any cholestatic disease
- A high bilirubin (mg/dL) to alkaline phosphatase (IU/L) ratio (> 2) is predictive of Wilson's disease
- Do not treat with penicillamine acutely, as there is a risk of hypersensitivity
- Treatment is with albumin dialysis, continuous haemofiltration, plasmapheresis, or plasma exchange
- Unlike most other causes, in Wilson's disease, diagnosis of ALF can be made when patients show evidence of cirrhosis if rapid deterioration occurs.

Budd–Chiari syndrome

- Confirm the diagnosis with hepatic venography; transplant if in the setting of ALF
- Ensure that malignancy has been excluded as a cause of hypercoagulability.

Mushroom poisoning

- This is preceded by severe gastrointestinal symptoms of diarrhoea, vomiting, and abdominal cramps
- Penicillin G or intravenous milk thistle (silibinin) are antidotes that lack evidence
- Transplant is often needed.

Transplantation in ALF

- Survival rates are greater than 60% with transplant
- There is no widely available liver support system, outside of a trial setting.

Polson J and Lee WM. AASLD Position Paper. The management of acute liver failure. *Hepatology* 2005; 41: 1179–1197.

25. A. With regard to the prognosis of acute liver failure, a hyperacute onset is better than a subacute onset. If grade 3 or 4 encephalopathy is present, survival is 10–40 % without orthotopic liver transplantation. Poor prognostic indicators for non-paracetamol-induced acute liver failure (King's College criteria) are as follows:

PT > 100 seconds (INR 6.5), or three out of five of the following:

> age < 10 or > 40 years
> jaundice to encephalopathy > 7 days

PT > 50 seconds (INR 3.5)
bilirubin level > 300 µmol/L
drug-induced or indeterminate cause

(This was published in *Gastroenterology*, 97, 2, John G. O'Grady *et al.*, 'Early indicators of prognosis in fulminant hepatic failure', pp. 439–445, Copyright Elsevier 1989.)

Other clinical features include the following:

- **A**irway may become compromised secondary to hepatic encephalopathy
- **B**reathing may become compromised due to pneumonia or aspiration in patients with encephalopathy, and non-cardiogenic pulmonary oedema may occur, especially in the context of paracetamol overdose
- **C**irculatory effects can occur, with a tachycardia and falling mean arterial pressure
- **D**epressed GCS score, due to cerebral oedema or encephalopathy
- **E**lectrolyte disturbances occur due to acute tubular necrosis from a direct toxic effect of the cause (paracetamol), dehydration, or a rapid onset of hepatorenal syndrome. Lactic acidosis is common, due to hypoperfusion and inability to remove the lactate from the body
- **F**ungal infections, such as candida or aspergillus, can occur in this setting, as can bacterial infections. Patients may not always mount a temperature or have an elevated white cell count. Around 50% of deaths in ALF are due to sepsis
- Hypo**G**lycaemia is common
- **H**aematological abnormalities occur. Coagulopathy is the most useful indicator of the severity of ALF. The platelet count is less than 100 in 70% of cases.

Bloom S, Webster G and Marks D. *Oxford Handbook of Gastroenterology and Hepatology*, 2nd edition. Oxford: Oxford University Press; 2012.

Hauser S, Pardi D and Poterucha J. *Mayo Clinic Gastroenterology and Hepatology Board Review*, 3rd edition. New York: Mayo Clinic Scientific Press; 2008.

26. A. The metabolism of drugs can be divided into phase 1 and phase 2 reactions. The phase 1 reactions incorporate the cytochrome P450 family of enzymes. The end products of these reactions can be toxic if they are not removed from the body or metabolized further. The phase 1 reactions can be affected by a number of factors including age, concurrent medications and toxins, which can cause induction or inhibition of the cytochrome P450 family of enzymes. Other enzyme inhibitors include the following:

- Erythromycin
- Rabeprazole
- Pantoprazole
- Itraconazole
- Ketoconazole.

Phase 2 reactions can also be influenced by age and nutritional status. This phase consists of increasing water solubility by conjugation.

Bloom S and Webster G. *Oxford Handbook of Gastroenterology and Hepatology*, 1st edition. Oxford: Oxford University Press; 2006.

Hauser S, Pardi D and Poterucha J. *Mayo Clinic Gastroenterology and Hepatology Board Review*, 3rd edition. New York: Mayo Clinic Scientific Press; 2008.

Arundel C and Lewis JH. Drug-induced liver disease in 2006. *Current Opinion in Gastroenterology* 2007; 23: 244–254.

27. D. Drug-induced liver injury (DILI) is common both within and outside the hospital setting. Most cases occur within 1 year of starting the drug, and it is generally a diagnosis of exclusion.

Around 5–10% of hospitalizations for jaundice are due to DILI, and it is responsible for 50% of cases of acute liver failure. The drugs that are most commonly implicated (excluding paracetamol) are antibiotics, anticonvulsants, herbal therapies, anaesthetic agents, and NSAIDs. Predisposing factors include malnutrition, previous DILI, chronic liver disease, alcohol, multi-drug use (induction of cytochrome P450), and female gender.

DILI can be subdivided first on the basis of direct chemical toxicity, i.e. dose-related toxicity (e.g. paracetamol). Variable doses are required to cause toxicity, due to individual differences in drug metabolism.

Secondly, there are idiosyncratic reactions unrelated to dose. These are divided into:

- *Metabolic reactions*, involving the accumulation of toxic metabolites within the hepatocytes, causing inflammation (e.g. isoniazid, ketoconazole, sodium valproate)
- *Hypersensitivity reactions*, which normally occur 1–5 weeks after exposure to the drug. They are associated with rash, fever, and peripheral eosinophilia (which occurs in about 20% of cases), and recur after re-exposure (e.g. diclofenac, phenytoin, dapsone).

DILI can result in various patterns of liver injury, including hepatocellular (elevated ALT, around 50%), mixed (elevated ALP and ALT, around 40%), and cholestatic (elevated ALP, around 10%) patterns.

There are specific guidelines in some circumstances, such as the use of antituberculous therapy regimes, on how to monitor liver function tests.

The current accepted regime for active tuberculosis is 2 months of treatment with isoniazid, rifampicin, pyrazinamide, and ethambutol (if not fully sensitive), followed by 4 months of maintenance treatment with isoniazid and rifampicin. Hepatotoxicity due to isoniazid and pyrazinamide, ranging from mild liver function derangement to acute liver failure, is widely reported. It often occurs within 10 days of starting isoniazid or rifampicin, but may occur later than this with pyrazinamide. It is an idiosyncratic drug reaction that causes mainly hepatocellular injury. Approximately 50% of cases will resolve spontaneously.

The American Thoracic Society guidelines advise monitoring the ALT for patients who have chronic alcohol use, take concomitant hepatotoxic drugs, have chronic viral hepatitis, have pre-existing liver disease, or who are in the third trimester of pregnancy. Other experts advise monitoring the ALT level in any patient aged over 35 years, and discontinuing if the ALT is more than three times the upper limit of normal and there are symptoms of hepatitis or jaundice, *or* if the ALT is more than five times the upper limit of normal.

Bloom S, Webster G and Marks D. *Oxford Handbook of Gastroenterology and Hepatology*, 2nd edition. Oxford: Oxford University Press; 2012.

Hauser S, Pardi D and Poterucha J. *Mayo Clinic Gastroenterology and Hepatology Board Review*, 3rd edition. New York: Mayo Clinic Scientific Press; 2008.

Saukkonen JJ, Cohn DL, Jasmer RM et al. An official ATS statement: hepatotoxicity of antituberculosis therapy. *American Journal of Respiratory and Critical Care Medicine* 2006; 174: 935–952.

Arundel C and Lewis JH. Drug-induced liver disease in 2006. *Current Opinion in Gastroenterology* 2007; 23: 244–254.

28. B. Other examples of a predominantly cholestatic type of liver injury include co-amoxiclav, mirtazapine, and tricyclic antidepressants.

Many drugs will cause a rise in liver function tests, and most will settle spontaneously without necessitating cessation. In general, a rise of liver enzymes by more than five times the upper limit of normal, or impaired liver synthetic function, should be used as a guide to withdrawing the offending agent.

In DILI, histologically, the features of centrilobular necrosis, eosinophilic infiltration, and granulomas are non-specific and need clinical correlation. There are some drugs that can mimic features of autoimmune hepatitis on biopsy, and in some instances steroids may be used if the injury does not resolve spontaneously.

Other features may be specific to certain drugs. Granulomas may be seen more typically in carbamazepine, quinine, or quinidine induced DILI. Methotrexate can cause fibrosis or non-cirrhotic portal hypertension. Azathioprine and busulfan can cause veno-occlusive disease.

Treatment mainly consists of withdrawal of the offending agent and supportive care. Hepatocellular liver injury is often more serious than cholestatic liver injury, but recovery is likely to be quicker. Steroids may be used, as mentioned above, and although there is no evidence of clinical benefit, ursodeoxycholic acid may be used in cholestatic-type DILI.

Referral to a liver transplant centre is essential with a rising bilirubin level, worsening synthetic function, or hepatic encephalopathy, if the patient is a transplant candidate.

Bloom S and Webster G. *Oxford Handbook of Gastroenterology and Hepatology*, 1st edition. Oxford: Oxford University Press; 2006.

Hauser S, Pardi D and Poterucha J. *Mayo Clinic Gastroenterology and Hepatology Board Review*, 3rd edition. New York: Mayo Clinic Scientific Press; 2008.

Arundel C and Lewis JH. Drug-induced liver disease in 2006. *Current Opinion in Gastroenterology* 2007; 23: 244–254.

29. E. Paracetamol is mostly conjugated to glucuronide or sulphate. There is a portion which is oxidized to NAPQI (*N*-acetyl-*p*-benzoquinone imine), which is further detoxified by glutathione transferase. If glutathione becomes depleted or if there is an increased rate of metabolism of paracetamol to the toxic metabolite, hepatocellular necrosis occurs.

Increased levels of the toxic metabolite ensue with chronic alcohol use, malnutrition or fasting, late presentation (more than 16 hours since ingestion), and concurrent use of certain drugs that promote the conversion of paracetamol to toxic metabolites, such as phenobarbitone, isoniazid, zidovudine, and phenytoin (cytochrome P450 inducers).

Bloom S, Webster G and Marks D. *Oxford Handbook of Gastroenterology and Hepatology*, 2nd edition Oxford: Oxford University Press; 2012.

Hauser S, Pardi D and Poterucha J. *Mayo Clinic Gastroenterology and Hepatology Board Review*, 3rd edition. New York: Mayo Clinic Scientific Press; 2008.

Arundel C and Lewis JH. Drug-induced liver disease in 2006. *Current Opinion in Gastroenterology* 2007; 23: 244–254.

30. E. Herbal medication use should always be specifically asked for in the history. Common culprits include over-the-counter/Internet-purchased weight loss medications and hair nutritional supplements. Vitamin A can cause non-cirrhotic portal hypertension as well as hepatocellular injury.

Arundel C and Lewis JH. Drug-induced liver disease in 2006. *Current Opinion in Gastroenterology* 2007; 23: 244–254.

Bloom S and Webster G. *Oxford Handbook of Gastroenterology and Hepatology*, 1st edition. Oxford: Oxford University Press; 2006.

Hauser S, Pardi D and Poterucha J. *Mayo Clinic Gastroenterology and Hepatology Board Review*, 3rd edition. New York: Mayo Clinic Scientific Press; 2008.

31. A. Complications that arise after liver transplantation can be summarized as follows:

Early complications

- *Primary graft non-function*: this is defined as at least two of the following:
  - AST > 10 000 U/L
  - INR > 3.0
  - Serum lactate > 3.0 mmol/L
  - Absence of bile production occurring between days 0 and 7 after transplantation; it is often due to a fatty donor liver
- *Hepatic artery thrombosis*: this is most common in children or in live donor transplantation, and normally occurs within the first week. The graft often fails due to ischaemia, and often a re-transplant is the only option
- *Acute rejection*: this can occur up to 2 months after the operation. The treatment consists of corticosteroids in the first instance
- *Biliary strictures*: these can often be treated endoscopically with stents. They most commonly occur at the anastomosis. Non-anastomotic strictures can also occur due to hepatic artery thrombosis or ABO incompatibility
- *Infections*: these commonly include cytomegalovirus, *Candida*, *Aspergillus*, and *Pneumocystis*.

Late complications

- *Recurrent disease*: this includes, for example, hepatitis C. In cases of alpha-1-antitrypsin deficiency, the donor phenotype is expressed, so levels return to normal within a few weeks after transplantation
- *Cardiovascular complications*: the rate of hypertension, diabetes, renal failure, hypercholesterolaemia, and obesity is increased by treatment with certain immunosuppressive drugs
- *Malignancies*: common ones include skin cancers and lymphoproliferative disease
- Complications related to *immunosuppression*: these include cytopenias and renal impairment.

There are five groups of immunosuppressants used in liver transplantation:

- *Corticosteroids*: these are commonly used in the post-operative phase, but are likely to be tapered over time
- *Thiopurines*: azathioprine or mycophenolate
- *Calcineurin inhibitors*: tacrolimus or cyclosporin (these must be minimized in cases of renal impairment)
- *Sirolimus*
- *Intravenous antibody therapy* to treat acute rejection: antithymocyte globulin or muromonab CD3.

Hepatitis C is the leading reason for liver transplantation among adults. Recurrence of the virus occurs in almost 100% of patients after a transplant. Persistent hepatitis C viraemia is almost universal after transplantation, but may vary in the degree of liver injury that it causes. It may lead to fibrosis and cirrhosis in a small number of patients. Recurrent hepatitis C can be treated with interferon and ribavirin.

Recurrent hepatitis B is prevented by antiviral therapy and immunoglobulin post transplant.

Hauser S, Pardi D and Poterucha J. *Mayo Clinic Gastroenterology and Hepatology Board Review*, 3rd edition. New York: Mayo Clinic Scientific Press; 2008.

NHS Blood and Transplant and the Liver Advisory Group. *Protocols and Guidelines for Adults Undergoing Deceased Donor Liver Transplantation in the UK*. Watford: NHS Blood and Transplant; 2009.

Murray KF and Carithers RL Jr. AASLD practice guidelines: evaluation of the patient for liver transplantation. *Hepatology* 2005; 41: 1407–1432.

Said A, Einstein M and Lucey MR. Liver transplantation: an update 2007. *Current Opinion in Gastroenterology* 2007; 23: 292–298.

32. E. In order to prevent the complications of chronic hepatitis B and reduce the risk of resistance to certain treatments, hepatitis B virus (HBV) replication must be suppressed to a level of HBV DNA as low as possible. HBV DNA level has been found to be the strongest predictor of progression to cirrhosis. Although the ideal end point of treatment would be to lose HBsAg with or without the presence of anti-HBsAg, this end point is extremely rare, and is not an achievable objective of therapy.

HBV is the cause of 10–15% of chronic viral hepatitis, and is responsible for 5–10% of cases of liver transplants in the developed world. It may be present as HBeAg positive or HBeAg negative. The presence of HBsAg 6 months after initial infection is used to define an individual as a chronic carrier of hepatitis B.

HBV carriers carry a risk of hepatocellular carcinoma, and it is recommended that screening should occur with an ultrasound scan and alpha-fetoprotein every 6 to 12 months starting at the age of 40 years for Asian men, 50 years for Asian women, and 20 years for African adults and any patient with cirrhosis.

The interpretation of hepatitis B serology is complex, and is summarized as follows:

- **Susceptible**   HBsAg –ve, anti-HBc –ve, HBsAb -ve
- **Resolved infection**   HBsAg –ve, anti-HBc +ve, HBsAb +ve
- **Vaccinated**   HBsAg –ve, anti-HBc –ve, HBsAb +ve
- **Acute HBV infection** HBsAg +ve, anti-HBc +ve, HBsAb –ve, anti-HBc IgM +ve
- **Chronic HBV infection** HBsAg +ve, anti-HBc +ve, HBsAb –ve, anti-HBc IgM -ve

There are 5 phases during the natural history of chronic HBV:

- **Immune tolerance**   High DNA, normal ALT, HBeAg +ve
- **Immune reactive**   High DNA, raised ALT, HBeAg +ve: consider treatment
- **Immune control**   Low DNA, normal ALT, HBeAg –ve, HBeAb +ve
- **Immune escape**   High DNA, raised ALT, HBeAg –ve, HBeAb +ve: consider treatment
- **HBsAg negative**   Undetectable serum DNA, HBsAg –ve with or without HBsAb. At risk of reactivation if immunosuppressed and anti-HBc +ve

Tan J and Lok ASF. Update on viral hepatitis: 2006. *Current Opinion in Gastroenterology* 2007; 23: 263–267.

Lok ASF and McMahon BJ. Chronic hepatitis B: update 2009. *Hepatology* 2009; 50: 661–662.

Bloom S and Webster G. *Oxford Handbook of Gastroenterology and Hepatology*, 1st edition. Oxford: Oxford University Press; 2006.

Hauser S, Pardi D and Poterucha J. *Mayo Clinic Gastroenterology and Hepatology Board Review*, 3rd edition. New York: Mayo Clinic Scientific Press; 2008.

European Association for the Study of the Liver. EASL Clinical Practice Guidelines: management of chronic hepatitis B. *Journal of Hepatology* 2009; 50: 227–242.

33. A. Treatment for hepatitis B virus (HBV) is indicated if there is a risk of disease progression. This is identified by the following:

- Raised liver enzymes and/or high HBV DNA levels (> 2000 IU/mL), *and*
- Active disease identified by liver biopsy specimens or non-invasive tests, such as the Fibroscan.®

Treatment is either with interferon (subcutaneous) or with an oral agent such as lamivudine, adefovir, tenofovir, or entecavir. Only oral agents are indicated if the patient has cirrhosis. Treatment with oral agents can be complicated by resistant mutations. HBV resistance occurs after amino acid substitutions. This reduces drug efficacy, potentially resulting in treatment failure.

The ideal end point of therapy in HBeAg-negative and HBeAg-positive patients is to lose HBsAg, with or without the presence of HBsAb. Loss of HBeAg is the next most favourable outcome, followed by undetectable HBV DNA in those who are still HBeAg positive.

The European Association for the Study of the Liver (EASL) guidelines published in 2009 provide the following definitions:

- Primary non-response is defined as less than 1 $\log_{10}$ IU/mL decrease in HBV DNA level after 3 months of therapy from baseline
- Response is defined as an HBV DNA level of 1 $\log_{10}$ IU/mL, but with detectable HBV DNA
- HBV DNA should be checked after 24 weeks of therapy if using lamivudine or telbivudine, and after 48 weeks of therapy if using entecavir, adefovir, or tenofovir.

Therapy should continue for at least 6 months after seroconversion of HBeAg. If seroconversion does not occur, therapy should be continued indefinitely.

Another indication for therapy with an oral agent is in the context of immunosuppression or cytotoxic therapy. All such patients should have HBsAg and anti-HBc antibodies checked. If they are seronegative, they should be vaccinated against HBV. If they are HBsAg positive, HBV DNA levels should be checked and treatment with an oral agent commenced before therapy and continued for 12 months after cessation of therapy (EASL guidelines). If they are HBsAg negative but anti-HBc positive, close monitoring of HBV DNA and ALT levels should take place. Therapy should commence if reactivation occurs.

Tan J and Lok ASF. Update on viral hepatitis: 2006. *Current Opinion in Gastroenterology* 2007; 23: 263–267.

Lok ASF and McMahon BJ. Chronic hepatitis B: update 2009. *Hepatology* 2009; 50: 661–662.

Bloom S, Webster G and Marks D. *Oxford Handbook of Gastroenterology and Hepatology*, 2nd edition. Oxford: Oxford University Press; 2012.

Hauser S, Pardi D and Poterucha J. *Mayo Clinic Gastroenterology and Hepatology Board Review*, 3rd edition. New York: Mayo Clinic Scientific Press; 2008.

European Association for the Study of the Liver. EASL Clinical Practice Guidelines: management of chronic hepatitis B. *Journal of Hepatology* 2009; 50: 227–242.

34. D. The complications of chronic hepatitis C are those of cirrhosis and portal hypertension, including development of hepatocellular carcinoma (HCC). The combination of pegylated interferon and ribavirin is the current standard treatment for hepatitis C genotypes 2 and 3, with a response rate of over 80%. Current best practice is to use boceprevir or telaprevir in combination with pegylated interferon and ribavirin for genotype 1 infection.

A liver biopsy could be considered if the patient or the treating clinician wishes to have information about the fibrosis stage for prognostic reasons or to make a decision regarding treatment. It is not essential prior to starting antiviral therapy. There are non-invasive tests available, such as the Fibroscan®, which may be useful for defining the presence or absence of advanced fibrosis.

The risk of HCC in hepatitis C is highest among those with established cirrhosis. Six-monthly surveillance with ultrasound and serum alpha-fetoprotein is recommended in these patients, whether the hepatitis C has been treated successfully or not.

Genotype 1 treatment (without protease inhibitor)

The HCV RNA level should be checked after 12 weeks of therapy. If there is a 2 $\log_{10}$ decrease in viral load from pre-treatment or an undetectable viral load (EVR = early virological response), therapy should continue. If not, therapy should cease, as there is a very low likelihood of sustained virological response (SVR = undetectable viral load 6 months after completion of treatment). Those who continue treatment should have their HCV RNA level re-checked at 24 weeks. If it is positive, therapy should stop, and if it is negative, therapy should continue for 48 weeks.

Genotype 2 and 3 treatment

The treatment should continue for 24 weeks. In some units the viral load is checked at 4 weeks to see whether there is a rapid virological response (undetectable viral load at 4 weeks after starting therapy). In this case, treatment may be shortened to 16 weeks.

Treatment side effects

- Haemolysis secondary to ribavirin, which is reversible. The dose may need to be reduced or erythropoietin administered to maintain haemoglobin levels
- Neutropenia due to pegylated interferon, which rarely requires intervention
- Neuropsychiatric symptoms secondary to pegylated interferon—these are more common in patients with pre-existing mental health problems.

Bloom S and Webster G. *Oxford Handbook of Gastroenterology and Hepatology*, 2nd edition. Oxford: Oxford University Press; 2012.

Hauser S, Pardi D and Poterucha J. *Mayo Clinic Gastroenterology and Hepatology Board Review*, 3rd edition. New York: Mayo Clinic Scientific Press; 2008.

Ghany MG, Strader DB, Thomas DL *et al*. Diagnosis, management, and treatment of hepatitis C: an update. *Hepatology* 2009; 49: 1335–74.

Tan J and Lok ASF. Update on viral hepatitis: 2006. *Current Opinion in Gastroenterology* 2007; 23: 263–267.

35. D. The radiological findings are consistent with a hepatic adenoma with a well-demarcated lesion that enhances early in the arterial phase due to blood supply from the hepatic artery. Hepatic adenomas are benign liver tumours that are at risk of malignant transformation or rupture and intra-abdominal bleeding. They are strongly associated with the oral contraceptive pill, anabolic steroid use, and glycogen storage disease, and less so with pregnancy and diabetes mellitus.

It can be argued that in small adenomas (< 5 cm) in asymptomatic patients, stopping the oral contraceptive pill and monitoring the size of the adenoma with radiological and alpha-fetoprotein surveillance is satisfactory, as complete regression has been observed. However, malignant transformation or rupture has been documented in adenomas despite a regression in size. In this symptomatic patient, surgical referral is indicated. Liver biopsy is not usually advised, due to the high risk of bleeding. Liver transplantation is reserved for adenomas that are unresectable due to location, size, or adenomatosis.

Hauser S, Pardi D and Poterucha J. *Mayo Clinic Gastroenterology and Hepatology Board Review*, 3rd edition. New York: Mayo Clinic Scientific Press; 2008.

Rodes J, Benhamou J and Mizzetto M. *The Textbook of Hepatology: from basic science to clinical practice*, 3rd edition. Malden, MA: Blackwell Publishing Ltd; 2007.

Shortell CK and Schwartz SI. Hepatic adenoma and focal nodular hyperplasia. *Surgery, Gynecology & Obstetrics* 1991; 173: 426–431.

Dokmak S, Paradis V, Vilgrain V *et al.* A single-center surgical experience of 122 patients with single and multiple hepatocellular adenomas. *Gastroenterology* 2009; 137: 1698–1705.

36. D. The presence of a raised IgG in the context of high titres of antimitochondrial antibody raises the suspicion of overlap syndrome of primary biliary cirrhosis with autoimmune hepatitis; the investigation of choice is a liver biopsy. Treatment when the diagnosis is confirmed is with ursodeoxycholic acid and corticosteroids, usually prednisolone 0.5 mg/kg/day, with tapering of the corticosteroid when the ALT level responds. Starting ursodeoxycholic acid treatment and adding corticosteroids if there is no response may be suitable in certain patients. Azathioprine should be considered if long-term steroid therapy is required. In all patients with ursodeoxycholic acid-treated primary biliary cirrhosis who sequentially develop autoimmune hepatitis, immunosuppression must be started.

European Association for the Study of the Liver. EASL Clinical Practice Guidelines: management of cholestatic liver diseases. *Journal of Hepatology* 2009; 51: 237–267.

37. B. Good response at 1 year can be assessed by either the Paris criteria or the Barcelona criteria.

Paris criteria

- Bilirubin < 17 μmol/L
- Alkaline phosphatase less than three times the upper limit of normal
- Serum alanine transaminase less than twice the upper limit of normal.

(Reprinted from *Clinical Gastroenterology and Hepatology*, 8, 6, EMM Kuiper *et al.*, 'Paris criteria are effective in diagnosis of primary biliary cirrhosis and autoimmune hepatitis overlap syndrome', pp. 530–534. Copyright 2012, with permission from Elsevier.)

Barcelona criteria

- Normalization or 40% reduction in alkaline phosphatase.

(Reprinted from *Journal of Hepatology*, 35, 3, Jordi Bruix *et al.*, 'Clinical Management of Hepatocellular Carcinoma. Conclusions of the Barcelona-2000 EASL Conference', pp. 421–430. Copyright 2001, with permission from European Association for the Study of the Liver.)

A good response, according to the Barcelona criteria, identifies patients with transplant-free survival equivalent to 95% of that of a normal population at 14 years.

Ursodeoxycholic acid at 15 mg/kg/day is the initial treatment of choice. It improves biochemistry and protects damaged cholangiocytes against the effect of bile acids.

There is no consensus on how to treat patients with a suboptimal response to treatment. The addition of budesonide 6–9 mg/day has been suggested in non-cirrhotic patients, but further trials are needed. As there is an increased risk of portal vein thrombosis, budesonide should not be used in cirrhotic patients.

Immunomodulators such as azathioprine, mycophenolate mofetil, and methotrexate are minimally effective and potentially harmful.

Referral for liver transplantation should be considered when the bilirubin level is > 103 µmol/L, the Mayo risk score is ≥ 7, and the latest MELD score is 12. Complications include nodular regenerative hyperplasia, and portal hypertension (which can occur early in PBC). The caveat to this is that in early pre-cirrhotic patients, where nodular regenerative hyperplasia has developed, varices may develop earlier. Patients should be screened for HCC if they are cirrhotic. All patients should have a baseline DEXA scan, vitamin D and calcium supplements, and be considered for bisphosphonates (although this should be reviewed if gastro-oesophageal reflux disease is present).

European Association for the Study of the Liver. EASL Clinical Practice Guidelines: management of cholestatic liver diseases. *Journal of Hepatology* 2009; 51: 237–267.

38. E.   This patient's presentation with cholestasis and positive ANA and SMA suggests a diagnosis of primary sclerosing cholangitis.

- The most frequently positive autoantibodies are p-ANCA, ANA, SMA, elevated IgG (61%), and elevated IgM (45%)
- Around 80% of patients with PSC have associated IBD; 80% have ulcerative colitis, 10% have Crohn's disease, and 10% have indeterminate colitis
- The investigation of choice is MRCP. ERCP is reserved for cases with therapeutic intention, due to the risks associated with ERCP
- ERCP and MRCP typically demonstrate a beaded appearance of the biliary tree.
- Ultrasonography is non-diagnostic and often normal
- Liver biopsy may support the diagnosis, but is non-specific; it may aid assessment of disease activity and staging. Periductal concentric fibrosis is suggestive of PSC, but is an infrequent finding on needle biopsy, and is associated with other conditions
- Abdominal CT is non-specific.

European Association for the Study of the Liver. EASL Clinical Practice Guidelines: management of cholestatic liver diseases. *Journal of Hepatology* 2009; 51: 237–267.

39. A. There is a therapeutic role for ERCP in dominant bile duct strictures (< 1.5 mm in the common bile duct and < 1 mm in the left and right hepatic duct) with cholestasis. Worsening jaundice in patients with primary sclerosing cholangitis (PSC) can be secondary to calculi in the biliary tree, as opposed to worsening disease. Biliary dilatation should be performed with stent insertion for patients in whom stricture dilatation and bile drainage are suboptimal, with prophylactic antibiotics when a stent has been placed. There is no effective treatment for PSC. Ursodeoxycholic acid improves liver biochemistry, but there is no proven benefit in terms of survival. Patients with late-stage PSC should be referred for transplantation. Colectomy in patients with advanced colitis or dysplasia pre-transplantation reduces the risk of recurrence post orthotopic liver transplantation.

European Association for the Study of the Liver. EASL Clinical Practice Guidelines: management of cholestatic liver diseases. *Journal of Hepatology* 2009; 51: 237–267.

40. A. Gallbladder masses in primary sclerosing cholangitis (PSC) are frequently (> 50%) adenocarcinomas irrespective of size, and subsequently cholecystectomy is the treatment of choice. Liver transplantation is recommended in patients with end-stage PSC, and considered in severe recurrent cholangitis and cholangiocyte dysplasia on brushings. Ten-year survival rates post transplantation are up to 80%. Recurrence of PSC in the allograft can occur and is thought to be associated with steroid-resistant rejection, ABO incompatibility, gender mismatch, CMV infection, and male gender.

European Association for the Study of the Liver. EASL Clinical Practice Guidelines: management of cholestatic liver diseases. *Journal of Hepatology* 2009; 51: 237–267.

41. A. The presence of hypergammaglobulinaemia with markedly elevated aminotransferases and interface hepatitis on liver biopsy points to the likely diagnosis of autoimmune hepatitis. Recommended treatment is with prednisolone 30 mg/day with the addition of azathioprine 1 mg/kg within 2 weeks. Alcohol cessation is also advised.

Diagnostic criteria of the International Autoimmune Hepatitis Group

	Definite	Probable
Liver histology	Interface hepatitis of moderate or severe activity with or without lobular hepatitis or central portal bridging necrosis, but without biliary lesions or well-defined granulomas or other prominent changes suggestive of a different aetiology	As for definite
Biochemistry	Any abnormality in serum aminotransferases, especially if the serum alkaline phosphatase is not markedly elevated. Normal serum concentrations of alpha antitrypsin, copper, and caeruloplasmin	Patients with abnormal serum concentrations of copper or caeruloplasmin may be included, provided that Wilson's disease has been excluded by appropriate investigations
Immunoglobulins	Total serum globulin or c globulin or IgG concentrations greater than 1.5 times the upper limit of normal	Total serum globulin or gamma globulin or IgG concentrations greater than 1.5 times the upper limit of normal
Autoantibodies	Seropositivity for ANA, SMA, or anti-LKM 1 antibodies at titres greater than 1:80. Lower titres (particularly of anti-LKM 1) may be significant in children. Seronegativity for AMA	Titres of 1:40 or greater. Patients who are seronegative for these antibodies but who are seropositive for other antibodies specified in the text may be included
Viral markers	Seronegativity for markers of current infection with hepatitis A, B, and C viruses	As for definite

	Definite	Probable
Other aetiological factors	Average alcohol consumption less than 25 g/day. No history of recent use of known hepatotoxic drugs	Alcohol consumption less than 50 g/day and no recent use of known hepatotoxic drugs. Patients who have consumed larger amounts of alcohol or who have recently taken potentially hepatotoxic drugs may be included, if there is clear evidence of continuing liver damage after abstinence from alcohol or withdrawal of the drug

Adapted from *Journal of Hepatology*, 31, 5, Alvarez F, Berg PA, Bianchi FB, *et al.*, 'International Autoimmune Hepatitis Group Report: review of criteria for diagnosis of autoimmune hepatitis', pp. 929–938. Copyright 1999, with permission from European Association for the Study of the Liver, published by Elsevier.

Other diagnosis scoring systems include the International Autoimmune Hepatitis Group (IAIHG) scoring system, in which a composite score of > 15 before treatment or > 17 after treatment indicates definite AIH, whereas a score of 10–15 suggests probable AIH.

Feature	Score
Female gender	+2
ALP:AST (or ALT) ratio	
3	+2
1.5–3	0
> 3	–2
Serum globulins or IgG above normal	
> 2.0	+3
1.5–2.0	+2
1.0–1.5	+1
< 1.0	0
ANA, SMA, or LKM-1	
> 1:80	+3
1:80	+2
1:40	+1
< 1:40	0
AMA negative	–4
Hepatitis viral markers	
Positive	–3
Negative	+3
Drug history	
Positive	–4
Negative	+1
Average alcohol intake	+2
60 g/day	–2
Liver histology	
Interface hepatitis	+3
Predominantly lymphoplasmacytic infiltrate	+1
Rosetting of liver cells	+1
None of the above	–5
Biliary features	–3
Atypical changes	–3

(Continued)

Feature	Score
Other autoimmune diseases	
In patient or first-degree relatives	+2
Optimal additional parameters	
Seropositive for other defined antibodies	+2
HLA DR3 or DR4	+1
Response to therapy	
Remission alone	+2
Remission with relapse	+3
Interpretation of aggregate scores	
Pre-treatment	
Definite AIH	> 15
Probable AIH	10–15
Post-treatment	
Definite AIH	> 17
Probable AIH	12–17

Adapted from *Journal of Hepatology*, 31, 5, Alvarez F, Berg PA, Bianchi FB, *et al.*, 'International Autoimmune Hepatitis Group Report: review of criteria for diagnosis of autoimmune hepatitis', pp. 929–938. Copyright 1999, with permission from European Association for the Study of the Liver, published by Elsevier.

Gleeson D and Heneghan MA. British Society of Gastroenterology (BSG) guidelines for management of autoimmune hepatitis. *Gut* 2011; 60: 1611–1629.

Alvarez F, Berg PA, Bianchi FB et al. International Autoimmune Hepatitis Group Report: review of criteria for diagnosis of autoimmune hepatitis. *Journal of Hepatology* 1999; 31: 929–938.

42. C. Although there are no histological findings pathognomonic for autoimmune hepatitis, interface hepatitis (inflammation of the hepatocytes at the junction of the hepatic parenchyma and the portal tracts), plasma cell infiltration, and perilobular necrosis can all be found on biopsy.

Florid duct lesions are consistent with PBC, the stages of which are as follows:

Stage 1	Florid bile duct lesions
Stage 2	Ductular proliferation
Stage 3	Septal fibrosis and bridging
Stage 4	Cirrhosis

Perls' Prussian blue stains iron, looking for overload. Steatosis with hepatocyte balloon degeneration is consistent with both alcoholic steatohepatitis and non-alcoholic steatohepatitis.

Gleeson D and Heneghan MA. British Society of Gastroenterology (BSG) guidelines for management of autoimmune hepatitis. *Gut* 2011; 60: 1611–1629.

European Association for the Study of the Liver. EASL Clinical Practice Guidelines: management of cholestatic liver diseases. *Journal of Hepatology* 2009; 51: 237–267.

43. A. In patients with a poor response, treatment can be altered to azathioprine 2 mg/kg with an increased prednisolone dose as tolerated. Other options include tacrolimus and prednisolone; expert advice should be considered. Remission is defined as the disappearance of symptoms, normal bilirubin and GGT, AST levels less than twice the normal value, and normal liver histology or minimal inflammation with no interface hepatitis.

Patients in remission should remain on treatment with azathioprine 1 mg/kg and 10–15 mg of prednisolone for 2 years or 12 months after transaminases have normalized. Approximately 70% of patients relapse within the first year of treatment cessation. Patients who have a relapse (ALT level more than three times the upper limit of normal) should be treated as initial presentation of AIH followed by maintenance azathioprine 1 mg/kg. Further relapses while taking azathioprine can be treated with reintroduction of steroid therapy.

Gleeson D and Heneghan MA. British Society of Gastroenterology (BSG) guidelines for management of autoimmune hepatitis. *Gut* 2011; 60: 1611–1629.

44. C. Treatment in older patients with mild autoimmune hepatitis has limited evidence of survival benefit. It is important to weigh up the risks versus the benefits of immunosuppression, especially in patients with diabetes, osteoporosis, and previous psychosis, due to the risk of adverse reactions to steroid therapy. In this asymptomatic patient, monitoring the liver function tests 3-monthly would be appropriate. Treatment should be considered for patients who are symptomatic, young, or have proven cirrhosis on biopsy.

Common first-line treatment regimens are prednisolone 60 mg as monotherapy or prednisolone 30 mg and azathioprine 1–2 mg/kg/day.

Gleeson D and Heneghan MA. British Society of Gastroenterology (BSG) guidelines for management of autoimmune hepatitis. *Gut* 2011; 60: 1611–1629.

45. D. This is likely to be hepatocellular carcinoma (HCC) in a non-cirrhotic patient, in view of the radiological findings and high α-fetoprotein (AFP) level. Patients should have a CT chest and abdomen to assess for metastases. Non-invasive diagnosis is not suitable in non-cirrhotic patients, and a pathological diagnosis must be sought with biopsies, which should be examined by an expert histopathologist.

The primary therapy in non-cirrhotic patients is resection, and discussion with a transplant centre should be considered. HCC in non-cirrhotic patients is usually fibrolamellar variant (young patients with an average age of 30 years at diagnosis) or HCC *de novo* in elderly patients. Transplantation for extensive tumours has been trialled, although the results have been poor. Non-cirrhotic patients with HCC often present with symptoms of more advanced disease, and survival is 25% at 5 years following resection, compared with 11% at 5 years following transplantation. Treatment allocation is driven by the Barcelona Clinic Liver Cancer classification, described in the answer to Question 15 (see p. 192).

It is important to note that sorafenib is not currently approved by the National Institute for Health and Clinical Excellence (NICE) as a treatment for advanced HCC in the UK.

Iwatsuki S and Starzl TE. Personal experience with 411 hepatic resections. *Annals of Surgery* 1988; 208: 421–434.

Ryder SD. Guidelines for the diagnosis and treatment of hepatocellular carcinoma (HCC) in adults. *Gut* 2003; 52 (Suppl. III): iii1–8.

European Association for the Study of the Liver. EASL–EORTC clinical practice guidelines: management of hepatocellular carcinoma. *Journal of Hepatology* 2012; 56: 908–943.

Houben KW and McCall JL. Liver transplantation for hepatocellular carcinoma in patients without underlying liver disease: a systematic review. *Liver Transplantation and Surgery* 1999; 5: 91–95.

46. B. This is HCC in a cirrhotic patient; patients should be assessed with a CT or MRI scan. In lesions greater than 2 cm which bear the hallmarks of HCC on imaging (hypervascular in the arterial phase, followed by washout in the venous phase), biopsy is not required. The diagnostic algorithm proposed by the EASL is shown in Figure 5.7.

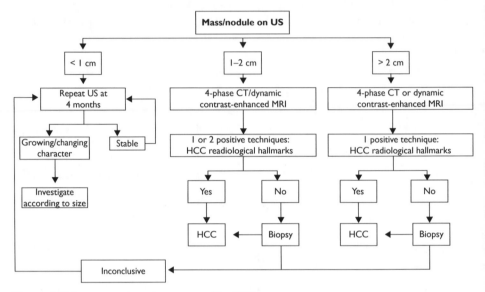

Figure 5.7 Diagnostic algorithm proposed by EASL.

Reprinted from *Journal of Hepatology*, 56, 4, European Association for the Study of the Liver, European Organisation for Research and Treatment of Cancer, 'EASL–EORTC Clinical Practice Guidelines: Management of hepatocellular carcinoma', pp. 908–943. Copyright 2012, with permission from European Association for the Study of the Liver, published by Elsevier.

The radiological hallmarks are hypervascular in the arterial phase, followed by washout in the venous phase on quadruple-phase CT or dynamic-contrast MRI.

Transplantation should be considered in cirrhotic patients (Child–Pugh class A or B) with a small HCC (lesion less than 5 cm in size or three lesions of 3 cm or less); it will also cure the underlying liver disease. Resection can be performed in selected patients with well-preserved hepatic function (Child–Pugh class A) with normal portal pressures and bilirubin levels. Radiofrequency ablation involves placement of a probe percutaneously, and can destroy lesions up to 3 cm with a single probe or 6 cm with multi-tipped probes by means of high-frequency ultrasound. In transarterial chemoembolization (TACE), a chemotherapy agent is injected into the hepatic artery (as most HCC is fed by the hepatic artery) to maximize delivery of chemotherapy to the tumour. Supportive management and palliative care input can be considered for patients who are unfit for any other treatments.

European Association for the Study of the Liver. EASL–EORTC clinical practice guidelines: management of hepatocellular carcinoma. *Journal of Hepatology* 2012; 56: 908–943.

47. B. This patient has polycythaemia vera and Budd–Chiari syndrome (hepatic vein thrombosis). In one-third of patients the cause is unknown. However, other causes of hepatic vein thrombosis include thrombophilia (myeloproliferative disorders, such as polycythaemia vera and factor V Leiden), hepatocellular carcinoma, the oral contraceptive pill, and leukaemia.

Unlike other hepatic causes of ascites, the ascitic fluid is an exudate with an SAAG of < 11 g/L. The diagnosis is made with either a Doppler ultrasound or CT. Treatment includes management of the underlying cause as well as anticoagulation (thrombolysis in acute liver failure). TIPSS has been used with good effect, and liver transplant may be required; this carries a better prognosis than surgical porto-caval shunting.

Bloom S, Webster G and Marks D. *Oxford Handbook of Gastroenterology and Hepatology*, 2nd edition. Oxford: Oxford University Press; 2012.

48 B. The coeliac artery arises from the anterior aspect of the aorta at the level of T12. After 1 cm it trifurcates into the left gastric, common hepatic, and splenic arteries. The common hepatic artery then gives off the branch of the gastroduodenal artery before dividing into branches into the right and left hepatic arteries which supply their respective lobes of the liver. The right hepatic artery supplies segments I, V, VI, VII, and VIII, and the left hepatic artery supplies segments II, III, and IV (A and B).

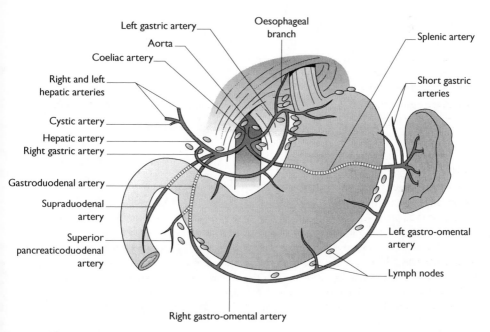

Figure 5.8 Arterial blood supply to the upper GI tract.

49. C. This patient has a resolved infection as she is HBsAg negative, and HBsAb and HBcAb positive (for a more detailed explanation, see the answer to Question 35 on p. 208). Her liver biochemistry is normal, which is to be expected with a resolved infection. Hepatitis B can be transmitted perinatally from infected mothers, or horizontally through minor breaks in the skin, mucous membranes, or close contact with body fluids. Vertical transmission and horizontal transmission below the age of 5 years have a greater than 95% chance of chronic infection. If hepatitis B is acquired in adulthood, less than 5% will develop a chronic infection unless they are immunocompromised; the majority will clear the virus spontaneously.

Ko HH, Wong DKH and Heathcote J. Management of hepatitis B. *Clinical Gastroenterology and Hepatology* 2011; 9: 385–391.

50. B. Predictors of response (HBe seroconversion) to therapy include the following:

Pre-treatment factors

- Low viral load (HBV DNA below 10^8 IU/mL or 8 log10 IU/mL)
- High serum ALT levels (above three times the upper limit of normal)
- High activity scores on liver biopsy.

Interferon (during treatment)

- HBV DNA decrease to less than 20 000 IU/mL at 12 weeks
- HBeAg decrease at week 24 may predict HBe seroconversion
- HBV genotype has a poor individual predictive value.

Nucleoside analogue (during treatment)

- A virological response at 24 or 48 weeks (undetectable HBV DNA in a real-time PCR assay) is associated with a lower incidence of resistance.
- HBV genotype does not influence the response.

European Association for the Study of the Liver. EASL Clinical Practice Guidelines: management of chronic hepatitis B virus infection. *Journal of Hepatology* 2012; 57: 167–185.

51. C. Hydatid liver disease is caused by the tapeworm *Echinococcus granulosis*. It is most commonly seen in people from North and East Africa, the Middle East, and Australia, in farming or rural communities. Transmission is via a faeco-oral route from food contaminated with infected dog faeces. The eggs penetrate the intestinal wall, enter the portal system, and are then carried to the liver. Further dissemination can occur to the lungs, brain, and kidneys. Symptoms include abdominal discomfort, jaundice, and fever. Diagnosis is with Echinococcus ELISA; alternatively, CT scanning shows characteristic daughter cysts. Eosinophilia only occurs in approximately 25% of cases. Treatment of the hepatic disease is with surgery, as medical treatment (mebendazole) alone is only effective in 30% of patients.

Bloom S and Webster G. *Oxford Handbook of Gastroenterology*, 1st edition. Oxford: Oxford University Press; 2006.

52. A. Beta-carotene (water-soluble vitamin A) has been shown to reduce the ALT and AST levels in rats with alcohol-induced steatohepatitis, but there is no convincing evidence that supplementation in humans will lead to a similar reduction. The other therapies have all been shown to have some benefit in the treatment of NASH. The pharmacotherapy with the most evidence in patients with diabetes is metformin. The most effective treatment for this man would be weight loss.

Mouralidarane A, Lin Ching-I, Suleyman N *et al*. Practical management of the increasing burden of non-alcoholic fatty liver disease. *Frontline Gastroenterology* 2010; 1: 149–155.

53. D. The liver biopsy in Figure 5.9/Colour Plate 4 is from a patient with non-alcoholic steatohepatitis. It shows the following features:
- Steatosis
- Hepatocyte ballooning degeneration
- Mild diffuse lobular acute and chronic inflammation
- Perivenular collagen deposition

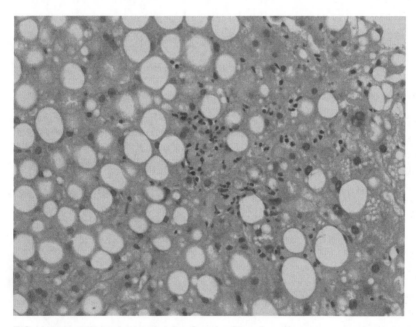

Figure 5.9 Haematoxylin and eosin staining. See also Plate 4.

Reproduced with permission from Dr Michael L Texler, PathWest, Australia.

Other features include Mallory's hyaline, vacuolated nuclei in periportal hepatocytes, and pericellular fibrosis (see Figure 5.10/Colour Plate 5), which is seen in the advanced stages of fibrosis or cirrhosis. Anti-smooth muscle antibody is present in 3–5% of the general population.

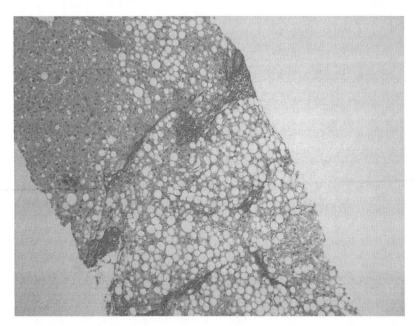

Figure 5.10 Van Gieson stain; red = fibrous tissue. See also Plate 5.

Reproduced with permission from Dr Michael L Texler, PathWest, Australia.

54. D. Wilson's disease

- Is an autosomal recessive disorder that affects the ATP7A gene on chromosome 13
- It causes retention of copper in the liver and impaired incorporation of copper into caeruloplasmin
- It usually presents between 5 and 40 years of age
- It presents with gallstones due to haemolytic anaemia, neuropsychiatric disorders, complications of cirrhosis, or renal calculi
- Biochemical abnormalities include a raised ALT, with low serum copper and caeruloplasmin levels
- Patients usually have raised urinary copper levels
- There is a diagnostic rise in urinary copper levels of > 25 mmol in 24 hours after 500 mg of penicillamine are administered at 24 and 36 hours
- Treatment includes penicillamine or trientine to increase copper excretion, and zinc to reduce gastrointestinal absorption.

Foods that have a high copper content should be avoided. These include liver, shellfish, chocolate, nuts, mushrooms, dried fruit, and peas.

Ala A, Walker AP, Ashkan K et al. Wilson's disease. *Lancet* 2007; 369: 397–408.

Bloom S, Webster G and Marks D. *Oxford Handbook of Gastroenterology and Hepatology*, 2nd edition. Oxford: Oxford University Press; 2012.

55. A. Around 80% of patients with haemochromatosis are homozygous for the C282Y polymorphism in the HFE gene, and around 5% are heterozygous for C282Y and H63D. Homozygosity for H63D alone is not a sufficient genetic cause of iron overload. The majority of the remaining haemochromatosis cases are as a result of C282Y heterozygosity along with another rarer genetic mutation; this includes S65C, hepcidin gene (HAMP), and transferrin receptor 2 gene. If a patient is found to be homozygous for C282Y with no evidence of iron overload, follow up once a year with a serum ferritin measurement is a reasonable approach.

Family screening should be considered for autosomal-recessive inheritance. Siblings of a haemochromatosis patient should undergo screening with ferritin, transferrin saturations, and ideally an HFE gene mutation analysis. With regard to children of a patient with haemochromatosis, HFE genotyping of the unaffected partner is useful for calculating the risk to the offspring. If a partner is homozygous for C282Y, the risk is increased and the genotype of the child should be measured. If the partner does not have a C282Y mutation, the child is at most heterozygous for C282Y, and therefore screening for iron overload is unnecessary.

Bacon BR, Adams PC, Kowdley VC et al. Diagnosis and management of hemochromatosis: 2011 practice guideline by the American Association for the Study of Liver Diseases. *Hepatology* 2011; 54: 328–343.

Hashem B, Inadomi JM and Kowdley KV. Screening for hereditary hemochromatosis in siblings and children of affected patients: a cost-effectiveness analysis. *Annals of Internal Medicine* 2000; 132: 261–269.

56. D. Management of haemochromatosis

- Individuals who are homozygous for C282Y should have a fasting glucose level checked, and HbA1c, ALT, and AST levels measured
- Symptoms may warrant further investigation with an echocardiogram, serum testosterone, thyroid function, and joint X-ray
- Definitive treatment is with therapeutic venesection (weekly or fortnightly) to a target serum ferritin of < 50 µg/L (15–300) and 50–100 mcg/L for maintenance. If the serum ferritin > 1000 µg/L (15–300) µg/L at diagnosis then assess for liver cirrhosis with either a liver biopsy or transient elastography
- In haemochromatosis and cirrhosis there is an 100-fold greater likelihood of developing HCC. This group warrants 6-monthly ultrasound scanning and alpha-fetoprotein measurements
- Dietary adjustment is not required for patients undergoing venesection
- Alcohol intake should be kept to a minimum.

Bloom S and Webster G. *Oxford Handbook of Gastroenterology*, 1st edition. Oxford: Oxford University Press; 2006.

European Association for the Study of the Liver. EASL Clinical Practice Guidelines: management of chronic hepatitis B. *Journal of Hepatology* 2009; 50: 227–242.

57. B. Ferritin is a highly sensitive test for iron overload. However, it lacks specificity. Inflammation, cancer, diabetes mellitus, alcohol, non-alcoholic fatty liver disease, and cell necrosis can result in higher levels of ferritin. Serum iron concentration does not quantitatively reflect iron stores, and therefore should not be used. A fasting transferrin saturations should be measured, and if it is higher than 45%, genetic testing for haemochromatosis should take place.

MRI imaging can be used to detect hepatic iron excess with 88% sensitivity and 90% specificity. Liver biopsy is rarely needed to make the diagnosis of haemochromatosis, but may still be required to assess for fibrosis.

European Association for the Study of the Liver. EASL clinical practice guidelines for HFE hemochromatosis. *Journal of Hepatology* 2010; 53: 3–22.

58. D. Adverse events occur in up to 20% of patients who take azathioprine, and the commonest are allergic reactions (e.g. fever, arthralgia, rash). Profound leucopenia can develop suddenly in approximately 3% of patients. Hepatotoxicity and pancreatitis are uncommon (less than 5%). Patients should be advised to report promptly if they develop a sore throat or any other evidence of infection. Although many patients experience adverse effects from azathioprine, these effects usually disappear within 3 weeks.

Organ transplant recipients who are receiving thiopurines have an up to fivefold increase in lymphoproliferative disorders. In absolute terms, the risk remains very small (less than 1% after 10 years of thiopurine use). There is an increased risk of non-melanoma skin cancer in patients who are treated with thiopurines. Patients should be advised to avoid excessive sun exposure and to use a high-strength sun block.

Mowat C, Cole A, Windsor A *et al.* Guidelines for the management of inflammatory bowel disease in adults. *Gut* 2011; 60: 571–607.

Austin AS and Spiller RC. Inflammatory bowel disease, azathioprine and skin cancer:case report and literature review. *European Journal of Gastroenterology and Hepatology* 2001; 13: 193–194.

1. **A 59-year-old man presented with acute severe central abdominal pain and vomiting. He rarely consumed alcohol and had no significant past medical history. A clinical diagnosis of acute pancreatitis was made. He was treated with intravenous fluid resuscitation and analgesia. A day after initial presentation he had blood tests performed.**

Investigations:

white cell count	8.3×10^9/L (4.0–11.0)
serum urea	7.2 mmol/L (2.5–7.0)
serum creatinine	103 µmol/L (60–110)
serum albumin	34 g/L (37–49)
serum total bilirubin	20 µmol/L (1–22)
serum alanine aminotransferase	55 U/L (5–35)
serum alkaline phosphatase	140 U/L (45–105)
serum amylase	829 U/L (60–180)
pH	7.40 (7.35–7.45)
PCO_2	5.0 kPa (4.7–6.0)
PO_2	11.7 kPa (11.3–12.6)
bicarbonate	24 mmol/L (21–29)
base excess	+ 1.8 mmol/L (±2)
serum C-reactive protein	22 mg/L (< 10)
abdominal ultrasound	several gallstones < 5 mm in size in a thin walled gallbladder; the common bile duct (CBD) measured 0.6 cm in diameter

His symptoms improved with fluid and analgesia. What is the most appropriate management plan for this patient?

A. Discharge once his symptoms have improved, laparoscopic cholecystectomy within 2 weeks

B. Discharge once his symptoms have improved, no follow-up required

C. ERCP with sphincterotomy within 72 hours of presentation

D. Laparoscopic cholecystectomy within 72 hours of presentation

E. MRCP within 72 hours of presentation

2. **A 74-year-old woman presented with a fever of 38°C, jaundice, and 4 kg weight loss in the previous 4 months.**

Investigations:

serum albumin	33 g/L (37–49)
serum total bilirubin	89 µmol/L (1–22)
serum alanine aminotransferase	75 U/L (5–35)
serum alkaline phosphatase	210 U/L (45–105)
serum CA 19–9	27 000 U/mL (< 33)
abdominal ultrasound	mass lesion in the common hepatic duct with proximal dilatation. Four peripheral liver lesions suspicious for metastatic deposits in segments I, III, and VII of the liver
CT thorax, abdomen, and pelvis	no other abnormality

She was treated with intravenous antibiotics and her fever settled.

What is the next step in the management of her mass lesion?

A. ERCP and brush biopsy of lesion

B. ERCP and metal stent

C. ERCP and plastic stent

D. Ultrasound-guided percutaneous biopsy of peripheral liver lesion

E. Ultrasound-guided percutaneous biopsy of the hilar mass

3. **A 42-year-old woman presented to your clinic with an incidental finding of gallstones in a thin walled gallbladder on ultrasound scanning undertaken for another reason. She denied fever, rigors, or pain, and was slightly overweight. She had a moderate alcohol intake but denied any other medical problems.**

Investigations:

serum albumin	39 g/L (37–49)
serum total bilirubin	17 µmol/L (1–22)
serum alanine aminotransferase	42 U/L (5–35)
serum alkaline phosphatase	104 U/L (45–105)
serum C-reactive protein	6 mg/L (< 10)
abdominal ultrasound	gallstones in a thin walled gallbladder

Which of the following most accurately reflects her prognosis over the next 10 years?

A. 20% chance of developing biliary colic

B. 50% chance of developing Mirizzi syndrome

C. Cholecystectomy is indicated to prevent symptomatic gallstones from developing

D. Less than 1% chance of developing pancreatitis, cholecystitis, and biliary obstruction

E. More than 90% chance of remaining asymptomatic

4. **A 50-year-old man underwent an abdominal ultrasound examination for upper abdominal pain. The report suggested that although the liver architecture was normal and the common bile duct of normal calibre, there was debris in the gallbladder and one large lesion adjacent to the gallbladder wall which may have been either a gallbladder stone or a polyp.**

   Which of the following statements about gallbladder polyps is most accurate?

   A. Cholecystectomy is recommended for all gallbladder polyps
   B. In the presence of PSC the malignant potential is increased
   C. Most commonly these are adenomatous polyps
   D. Symptomatology does not dictate the need for cholecystectomy
   E. They have significant malignant potential irrespective of size

5. **A 45-year-old man presented with severe sudden onset of epigastric pain associated with vomiting. He drank 38 units of alcohol a week and smoked 40 cigarettes a day.**

   Investigations at 24 hours:

white cell count	21×10^9/L (4.0–11.0)
serum urea	9 mmol/L (2.5–7.0)
serum calcium	1.8 mmol/L (2.20–2.60)
serum albumin	34 g/L (37–49)
serum alanine aminotransferase	84 U/L (5–35)
serum lactate dehydrogenase	450 U/L (10–250)
plasma glucose	8 mmol/L (3.0–6.0)
serum amylase	1012 U/L (60–180)
PO_2	10.5 kPa (11.3–12.6)
serum C-reactive protein	120 mg/L (< 10)

   What is the Glasgow acute pancreatitis score for this patient?

   A. 2
   B. 3
   C. 4
   D. 5
   E. 6

6. **A 60-year-old woman was referred to clinic to discuss an incidental finding of a cystic lesion in the head of pancreas while undergoing a CT thorax and abdomen for assessment of a thyroid goitre. She went on to have an endoscopic ultrasound examination with biopsy. This, together with CT findings, confirmed a serous cystic tumour.**

   Which of the following CT findings is pathognomonic of a pancreatic serous cystic tumour?

   A. A cystic lesion lined by a mucinous epithelium
   B. A cystic lesion with multiple contrast-enhancing septations
   C. A mixed solid and cystic pancreatic lesion
   D. A poorly defined lesion with central fat sparing
   E. A well-demarcated lesion with sunburst central calcification

7. **An 80-year-old man presented with painless jaundice and significant weight loss.**

   Investigations:
   CT abdomen and pelvis   intra- and extrahepatic biliary dilatation down to the level of pancreas, with the impression of a mass in the pancreatic head

   Which of the following has the strongest aetiological association with the development of pancreatic cancer?

   A. Adult-onset diabetes
   B. Chronic pancreatitis
   C. Excess alcohol
   D. Hereditary pancreatitis
   E. Smoking

8. **A 45-year-old man presented with abdominal pain and vomiting on a background of long-standing alcohol misuse. He took no regular medications.**

   Investigations:
   serum amylase   1200 U/L (60–180)
   abdominal ultrasound   normal

   He made slow progress, and during week 5 of his inpatient stay a CT scan was performed due to continuing pain associated with dyspepsia and bloating.

   CT abdomen   a large fluid-filled mass around the head of pancreas

   Which of the following statements about the management of pancreatic pseudocysts is most accurate?

   A. All pseudocysts over 6 cm in diameter require treatment
   B. Complication rates are comparable for endoscopic and surgical treatments
   C. If infection is suspected, endoscopic drainage is not appropriate
   D. Surgery is always the treatment of choice
   E. Symptomatology is the most important factor

9. **A 60-year-old woman presented with a history of severe postprandial epigastric pain and loose bowel motions four times daily for 6 months. She was previously alcohol dependent, with repeated bouts of abdominal pain secondary to acute pancreatitis. However, she had been reliably abstinent from alcohol for 6 years.**

Investigations:

serum vitamin B_{12} 130 ng/L (160–760)

serum amylase   192 U/L (60–180)

She was under investigation for diabetes by her GP following a high random glucose level on routine bloods.

Which of the following is the most appropriate treatment for her low vitamin B_{12} level?

A. Oral hydroxycobalamin and dietary advice

B. Pancreatic enzymes and oral hydroxycobalamin

C. Pancreatic enzymes and parenteral hydroxycobalamin

D. Pancreatic enzymes and proton pump inhibitor

E. Pancreatic enzymes, dietary advice, and re-checking vitamin B_{12} levels in 1 month

10. **A 75-year-old man presented with acute pancreatitis; he was abstinent from alcohol. The aetiology of his acute pancreatitis had not yet been identified. He had been treated in the community for recurrent urinary tract infections.**

Investigations:

abdominal USS   normal

CT abdomen   normal

Which of the following is most likely to be causal in the development of acute pancreatitis?

A. Amoxicillin

B. Cefalexin

C. Ciprofloxacin

D. Nitrofurantoin

E. Tetracycline

11. **A 32-year-old woman presented with RUQ pain. She had been diagnosed with biliary colic a few months ago, and was awaiting an outpatient cholecystectomy.**

Investigations:

white cell count	6.2 x 10⁹/L (4.0–11.0)
serum urea	5.1 mmol/L (2.5–7.0)
serum creatinine	61 μmol/L (60–110)
serum albumin	37 g/L (37–49)
serum total bilirubin	31 μmol/L (1–22)
serum alanine aminotransferase	78 U/L (5–35)
serum aspartate aminotransferase	67 U/L (1–31)
serum amylase	56 U/L (60–180)
serum C-reactive protein	12 mg/L (< 10)
abdominal ultrasound scan	gallstones in a thin walled gallbladder with a fatty liver

What is the most appropriate next step?

A. CT abdomen
B. ERCP
C. EUS
D. Laparoscopic cholecystectomy
E. MRCP

12. **A 30-year-old woman presented with severe biliary-type pain. She had had multiple admissions with similar pain in the past 18 months, despite having had a cholecystectomy 2 years ago when the resected gallbladder was acalculous.**

Investigations:

serum albumin	40 g/L (37–49)
serum total bilirubin	45 μmol/L (1–22)
serum alanine aminotransferase	54 U/L (5–35)
serum alkaline phosphatase	132 U/L (45–105)
serum amylase	72 U/L (60–180)
serum C-reactive protein	9 mg/L (< 10)
abdominal ultrasound	normal liver, unable to visualize CBD
MRCP	slightly dilated intrahepatic ducts. CBD 9 mm. No stones or masses seen

The pain settled with analgesia, and 48 hours later the patient's LFTs had returned to normal. A diagnosis of sphincter of Oddi dysfunction was made.

Which is the most appropriate next step in this patient's management?

A. ERCP and intrasphincteric injection of botox
B. ERCP and manometry
C. ERCP and permanent pancreatic stent
D. ERCP and sphincteroplasty
E. ERCP and sphincterotomy

13. **A 60-year-old man presented to the emergency clinic with painless jaundice. His USS and CT supported a diagnosis of pancreatic carcinoma, and biopsies obtained via ERCP confirmed adenocarcinoma. He was keen to have surgical treatment if possible, and was discussed by the upper GI MDT.**

    In the case of a tumour of the head of pancreas, which of the CT findings has the most promising likelihood of cure with surgical intervention?

    A. Aortic encasement
    B. Bulky tumour with local lymph nodes
    C. Coeliac axis abutment
    D. Distant metastases
    E. Portal vein encasement

14. **A 30-year-old woman who was 34 weeks pregnant presented with right upper quadrant pain and deranged liver function tests. She was pyrexial at 38.2°C and tachycardic. Her abdominal USS showed a dilated distal CBD with no obvious filling defect, together with dilated intrahepatic ducts and stones within a thin walled gallbladder.**

    Investigations:

haemoglobin	110 g/L (115–165)
white cell count	18.3 x 10⁹/L (4.0–11.0)
platelet count	162 x 10⁹/L (150–400)
prothrombin time	12.5 seconds (11.5–15.5)
serum total bilirubin	73 µmol/L (1–22)
serum alanine aminotransferase	67 U/L (5–35)
serum aspartate aminotransferase	56 U/L (1–31)
serum alkaline phosphatase	210 U/L (45–105)
serum C-reactive protein	93 mg/L (< 10)
urine dipstick	no abnormality detected
blood pressure	110/65 mmHg

    What is the most appropriate next step in the management of this patient?

    A. CT abdomen
    B. ERCP
    C. MRCP
    D. Non-invasive liver screen
    E. Watch and wait

15. **A 30-year-old woman was reviewed in clinic after a recent inpatient stay with cholangitis. She originally presented with jaundice, rigors, and right upper quadrant pain. She was treated with antibiotics, and after an abdominal ultrasound scan which suggested a dilated CBD, she went on to have an ERCP. The ERCP did not reveal stone disease, but showed fusiform dilatation of the CBD. She made a good recovery and was discharged.**

    An MRCP was arranged as an outpatient, which confirmed spindle-like dilatation along the length of the CBD. A diagnosis of choledochal cyst type I was made.

    What is the most appropriate management for a type I choledochal cyst?

    A. Cholecystoenterostomy
    B. Sequential scanning with a view to surgical excision if progression occurs
    C. Surgical excision even if asymptomatic
    D. Surgical excision if complications are problematic
    E. Treatment of complications as and when they arise

1. A. This patient has presented with mild pancreatitis, based on the Glasgow pancreatitis severity score; he scores 1 for age. In the absence of an alcohol history the most likely cause is stone disease, as suggested by the mildly deranged LFTs and the presence of gallstones on ultrasound. According to BSG guidelines, appropriate treatment for mild gallstone pancreatitis is to provide supportive care and perform an elective cholecystectomy within 2 weeks of initial presentation.

If the patient has severe pancreatitis with evidence of gallstones, it is recommended that they should undergo ERCP and stone extraction within 72 hours of presentation. Cholangitis, jaundice, and a dilated common bile duct (CBD) are other reasons to consider urgent ERCP during an attack of acute gallstone pancreatitis.

Endoscopic ultrasound (EUS) or MRCP are both useful imaging modalities in the investigation of CBD stones where they have not been identified by ultrasound. They should be reserved for the investigation of CBD stones in patients with biliary symptoms, normal ultrasound findings in the gallbladder, and no other aetiology for pancreatitis.

Glasgow criteria for the classification of severity in acute pancreatitis

Age	> 55 years
White cell count	> 15 x 10^9/L
Glucose	> 10 mmol/L
Urea	> 16 mmol/L
PO$_2$	< 8 kPa
Calcium	< 2 mmol/L
Albumin	< 32 g/L
Lactate dehydrogenase	> 600 U/L
Aspartate/alanine transferase	> 100 U/L

Reprinted from *The Lancet*, 326, A. P. Corfield *et al.*, 'Prediction of severity in acute pancreatitis: prospective comparison of three prognostic indices', pp. 403–407. Copyright 1985, with permission from Elsevier.

A Glasgow score of ≥ 3 during the first 48 hours should be managed as a severe attack.

Williams EJ, Green J, Beckingham I *et al.* UK guidelines for the management of acute pancreatitis. *Gut* 2008; 57: 1004–1021.

BSG Working Party. UK Guidelines for the management of acute pancreatitis. *Gut* 1998; 42: S1–13.

2. B. The patient has a clinical and radiological diagnosis of probable metastatic cholangiocarcinoma affecting the common hepatic duct, also known as a Klatskin or perihilar tumour. The Bismuth classification is commonly used to assess the extent of duct involvement in these tumours. Type I remain below the confluence of the right and left hepatic ducts, type II reach the confluence but do not involve the right or left hepatic duct, and types III and IV involve the confluence and extend into either, or both, of the hepatic ducts, respectively.

There are no alternative primaries seen on the CT, although local spread is apparent, and the cholangiocarcinoma is associated with probable biliary sepsis. Correct management consists of treating the sepsis, relieving the obstructed biliary system, and attempting a tissue diagnosis. A staging CT should be undertaken before the placement of any stents, to ensure that the images are not degraded.

Unfortunately, the prognosis in hilar cholangiocarcinoma is poor. In such patients, metal stents provide palliation but do not prolong survival. In this scenario the patient has metastatic liver involvement which is non-resectable, and palliation is the aim. In such patients, plastic stenting is equally effective in the short term, but is likely to require further intervention if patient survival extends beyond 6 months.

Stenting via ERCP is generally thought to be feasible for Bismuth type I tumours. Type II, III, and IV Bismuth tumours are better suited to percutaneous stenting, but each case must be looked at individually and management should be decided in the context of a multidisciplinary team (MDT) meeting.

An attempt to obtain histological material should be made at the time of stenting, to confirm the diagnosis. However, it should be avoided in potentially resectable disease, due to the risk of tumour seeding. Resectability should be assessed by the regional hepatobiliary MDT prior to obtaining tissue.

Treatment with chemotherapy has not been shown to prolong life in randomized controlled trials, but patients should be encouraged to take part in clinical trials of chemotherapy, radiotherapy, biotherapy, or photodynamic therapy.

Khan SA, Davidson BR, Goldin R et al. Guidelines for the diagnosis and treatment of cholangiocarcinoma: consensus document. Gut 2002; 51 (Suppl. 6): vi1–9.

3. A. Asymptomatic gallstones generally do not require therapy, and can be found in approximately 15% of the population in the USA and the UK. Patients with asymptomatic gallstones have an approximately 20% chance of developing biliary colic within 10 years, and 80% remain asymptomatic.

Pain associated with gallstones indicates a higher chance of complications. Patients with asymptomatic gallstones have a 2–3% chance of developing pancreatitis, cholecystitis, and biliary obstruction. Cholecystectomy should be offered if symptoms develop, depending on the operation risk.

Cholecystectomy is not recommended for patients with asymptomatic stones.

However, there are special situations where asymptomatic gallstones might increase the risk of gallbladder carcinoma and cholecystectomy should be considered. These are patients with coexisting primary sclerosing cholangitis (PSC), choledochal cysts, Caroli's disease, or porcelain gallbladder.

Mirizzi's syndrome is a rare complication of gallstones. It refers to biliary obstruction with jaundice either as a direct consequence of stone impaction or from inflammation when a large stone resides in Hartmann's pouch of the gallbladder. This causes pressure on the common bile duct and thus obstructive jaundice. Treatment is surgical, by cholecystectomy.

Williams EJ, Green J, Beckingham I et al. Guidelines on the management of common bile duct stones (CBDS). Gut 2008; 57: 1004–1021.

4. B. Gallbladder polyps are becoming more prevalent with the increased availability of high-quality ultrasound imaging. They are a common incidental finding on ultrasound scanning that is being undertaken for other reasons. No association has been found between any risk factors that are generally believed to be associated with gallstone formation.

Most commonly gallbladder polyps consist of cholesterol, with adenomatous change being the most common neoplastic lesion. The malignant potential of gallbladder polyps is a controversial subject.

It is commonly considered that polyps over 1 cm in diameter have an increase in malignant potential and that cholecystectomy should be considered in these cases.

Monitoring for a change in size with sequential ultrasound is recommended, usually at least one further scan 3 months after index diagnosis, and then discontinuation if the polyp size remains unchanged. There is no clear consensus on the timing and duration of surveillance.

Surgical management of gallbladder polyps is generally recognized as the treatment of choice for polyps that reach over 1 cm in diameter or are symptomatic. Symptoms can include right upper quadrant pain, nausea, vomiting, and dyspepsia. At cholecystectomy up to 50% of these symptomatic polyps turn out to be stones.

Advancing age (over 50 years), increasing size on sequential scanning, co-existent gallstones, and solitary polyps are all thought to be risk factors for malignancy, and should be considered when making a treatment plan. In particular, there has been some interest in gallbladder polyps in the setting of primary sclerosing cholangitis. It is thought that this may be a high-risk group, and some authorities recommend aggressive surgical treatment in this setting.

Leung UC, Wong PY, Roberts RH *et al*. Gallbladder polyps in sclerosing cholangitis: does the 1-cm rule apply? *ANZ Journal of Surgery* 2007; 77: 355–357.

Myers RP, Shaffer EA and Beck PL. Gallbladder polyps: epidemiology, natural history and management. *Canadian Journal of Gastroenterology* 2002; 16: 187–194.

5. A. The UK guidelines on the management of acute pancreatitis suggest that a diagnosis should be made by correlating clinical symptoms with raised amylase or lipase levels within 48 hours of admission. There are scoring systems which are used to assess the severity of the attack and hence the prognosis in acute pancreatitis.

Initial assessment should be clinical and should use the APACHE II score. This will give an idea of whether the episode will become severe.

After 24 hours the Glasgow score and CRP are accurate assessment tools and should be used. A Glasgow score of ≥ 3 between 24 and 48 hours after admission should be managed as a severe attack.

The CRP has independent prognostic value. The current guidelines use a cut-off value of 150 mg/L more than 48 hours after the onset of symptoms as a marker of a severe attack.

Details of the Glasgow criteria can be found in the answer to Question 1 (see p. 229).

Williams EJ, Green J, Beckingham I *et al*. UK guidelines for the management of acute pancreatitis. *Gut* 2008; 57: 1004–1021.

BSG Working Party. UK guidelines for the management of acute pancreatitis. *Gut* 1998; 42: S1–13.

6. E. Cystic lesions of the pancreas are classified according to the WHO classification. The four main subtypes are serous cystic tumours, mucinous cystic neoplasms, intraductal papillary mucinous neoplasms, and solid pseudopapillary neoplasms. The importance of identifying the subtype of a lesion is to assess malignant potential and therefore to decide whether operative treatment is required.

Serous cystic tumours have very little malignant potential, with reported transformation into a cystadenocarcinoma limited to a few case reports. CT findings typically show a well-demarcated multicystic lesion. The pathognomonic finding of a central scar or 'sunburst' calcification occurs in up to 20% of serous cystic tumours.

Mucinous cystic neoplasms (MCNs) and intraductal papillary mucinous neoplasms (IPMNs) are considered to be pre-malignant lesions, and can also be overtly malignant. MCNs usually have thick fibrotic walls and can be multiple. In contrast to IPMNs, the cysts do not communicate with the pancreatic ducts. The stroma of MCNs is often referred to as 'ovarian-like', and this is the hallmark on histology. The diagnosis of MCNs is important, as the treatment of choice for those patients in whom it is appropriate is surgical resection.

IPMNs usually involve the main pancreatic duct, but can affect the side branches, and there are many histological subtypes. These all produce mucin, and the presence of mucin draining from the ampulla of Vater is pathognomonic. Due to the malignant potential of main duct IPMNs, the treatment of choice is surgical resection. A select number of patients who are asymptomatic with small lesions affecting the branch ducts may be treated conservatively with careful radiological monitoring, due to the lower malignant potential in these cases.

Solid pseudopapillary tumours are a rare form of pancreatic cystic lesion. These lesions are most commonly found in young females, and present with non-specific gastrointestinal symptoms. Imaging usually reveals a mixed solid and cystic appearance with good vascularization. They also have malignant potential, and the finding of distant metastases is not unusual. Therefore surgical resection where possible is the recommended treatment.

Brugge WR, Lauwers GY, Sahani D et al. Cystic neoplasms of the pancreas. New England Journal of Medicine 2004; 351: 1218–1226.

Garcea G, Ong SL, Rajesh A et al. Cystic lesions of the pancreas. Pancreatology 2008; 8: 236–251.

7. E. According to the BSG guidelines on the management of patients with pancreatic cancer, cigarette smoking has the strongest association with the development of pancreatic cancer. It is thought to be responsible for approximately 25–30% of cases of pancreatic cancer. Patients with chronic pancreatitis (a 5- to 15-fold increase) and hereditary pancreatitis (a 50- to 70-fold increase) are also at special increased risk and may be considered for screening. Adult-onset diabetes, familial pancreatic cancer, obesity, and consumption of processed meats are other risk factors.

The Pancreatic Section of the British Society of Gastroenterology, Pancreatic Society of Great Britain and Ireland, Association of Upper Gastrointestinal Surgeons of Great Britain and Ireland et al. Guidelines for the management of patients with pancreatic cancer periampullary and ampullary carcinomas. Gut 2005; 54 (Suppl. 5): v1–16.

8. E. Pseudocyst formation complicates approximately 5% of episodes of acute pancreatitis. The most common symptoms include early satiety, pain, and gastric outlet obstruction. Other symptoms may include dyspepsia, nausea, vomiting, or a palpable mass. The likelihood of developing a pancreatic pseudocyst is not related to the severity of pancreatitis.

Small cysts can resolve spontaneously, but larger cysts may require endoscopic drainage with a transduodenal or transgastric stent, usually guided by luminal ultrasound. Cysts smaller than 4 cm in diameter tend to have a high rate of regression, and so may not require treatment unless a complication occurs. However, multiple cysts, wall thickness >1 cm, increasing size, and lack of communication with the pancreatic duct are all poor indicators for spontaneous regression.

The decision to drain a cyst depends on the symptoms that it causes and to a lesser extent on its size. For this reason there is no clear guidance on treatment.

Complications of pseudocyst formation include haemorrhage into the cyst, usually from a pseudoaneurysm, abscess formation, rupture, and pressure effects such as obstructive jaundice. Treatment of these complications can commonly be achieved with endoscopic procedures.

Transgastric and less commonly transduodenal routes are taken. Laparoscopic techniques are becoming more popular. However, open surgery is sometimes required. Open surgery carries with it a higher morbidity and mortality, so endoscopic and more recently laparoscopic procedures are favoured if technically possible.

Lerch MM, Stier A, Wahnschaffe U et al. Pancreatic pseudocysts: observation, endoscopic drainage, or resection? Deutsches Arzteblatt International 2009; 106: 614–621,

9. E. The three major complications of chronic pancreatitis are pain, exocrine and endocrine insufficiency. Pain is the most difficult symptom to treat, and usually requires a multidisciplinary team approach. Analgesics are the mainstay of treatment for pain, but mesenteric nerve block, diet, and surgery are effective and underused treatments. There is little evidence that pancreatic enzyme supplements help to relieve pain.

Exocrine insufficiency can complicate chronic pancreatitis and presents with steatorrhoea and malabsorption. Hypocalcaemia is common in the context of steatorrhoea, as calcium chelates to unabsorbed fat. Weight loss occurs as patients limit their food intake to reduce pain, but also because of protein catabolism. Serum vitamin B_{12} levels are low because of the lack of pancreatic enzymes. Poor absorption of vitamin B_{12} in chronic pancreatitis is likely to be multifactorial. Without pancreatic enzymes, vitamin B_{12} remains bound to R protein in the small bowel, and therefore is unable to bind with intrinsic factor in the usual way. Vitamin B_{12} supplementation is rarely required if adequate replacement with pancreatic enzymes is achieved. However, the neurological sequelae of vitamin B_{12} deficiency can be difficult to reverse. Therefore close monitoring is recommended.

Pancreatic enzyme supplements in the past required co-administration of a proton pump inhibitor for maximal effect, but this is not necessary with more modern preparations.

Glucose intolerance or frank diabetes occurs in approximately 30% of patients with chronic pancreatitis. This can be difficult to treat as hypoglycaemic attacks are common and, when insulin is required it needs to be titrated cautiously. A lack of glucagon stores further exacerbates this problem.

Allen RH, Seetharam B, Allen NC et al. Correction of cobalamin malabsorption in pancreatic insufficiency with a cobalamin analogue that binds with high affinity to R protein but not to intrinsic factor. In vivo evidence that a failure to partially degrade R protein is responsible for cobalamin malabsorption in pancreatic insufficiency. Journal of Clinical Investigation 1978; 61: 1628–1634.

Guéant JL, Djalali M, Aouadj R et al. In vitro and in vivo evidences that the malabsorption of cobalamin is related to its binding on haptocorrin (R binder) in chronic pancreatitis. American Journal of Clinical Nutrition 1986; 44: 265–277.

10. E. Drugs are reported as being a cause of pancreatitis after description in multiple case reports or series. The strongest evidence for such causality is when a drug thought to be responsible for pancreatitis causes a recurrent attack after being restarted in the same individual.

In an update of drug-induced pancreatitis published in 2005 it was shown that tetracycline and septrin (sulfamethoxazole/trimethoprim) both had a class 1 association, meaning that these drugs were implicated in over 20 cases of drug-induced pancreatitis, with at least one episode of pancreatitis following re-exposure.

Drugs reported to be implicated with a class 1 association include the following:

- Thiopurines: azathioprine and 6-mercaptopurine
- Corticosteroids

- Sulphasalazine and the 5-ASA group
- Furosemide
- Sulindac
- Valproic acid
- Opiates
- Tetracycline and septrin

Definite associations are difficult to prove, but it has been postulated that the drugs may be a trigger or cofactor in the development of acute pancreatitis.

Trivedi CD and Pitchumoni CS. Drug-induced pancreatitis: an update. *Journal of Clinical Gastroenterology* 2005; 39: 709–716.

11. E. The diagnosis is likely to be common bile duct stones, in view of the abnormal liver function tests, right upper quadrant pain, and known gallstones.

ERCP is an invasive procedure with significant risks. With the development of risk-free investigations, ERCP should be used for therapy and tissue sampling rather than as a diagnostic tool. Post-ERCP pancreatitis occurs in around 5% of patients undergoing ERCP, and has the potential to cause significant morbidity. Any patient undergoing ERCP should also be consented for the risks of bleeding, perforation, cholangitis, and procedure failure.

EUS is a good method for diagnosing CBD stones that are not seen at USS, but again is an invasive test with a risk of perforation.

CT alone for the investigation of CBD stones is not a sensitive test, but when combined with biliary contrast it can be useful. It has not been demonstrated to be as sensitive as ERCP, EUS, or MRCP in diagnosing CBD stones.

MRCP is currently thought to be the standard diagnostic test for CBD stones that are not seen on USS. It is recognized that the sensitivity of MRCP is influenced by stone diameter. The sensitivity of MRCP declines from 100% for stones >1 cm in diameter to 71% for stones <5 mm in diameter. MRCP has the benefit of being a non-invasive test with no ionizing radiation.

An alternative treatment option would be for the patient to undergo a laparoscopic cholecystectomy with an on-table cholangiogram. This would deal with the underlying problem and also look into whether a CBD stone is present. A laparoscopic cholecystectomy alone would not address the issue of a possible CBD stone. This option depends on local availability and surgical expertise.

Williams EJ, Green J, Beckingham I *et al*. Guidelines on the management of common bile duct stones (CBDS). *Gut* 2008; 57: 1004–1021.

Johanson JF, Schmitt CM, Deas TM *et al*. Quality and outcomes assessment in gastrointestinal endoscopy. *Gastrointestinal Endoscopy* 2000; 52: 827–830.

Green J. *Guidelines on Complications of Gastrointestinal Endoscopy*. BSG Guidelines in Gastroenterology. London: British Society of Gastroenterology; 2006.

12. E. Sphincter of Oddi dysfunction—also known as biliary dyskinesia—is a disorder that presents in its classic form (type 1) as recurrent biliary colic-type pain, variable degrees of biliary obstruction, and transient abnormality in liver function tests.

Less commonly, patients present with pancreatic pain with elevated lipase activity caused by spasm of the pancreatic sphincter.

Three types of biliary sphincter dysfunction have been described in the Milwaukee classification, and require the following criteria to be met on two or more occasions:

- Type I—biliary pain with abnormal LFTs *and* dilated ducts
- Type II—biliary pain with abnormal LFTs *or* dilated ducts
- Type III—biliary pain with no evidence of biliary obstruction or abnormal LFTs.

(Reproduced from Hogan WJ and Geenen JE, 'Biliary dyskinesia', *Endoscopy*, 20, S1, pp. 179–183, 1988, Thieme Publishing Group, with permission.)

Initial investigations should include LFTs and an ultrasound scan looking for duct dilatation, which is often provoked after a fatty meal or opioid analgesia.

Endoscopic manometry is available at specialist centres and shows increased baseline pressure of the sphincter of Oddi (over 40 mmHg). There is a significant risk of procedure-related pancreatitis, which can be reduced by placement of a prophylactic pancreatic stent.

ERCP and sphincterotomy is a successful treatment in 90% of patients with type I, with a 5% risk of pancreatitis after pancreatic stent placement. Manometry and secretin-stimulated ERCP are not required.

The majority of patients with suspected sphincter of Oddi dysfunction are classified as type II. A straight-to-treatment strategy results in 60% symptomatic improvement at a cost of a 15% rate of pancreatitis. It is recommended that such patients should only be considered for sphincterotomy after positive analysis by secretin-stimulated MRCP and/or biliary manometry if available.

Extreme caution should be exercised before undertaking any intervention in patients with type III syndrome.

Management with intra-sphincter injection with botulinum toxin or medical treatment with tricyclic antidepressants or nifedipine results in a variable and unsustained response.

Hogan WJ and Geenen JE. Biliary dyskinesia. *Endoscopy* 1988; 20: 179–183.

Baillie J. Sphincter of Oddi dysfunction: due for an overhaul. *American Journal of Gastroenterology* 2005; 100: 1217–1220.

Bistritz L and Bain VG. Sphincter of Oddi dysfunction: managing the patient with chronic biliary pain. *World Journal of Gastroenterology* 2006; 12: 3793–3802.

13. B. The most appropriate curative surgical procedure for a head of pancreas tumour is a pancreaticoduodenectomy (Whipple's procedure). Distant metastases and aortic or coeliac axis involvement render tumours non-resectable. Most surgeons would agree that venous encasement is non-resectable. Size of tumour and local lymph nodes are not clear indications to avoid surgery.

The Pancreatic Section of the British Society of Gastroenterology, Pancreatic Society of Great Britain and Ireland, Association of Upper Gastrointestinal Surgeons of Great Britain and Ireland et al. Guideline for the management of patients with pancreatic cancer periampullary and ampullary carcinomas. *Gut* 2005; 54 (Suppl. 5): v1–16.

14. B. In this case there is a high probability that the cause of symptoms is ascending cholangitis requiring either ERCP-directed stenting or stone extraction, should time permit. USS is useful for looking at dilated ducts, but does not always accurately identify stones within the common bile duct. Patients with ascending cholangitis should undergo ERCP to relieve the obstruction as soon as possible; waiting for further imaging will not only be unhelpful but will also delay life-saving treatment.

Liver function tests during pregnancy can become deranged for a number of reasons, but the only physiological alteration in LFTs is a raised alkaline phosphatase from placental tissue. Pregnancy should not deter one from performing ERCP when it is indicated, as despite the radiation exposure, in the context of ascending cholangitis it is life-saving. Positioning of the patient may be more challenging during ERCP, but is not impossible. Radiation exposure should be kept to a minimum, and a shield worn to protect the unborn baby.

Due to the technical difficulties of performing an ERCP during pregnancy, the definitive aim of duct clearance in CBD stone disease is often compromised. Temporary decompression with biliary stenting followed by a completion ERCP after delivery is an appropriate strategy. This also reduces the risk of pancreatitis at the index ERCP, which may compromise the pregnancy.

Cappell MS. Risks versus benefits of gastrointestinal endoscopy during pregnancy. *Nature Reviews. Gastroenterology & Hepatology* 2011; 8: 610–634.

15. C. In 1977, Todani described five types of choledochal cyst:

- *Type I*: this consists of dilatation of the common bile duct (CBD) which may be cystic (A), focal (B), or fusiform (C), and does not include the intrahepatic ducts
- *Type II*: this describes a diverticulum of the CBD
- *Type III*: commonly called a choledochocoele, this represents a dilatation of the distal CBD, which some believe is actually a duodenal diverticulum
- *Type IV*: this consists of multiple dilatations of the intra- and extrahepatic biliary tree (A) or just the extrahepatic ducts (B)
- *Type V*: this is also known as Caroli's disease, and involves multiple intrahepatic dilatations.

(Reprinted from *The American Journal of Surgery*, 134, 2, Todani et al., 'Congenital bile duct cysts: Classification, operative procedures, and review of thirty-seven cases including cancer arising from choledochal cyst', pp. 263–269. Copyright 1977, with permission from Elsevier.)

The most common category of choledochal cysts is type I, and type IVA is the second most common. The remaining categories are rare.

The presentation can be varied. The classical triad includes jaundice, RUQ mass and abdominal pain, but is rare and more likely to occur in children. When the diagnosis is delayed until adulthood they are most commonly diagnosed incidentally after imaging for another reason, but can present with the complications of the condition, such as cholangitis, pancreatitis, and biliary peritonitis from cyst rupture.

The gold standard investigation for diagnosing choledochal cysts is MRCP, although ultrasound may be more useful in paediatric cases. ERCP is a useful imaging modality and may be carried out for another reason, as in this clinical case, but should be used primarily as a therapeutic test rather than for diagnostic reasons alone. Radionucleotide scintigraphy has been used in the past and is thought to have a high sensitivity, especially for type I cysts, but has been somewhat eclipsed by MR scanning. CT is not a sensitive or specific imaging modality for diagnosing choledochal cysts, but may be useful in the post-operative period for defining the anatomy of the biliary–enteric anastomosis.

The treatment for choledochal cysts is still surgical excision, due to their malignant potential and the possibility of developing serious complications. The incidence of malignant change has been reported to be in the range 10–30%. This does depend somewhat on the type of choledochal cyst, particularly when considering type III cysts (choledochocoeles), which are thought to have a smaller malignant potential. Endoscopic sphincterotomy is a viable treatment option in this case.

Metcalf MS, Wemyss-Holden SA and Maddern GJ. Management dilemmas with choledochal cysts. *Archives of Surgery* 2003; 138: 333–339.

Yoon JH. Magnetic resonance cholangiopancreatography diagnosis of choledochal cyst involving the cystic duct: report of three cases. *British Journal of Radiology* 2011; 84: e18–22.

1. **A 67-year-old man attended for a gastroscopy. After consenting by a junior doctor while an inpatient previously, he had spoken to a friend regarding the quality of endoscopy in the hospital. He expressed concerns, and requested evidence of good practice.**

    Which of the following best demonstrates evidence of quality assurance in an endoscopy department?

    A. Audits
    B. Endoscopy governance meetings
    C. Global Rating Scale assessments
    D. Joint Advisory Group approval
    E. Patient feedback surveys

2. **A 38-year-old man presented to the Emergency Department with a 4-hour history of melaena. He was referred for upper gastrointestinal endoscopy.**

    For which of the following findings would endoscopic injection of adrenaline and thermal therapy be most appropriate?

    A. 1 cm duodenal ulcer with a clean base in the posterior duodenum
    B. 1 cm gastric ulcer with adherent clot in the pre-pyloric area
    C. 2 cm duodenal ulcer with a flat red spot in the anterior duodenal bulb
    D. 2 cm gastric ulcer with a flat black spot in the antrum
    E. 3 cm malignant gastric ulcer adjacent to a pool of fresh blood in the fundus

3.   **A 42-year-old woman presented to the Emergency Department with melaena and haematemesis on a background of cirrhosis, COPD, and congestive cardiac failure. Emergency gastroscopy was performed.**

Endoscopy identified the findings in Figure 7.1/Colour Plate 6.

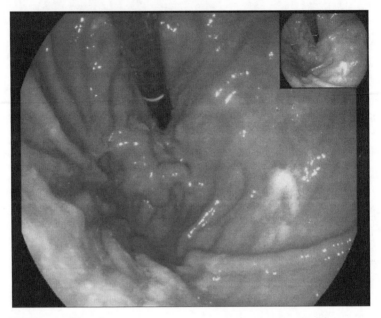

Figure 7.1 See also Plate 6.

Which of the following is the most appropriate initial treatment?

A. Alcohol injection

B. Cyanoacrylate injection

C. Endoscopic band ligation

D. Thrombin injection

E. Transjugular intrahepatic portosystemic stent shunt

4. An 87-year-old man attended an endoscopy list as a 2-week referral for dysphagia. The endoscope was introduced into the oesophagus with some difficulty, and the view shown in Figure 7.2/Colour Plate 7 was seen at 31 cm.

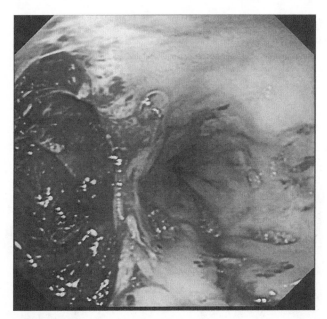

Figure 7.2 See also Plate 7.

Reprinted from *Journal of Gastrointestinal Endoscopy*, 4, Matull WR, Cross TJ, Yu D et al., 'A removable covered self-expanding metal stent for the management of Sengstaken-Blakemore tube-induced esophageal tear and variceal hemorrhage', pp. 767–768. Copyright 2008, with permission from Elsevier.

Management of the patient 'nil by mouth' and the provision of intravenous antibiotics is planned.

Which of the following is the most appropriate additional management?

A. Covered stent placement
B. Endoscopic clipping
C. Endoscopic gluing
D. Nasogastric tube placement
E. Surgical referral

5. **A 68-year-old woman attended for a gastroscopy having been referred by her GP with anaemia, 4 kg weight loss, and non-specific abdominal discomfort. No melaena had been witnessed, although she reported occasional dark stools.**

    Investigations:

haemoglobin	122 g/L (130–180)
white cell count	4.6 x 10⁹/L (4.0–11.0)
MCV	76 fL (80–96)
platelet count	209 x 10⁹/L (150–400)
serum ferritin	6 µg/L (15–300)
serum folate	2.6 µg/L (2.0–11.0)
serum vitamin B₁₂	178 ng/L (160–760)
serum C-reactive protein	16 mg/L (< 10)

    The endoscopic images demonstrated the findings shown in Figure 7.3/Colour Plate 8.

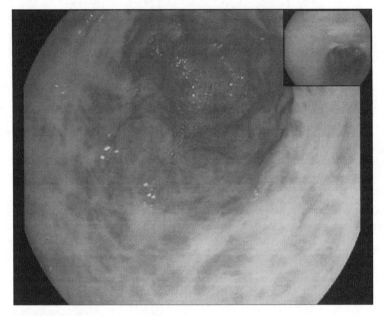

    Figure 7.3 See also Plate 8.

    Which of the following is the most appropriate next step?

    A. Antrectomy

    B. Argon plasma coagulation

    C. Iron supplementation

    D. Propranolol

    E. Transjugular intrahepatic portosystemic stent shunt

6. **A 69-year-old man with known Barrett's oesophagus attends for a surveillance gastroscopy. He was admitted by an endoscopy nurse who raised several concerns.**

   Which of the following is the most important risk factor for sedation-related complications?

   A. Diabetes mellitus
   B. Diuretic usage
   C. Hypokalemia
   D. Obesity
   E. Recent hip replacement

7. **A patient telephoned the endoscopy department for advice. In the past, they had been given antibiotic prophylaxis for a minor dental procedure, and developed a rash. They wished to know whether the antibiotic would be required on this occasion.**

   Which of the following endoscopic situations is most likely to require antibiotic prophylaxis?

   A. A 59-year-old woman undergoing an EUS and FNA for a solid lesion in the pancreas seen on a CT scan
   B. A 65-year-old man undergoing ERCP for jaundice secondary to a hilar cholangiocarcinoma
   C. A 68-year-old man with a previous history of an aortic valve replacement undergoing a colonoscopy and polypectomy
   D. A 69-year-old woman undergoing ERCP for stones within the common bile duct without intercurrent sepsis
   E. A 70-year-old woman undergoing a gastroscopy and oesophageal dilatation for a benign oesophageal stricture

8. **A 65-year-old man with a past medical history of insulin-dependent type 2 diabetes developed loose stools and was referred to the endoscopy department for a colonoscopy. He was normally well controlled on a basal bolus regime of NovoRapid 10 units three times a day with meals, and Lantus 25 units in the evening. He was scheduled for the first appointment on the afternoon list.**

   What is the most appropriate advice about the management of this man's diabetes before the procedure?

   A. Continue the normal doses of short-acting insulin, but omit the long-acting insulin on the day before and the day of the procedure
   B. Make no changes to the usual regime
   C. On the day before the procedure, take half the normal dose of short-acting insulin and the normal dose of long-acting insulin, and on the morning of the procedure take half the normal dose of short-acting insulin and omit the lunchtime dose of short-acting insulin
   D. On the day before the procedure, take the normal doses of short-acting and long-acting insulin, and on the day of the procedure take half the normal dose of short-acting insulin
   E. Stop all insulin the day before and the day of the procedure, and monitor blood sugar levels

9. **A 70-year-old man presented with recurrent episodes of melaena and was referred to gastroenterology. A gastroscopy and a colonoscopy were performed. The gastroscopy was normal. The colonoscopy showed the image in Figure 7.4/Colour Plate 9 in the caecum.**

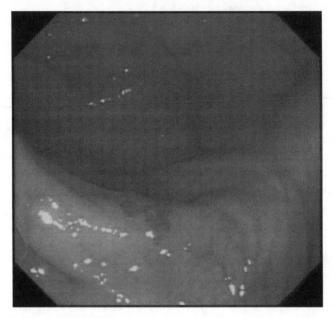

Figure 7.4 See also Plate 9.

Which of the following is the most appropriate management option for this condition?

A. Angiography and embolization

B. Argon plasma coagulation

C. Right hemicolectomy

D. Thalidomide

E. Tranexamic acid

10. **A 65-year-old man underwent a colonoscopy as part of the National Bowel Cancer Screening Programme. A 2.5 cm sessile polyp was found and removed from the ascending colon. Following the procedure, the patient was discharged from the endoscopy department. Two days later, the man presented through the surgical take with increasing abdominal pain. Clinical examination revealed tachycardia, with abdominal tenderness.**

Investigations:

haemoglobin	135 g/L (130–180)
white cell count	13.0 × 10⁹/L (4–11)
platelet count	450 × 10⁹/L (150–400)
serum C-reactive protein	34 mg/L (< 10)

What is the best next step in this patient's management?

A. Chest X-ray
B. Colonoscopy
C. CT scan
D. Laparoscopy
E. Laparotomy

11. **A 70-year-old man with a past medical history of gout, ischaemic heart disease, and atrial fibrillation was admitted on the acute medical take. He had a two day history of abdominal pain and multiple episodes of diarrhoea mixed with fresh blood.**

He was currently managed with ibuprofen 400 mg orally three times daily, and his general practitioner had recently provided a one week course of 5-aminosalicylic acid enemas.

Investigations:

haemoglobin	118 g/L (130–180)
white cell count	19.0 × 10⁹/L (4–11)
platelet count	450 × 10⁹/L (150–400)
serum C-reactive protein	156 mg/L (< 10)
flexible sigmoidoscopy	performed to the mid-sigmoid colon, showing severe colonic inflammation of the sigmoid colon to the limit of insertion with rectal sparing

Which of the following is the most likely diagnosis in this case?

A. Crohn's disease
B. Infective colitis secondary to *Campylobacter jejuni*
C. Ischaemic colitis
D. Non-steroidal anti-inflammatory drug (NSAID)-induced colitis
E. Ulcerative colitis

12. **A 54-year-old man with iron-deficiency anaemia was referred for further investigation. He had a history of ischaemic heart disease, and a coronary artery bare metal stent was placed three months ago. He had atrial fibrillation, but no evidence of valvular heart disease or peripheral vascular disease. His current medications included ramipril, aspirin, and clopidogrel.**

Investigations:

   barium enema   single polyp in the sigmoid colon measuring 1.5 cm

What is the best advice to give this man prior to colonoscopy and polypectomy, with regard to his antiplatelet therapy?

A. Continue both aspirin and clopidogrel

B. Liaise with a cardiologist

C. Stop aspirin but continue clopidogrel

D. Stop both aspirin and clopidogrel

E. Stop clopidogrel and continue aspirin

13. **A 45-year-old man was referred by his GP for further investigation of epigastric discomfort that had not resolved despite an adequate trial of proton pump inhibitor therapy. On upper gastrointestinal endoscopy a lesion was seen in the antrum. An endoscopic ultrasound examination was performed to further characterize the lesion.**

    The endoscopic ultrasonographic appearance of the lesion is shown in Figure 7.5/Colour Plate 10.

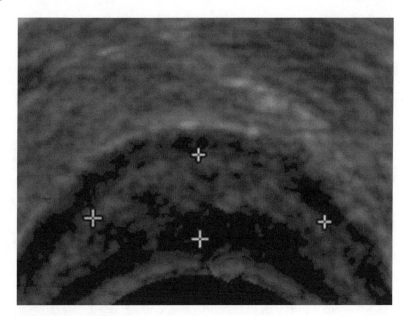

Figure 7.5 Radial endoscopic ultrasound of gastric antrum.

In which layer of the stomach does the lesion lie?

A. Interface

B. Mucosa

C. Muscularis propria

D. Serosa

E. Submucosa

14. **A 63-year-old woman with type 2 diabetes was admitted to hospital with central abdominal pain of sudden onset, radiating through to the back. She had a history of hypercholesterolaemia.**

    On examination she was not jaundiced, but was tachycardic with a pulse rate of 120 beats/minute; she had central and epigastric abdominal tenderness on palpation.

    Investigations:

white cell count	17.2 x 10^9/L (4.0–11.0)
serum albumin	30 g/L (37–49)
serum total bilirubin	45 μmol/L (1–22)
serum alanine aminotransferase	63 U/L (5–35)
serum alkaline phosphatase	103 U/L (45–105)
serum glucose	13 mmol/L
serum amylase	690 U/L (60–180)
serum C-reactive protein	23 mg/L (< 10)
abdominal ultrasound	common bile duct diameter of 6 mm; presence of a stone measuring 5 mm in the common bile duct, and several stones in the gallbladder

    What is the best next step in the management of this patient?

    A. Endoscopic retrograde cholangiopancreatogram, sphincterotomy, and clearance of the common bile duct stone
    B. Laparoscopic cholecystectomy and stone removal 6 weeks after recovery
    C. Laparoscopic cholecystectomy, on-table cholangiogram, and stone removal
    D. Magnetic resonance cholangiopancreatogram
    E. Percutaneous transhepatic cholangiogram with biliary drainage

15. **A 23-year-old woman presented to the Emergency Department with right upper quadrant pain following an endoscopic retrograde pancreatography. On examination she had a BMI of 32 kg/m^2, and a generally tender abdomen to deep palpation, with no guarding.**

    Investigations:

white cell count	12.5 x 10^9/L (4.0–11.0)
serum total bilirubin	21 μmol/L (1–22)
serum alanine aminotransferase	65 U/L (5–35)
serum alkaline phosphatase	134 U/L (45–105)
serum amylase	678 U/L (60–180)
serum C-reactive protein	32 mg/L (< 10)

    Which of the following is least likely to be a factor in pancreatitis after ERCP?

    A. Female gender
    B. Normal bilirubin
    C. Raised body mass index (BMI)
    D. Suspected sphincter of Oddi dysfunction
    E. Young age

16. A 42-year-old man presented to the Emergency Department with haematemesis and melaena. He had a past medical history of gout and had recently increased his dose of ibuprofen. On examination he was pale with mild epigastric tenderness. His pulse was 124 beats/minute and his blood pressure was 104/79 mmHg.

He had an upper gastrointestinal endoscopy demonstrating the lesion shown in Figure 7.6/Colour Plate 11.

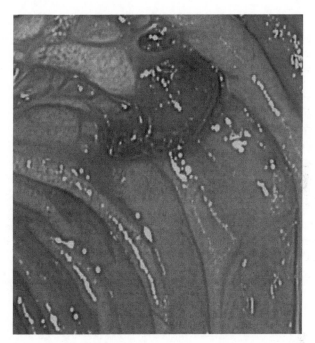

Figure 7.6 Endoscopic image of the second part of the duodenum. See also Plate 10.

Which Forrest classification best describes this lesion?

A. Ia

B. Ib

C. IIa

D. IIc

E. III

1. C. The Global Rating Scale (GRS) is the national web-based patient-centred assessment tool that allows endoscopy departments to fully assess all areas of their service. It is divided into four dimensions: clinical quality, quality of patient experience, workforce, and training. GRS assessment is submitted biannually to the Joint Advisory Group on GI Endoscopy (JAG). The JAG collates the submitted GRS scores, and provides accreditation of units based on successful attainment of standards. The JAG can also utilize a visiting team to assess the units, their data, evidence, and personnel when necessary.

Regular audit of the department has an important role. This includes British Society of Gastroenterology (BSG) auditable outcomes, adverse events, and endoscopist and nurse assessment of formal comfort scores. Patient feedback should be collated prospectively. It is recommended that audit and feedback data are fed back at least twice yearly to endoscopists, and to the department through governance meetings.

It is expected that all endoscopists and gastroenterology trainees will have a full understanding of local and national endoscopy departmental standards, as described on the GRS and JAG websites, and decontamination as described in the national endoscopy team standards.

JAG Accreditation System Incorporating GRS. www.jagaccreditation.org (accessed 7 January 2012).

Joint Advisory Group on GI Endoscopy: accreditation system. www.jagvisits.org.uk. (accessed 7 January 2012).

National Endoscopy Programme: decontamination standards for flexible endoscopes. Updated March 2009. www.bsg.org.uk/images/stories/docs/clinical/decontam_jag_2010.pdf (accessed 7 January 2012).

2. B. Resuscitation of patients with gastrointestinal (GI) bleeding with intravenous fluids can maintain tissue oxygenation, and should be performed prior to endoscopy to avoid cardiovascular and respiratory complications of endoscopy. Evidence suggests that the type of fluid is not important. Hypotension and tachypnoea suggest class 3 hypovolaemic shock; blood transfusion should be considered when this occurs. Proton pump inhibitor therapy prior to endoscopic diagnosis has not been shown to affect clinical outcome. Rockall scoring can be used to predict mortality prior to endoscopy, and both rebleeding and mortality after endoscopy.

Endoscopy for upper GI bleeding is recommended early (within 24 hours) in a dedicated endoscopy area, with appropriately trained staff, to reduce transfusion requirements, rebleeding, and surgery rates. The decision to perform therapeutic endoscopy is based on the presence of high-risk features predictive of a significant risk of rebleeding, namely active bleeding (80%), a visible vessel (40–50%), or adherent clot (35%). Ulcer size, site, and presumed malignancy are not factors; ulcers with a clean base and a black or red spot have an excellent prognosis without endoscopic therapy.

Rockall scoring

	0	1	2	3
Age (years)	< 60	60–79	≥ 80	
Shock	No shock SBP ≥ 100 mmHg Pulse < 100 beats/minute	Tachycardia SBP ≥ 100 mmHg Pulse ≥ 100 beats/minute	Hypotension SBP < 100 mmHg	
Comorbidity	No major comorbidity		Cardiac failure, IHD, major comorbidity	Renal failure, liver failure, disseminated malignancy
Diagnosis at endoscopy	Mallory–Weiss tear, no lesion identified and no stigmata of recent haemorrhage	All other diagnoses	Malignancy of upper GI tract	
Major stigmata of recent haemorrhage at endoscopy	None or dark spot only		Blood in upper GI tract, adherent clot, visible or spurting vessel	

SBP, systolic blood pressure; IHD, ischaemic heart disease; GI, gastrointestinal.
Reproduced from *Gut*, TF Rockall et al., 'Risk assessment after acute upper gastrointestinal haemorrhage', 38, 3, pp. 316–321.
Copyright 1996, with permission from BMJ Publishing Group Ltd.

Observed mortality by initial Rockall risk score

Rockall score	0	1	2	3	4	5	6	7
Death (%)	0.2	2.4	5.6	11.0	24.6	39.6	48.9	50.0

Several vessels supply the stomach. Of particular significance is the gastroduodenal artery, a short but large-volume branch of the right gastric artery that runs adjacent to the pylorus and supplies the posterior duodenal wall. Surgical therapy may be required for bleeding in this location.

Only in high-risk endoscopic features (active bleeding, a visible vessel, or adherent clot) is dual endoscopic therapy recommended; there is no evidence for endoscopic therapy when high-risk features are absent. Injection therapy is most commonly performed with 1 in 10 000 adrenaline, and recent guidelines suggest the use of over 13 mL. This tamponade effect reduces rebleeding from non-bleeding visible vessels from 50% to 15–20%, and from adherent clot from 35% to 10%.

Injection should be combined with a second therapy. Clipping has similar efficacy to coagulation, but is sometimes limited by difficult access or poor visualization. Coagulation with a heater probe or multipolar coagulation device should be applied until the area is black and cavitated; complications are rare, there is a low rate of perforation.

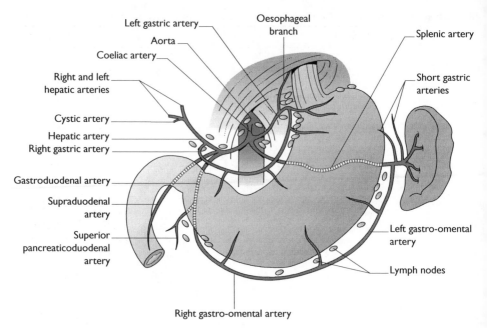

Figure 7.7 Gastric blood supply and anatomy.

Heater probe/multipolar coagulation device

- This is a bipolar circuit in which the two electrodes are close together within an accessory limiting tissue injury to the area in contact
- Low-level heat coagulates tissues
- The coagulation current is an intermittent wave form
- Bipolar devices are appropriate for those with a permanent pacemaker; automated implantable cardioverter–defibrillator (AICD) devices should be deactivated.

Polypectomy snare device

- This is a monopolar circuit in which the two electrodes (accessory and the return plate) are far apart
- A high-level thermal effect is achieved
- It requires a return plate; burns can occur at the return plate if contact is poor; cardiac leads require a 15 cm clearance
- The cutting current is a constant wave form that cuts and coagulates simultaneously.

After dual therapy for high-risk GI bleeding, intravenous proton pump inhibitor (PPI) treatment with omeprazole or pantoprazole as an 80 mg bolus followed by 8 mg/hour infusion for 72 hours is recommended. Low dose aspirin can be continued once haemostasis is achieved. Studies of tranexamic acid and somatostatin have failed to show a benefit. A repeat endoscopy within 24 hours is recommended when initial treatment is suboptimal or when rebleeding may be life-threatening. If rebleeding occurs despite endoscopic therapy, options include repeat endoscopic therapy, surgery, or radiological selective arterial embolization.

Prediction of rebleeding and mortality with the post-endoscopy Rockall score

Rockall score	0	1	2	3	4	5	6	7	≥ 8
Rebleeding (%)	4.9	3.4	5.3	11.2	14.1	24.1	32.9	43.8	41.8
Death (%)	0	0	0.2	2.9	5.3	10.8	17.3	27.0	41.1

Late recurrence of bleeding occurs in around a third of cases at 2 years, and half of cases by 10 years, if preventative measures are not taken. Repeat endoscopy to confirm healing of gastric ulcers may be undertaken to ensure that malignancy masquerading as peptic ulcer disease is identified. Following gastric or duodenal ulcer bleeding, *Helicobacter pylori* testing should be undertaken at endoscopy or by breath test; eradication should be undertaken and confirmed thereafter. Non-steroidal anti-inflammatory drugs (NSAIDs), COX-2 inhibitors, and aspirin should be reviewed, and stopped where possible. If causal medications must be restarted after healing has been confirmed, and *Helicobacter pylori* was not present, long-term concomitant PPI therapy is recommended. Selective serotonin reuptake inhibitors, corticosteroids, and oral anticoagulants may increase the risk of GI bleeding, and should be used with caution in those at risk of the latter, particularly with concurrent NSAIDs or aspirin.

Scottish Intercollegiate Guidelines Network. *Management of Acute Upper and Lower Gastrointestinal Bleeding: a national clinical guideline.* www.sign.ac.uk/pdf/sign105.pdf (accessed 7 July 2011).

Baskett PJF. ABC of major trauma. Management of hypovolaemic shock. *British Medical Journal* 1990; 300: 1453–1457.

Rockall TA, Logan RF, Devlin HB *et al.* Risk assessment after acute upper gastrointestinal haemorrhage. *Gut* 1996; 38: 316–321.

3. B. The endoscopic image is of gastric varices. Initial management of upper gastrointestinal (GI) bleeding due to all varices is with fluid resuscitation. Vasoactive treatment with intravenous terlipressin 2 mg 6-hourly should be instituted in suspected and confirmed variceal haemorrhage; octreotide or high-dose somatostatin for 3–5 days are alternatives after endoscopic therapy. Antibiotics, usually intravenous, are recommended for all causes of upper GI bleeding in chronic liver disease. The outcome of variceal bleeding can be predicted using the Child–Turcotte–Pugh (CTP) score.

Child–Turcotte–Pugh (CTP) score

	1	2	3
Encephalopathy	None	Mild (grade 1–2)	Severe (grade 3–4)
Ascites	None	Mild	Moderate/large
Bilirubin (µmol/L)	< 34	34–51	> 51
Albumin (g/L)	≥ 35	28–35	≥ 28
Prothrombin time (PT) prolongation (seconds)	< 4	4–6	> 6
or			
international normalized ratio (INR)	< 1.3	1.3–1.5	> 1.5

Reproduced from R. N. H. Pugh *et al.*, 'Transection of the oesophagus for bleeding oesophageal varices', *British Journal of Surgery*, 60, 8, pp. 646–649. Copyright 1973 with permission from Wiley and British Journal of Surgery Society Ltd.

Predicting mortality (after sclerotherapy for oesophageal varices)

- Child–Pugh grade A: score 5–6; mortality 32%
- Child–Pugh grade B: score 7–9; mortality 46%
- Child–Pugh grade C: score 10–15; mortality 79%.

Endoscopic management of varices depends on their site. Oesophageal varices (discussed in Chapter 5) are best managed with band ligation. Sclerotherapy can be used when banding is technically challenging, and a transjugular intrahepatic portosystemic shunt (TIPPS) is the recommended second-line option. Cyanoacrylate (glue) injection has the best evidence base in gastric varices; randomized controlled trial (RCT) evidence supports the use of glue over alcohol injection and ligation therapy; thrombin injection lacks RCT evidence. TIPPS has similar outcomes to cyanoacrylate injection, but is less cost-effective.

Balloon tamponade with a Sengstaken–Blakemore tube or similar device is reserved for uncontrolled variceal bleeding despite vasoactive drug and endoscopic therapy. Haemostasis is achieved in 80–95% of all forms of varices; complications include pneumonia, oesophageal perforation, and pain. Only the gastric balloon should be inflated, to avoid oesophageal necrosis. Once bleeding is controlled, second-line endoscopic treatment can be considered. TIPPS is recommended for uncontrolled haemorrhage rather than surgical shunts. Oesophageal stents may have a role in the future.

Variceal bleeding recurs in up to 50% of cases within 24 hours and 80% within 1 year. Octreotide has no role in prevention. Combined variceal band ligation and propranolol therapy is recommended for oesophageal varices; the combination of nitrates and propranolol is an alternative when band ligation is not possible. TIPPS can be considered when endoscopic or propranolol therapy is not possible. There are no placebo-controlled trials of propranolol in gastric varices, although one study showed that histoacryl glue was not more effective than propranolol. TIPPS is recommended to prevent gastric variceal rebleeding.

Scottish Intercollegiate Guidelines Network. *Management of Acute Upper and Lower Gastrointestinal Bleeding: a national clinical guideline.* www.sign.ac.uk/pdf/sign105.pdf (accessed 7 July 2011).

4. A. This view illustrates a full-thickness oesophageal perforation. Diagnostic gastroscopy is rarely associated with perforation; it occurs in 0.03% of cases and causes mortality in 0.001%. It is most commonly pharyngeal or oesophageal, and occurs more commonly at the site of pathology, or associated with blind intubation. It is associated with the presence of a pharyngeal pouch, eosinophilic oesophagitis, anterior cervical osteophytes, benign strictures (particularly caustic strictures), malignant strictures, and with inexperienced endoscopists.

Complications in gastroscopy are uncommon. Sore throats and abdominal discomfort occur in 2% of cases. Tooth damage, jaw dislocation, and scope impaction in a hiatus hernia are rare. Significant bleeding in diagnostic gastroscopy is very rare. Biopsy is safe when the platelet count is > 20 x 10⁹/L (150–400), and on any anticoagulants within the therapeutic range.

Aspiration is the most commonly recognized infectious complication of gastroscopy, particularly if the patient is over-sedated. Creutzfeldt–Jakob disease (CJD) is not destroyed by decontamination techniques, and dedicated scopes and quarantine of the scopes are mandated. Bacteraemia is uncommon and rarely of clinical significance. The following table lists the American Society of Gastrointestinal Endoscopy published rates of bacteraemia, combined with the British Society of Gastroenterology data for complications.

Published rates of bacteraemia and complications associated with GI endoscopy

Procedure	Rate of bacteraemia (%)	Rate of perforation (%)	Rate of mortality (%)
Oesophageal dilatation	12–22	2–3 Benign: 1–2 Malignant: 4–6 Achalasia: 3–4	1 Benign: 0.5 Malignant: 2–3 Achalasia: 1
Variceal sclerotherapy	14.6 (0–52)	2–5	2–5
Variceal ligation	8.8 (1–25)	0.7	1
Gastroscopy	4.4 (0–8)	0.03	0.001
Colonoscopy	4.4 (0–25)	0–0.19	0–0.07
Flexible sigmoidoscopy	0–1	0–0.09	
Percutaneous endoscopic gastrostomy			0–28
Brushing teeth	20–68		
Chewing food	7–51		

Data from Riley S, Alderson D. British Society of Gastroenterology Guidelines on Complications of Upper Gastrointestinal Endoscopy. www.bsg.org.uk/images/stories/docs/clinical/guidelines/endoscopy/complications.pdf (accessed 7 July 2011). Green J. Complications of Gastrointestinal Endoscopy. British Society of Gastroenterology, 2008. www.bsg.org.uk/images/stories/docs/clinical/guidelines/endoscopy/complications.pdf (accessed 29 January 2012). Banerjee S, Shen B, Baron T et al. Antibiotic Prophylaxis for GI endoscopy. American Society for Gastrointestinal Endoscopy. Gastrointestinal Endoscopy 2008; 67(6): 791–8.

Successful management of oesophageal perforation and avoidance of mortality is achieved by early recognition. Nil by mouth and intravenous antibiotics are first-line measures. These can be combined with mediastinal or pleural cavity drainage for non-operative management of perforations detected early or with a contained leak, where the oesophagus is not malignant, no septicaemia has occurred, and drainage into the oesophageal lumen is demonstrated. For those cases that do not meet these criteria, surgical treatment of oesophageal perforation has the largest evidence base, and includes drainage for cervical perforations and exploration with a view to surgical repair for thoracic and abdominal perforations.

Non-surgical treatments of oesophageal perforation have an emerging role. Clipping is not uncommonly used for post-polypectomy perforations of the colon. However, due to technical difficulties with clip application in a narrow lumen such as the oesophagus, it is rarely performed unless surgery and stenting are inappropriate. Gluing has been successfully described in case reports, but is not widely adopted. Nasogastric tubes, although potentially useful for drainage and provision of feeding, can promote gastrointestinal reflux and increase mediastinal contamination, and are therefore best avoided. In this age group intrathoracic surgery would be high risk, and therefore a covered stent would be a good option.

Oesophageal stents are useful in the palliation of malignancy-related dysphagia (see Figure 7.8/Colour Plate 12). Despite having fewer procedure-related complications than rigid stents, self-expanding metal stents have a complication rate of 20–40%, with a mortality of 3%. Perforation is more common with rigid (5%) compared with self-expanding metal stents (1–2%). Oesophageal stent complications include stent migration (5–15%), tumour ingrowths (10–20%), food bolus obstruction (5–15%), and gastro-oesophageal reflux.

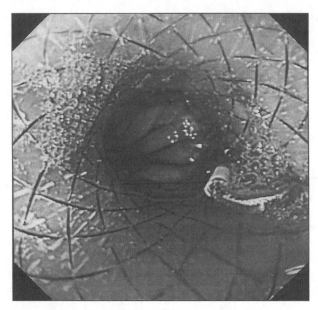

Figure 7.8 Oesophageal stent *in situ*. See also Plate 11.

Reprinted from *Journal of Gastrointestinal Endoscopy*, 68, 4, Matull WR, Cross TJ, Yu D *et al.*, 'A removable covered self-expanding metal stent for the management of Sengstaken–Blakemore tube-induced oesophageal tear and variceal hemorrhage', pp. 767–768. Copyright 2008, with permission from Elsevier.

Riley S and Alderson D. Complications of upper gastrointestinal endoscopy. In: *Guidelines on Complications of Gastrointestinal Endoscopy*. London: British Society of Gastroenterology; 2006. www.bsg.org.uk/images/stories/docs/clinical/guidelines/endoscopy/complications.pdf (accessed 7 July 2011).

Green J. *Complications of Gastrointestinal Endoscopy*. London: British Society of Gastroenterology; 2008. www.bsg.org.uk/images/stories/docs/clinical/guidelines/endoscopy/complications.pdf (accessed 29 January 2012).

American Society for Gastrointestinal Endoscopy. Guideline on antibiotic prophylaxis for GI endoscopy. *Gastrointestinal Endoscopy* 2008; 67: 791–798.

Brinster CJ, Singhal S, Lee L *et al.* Evolving options in the management of oesophageal perforation. *Annals of Thoracic Surgery* 2004; 77: 1475–1483.

Fischer A, Schrag HJ, Goos M *et al.* Nonoperative treatment of four oesophageal perforations with hemostatic clips. *Diseases of the Esophagus* 2007; 20: 444–448.

5. C. This image illustrates gastric antral vascular ectasia (GAVE). Endoscopic appearances are characterized by red areas; on close inspection tiny blood vessels may be visible. These often appear as streaks, hence the term 'watermelon stomach.' Histology is rarely necessary, but can demonstrate dilated capillaries in the lamina propria. The aetiology has not been established. GAVE is most common in women over 70 years of age. It is associated with autoimmune disease, most commonly systemic sclerosis, renal failure, and heart disease. Less than 30% of GAVE cases are associated with liver cirrhosis; in cirrhosis GAVE can be mistaken for portal hypertensive gastropathy (PHG) and therefore can be mistaken for portal hypertensive gastropathy (PHG).

Gastrointestinal angiodysplasia is not uncommon, and is most frequently found in the right colon, particularly the caecum. Asymptomatic angiodysplasia does not warrant treatment. However, if associated with significant bleeding, or found to be the cause of iron-deficiency anaemia that is unresponsive to iron replacement, treatment may be considered. Heyde's syndrome describes a combination of aortic valve stenosis and gastrointestinal angiodysplasia, usually colonic. An acquired von Willebrand's syndrome occurs, leading to bleeding from the angiodysplasia. Argon plasma coagulation treatment may be of benefit, and aortic valve replacement provides a definitive treatment. Regular blood transfusion is reserved for those unfit for surgery.

Cases of GAVE often present with chronic blood loss resulting in anaemia, although up to 4% of acute bleeds may relate to GAVE. Treatment of GAVE is often endoscopic, involving treatment with argon plasma coagulation at endoscopy; this may have to be performed repeatedly. Antrectomy can be considered in severe cases that are unresponsive to endoscopic management. Treatment of portal hypertension is not helpful.

PHG is differentiated from GAVE by its diffuse distribution rather than streaks, and its location predominantly in the fundus and body of the stomach. There are four features; early signs include a mosaic-like pattern; in more advanced cases red point lesions, cherry red spots, and black-brown spots can occur. PHG occurs in around 65% of cirrhotic individuals, and can be considered a marker of severe liver disease. It has been found to be an independent risk factor for variceal bleeding. PHG is thought to account for up to 8% of non-variceal bleeding in liver patients. It is often associated with varices, and responds to lowering of the portal pressures with propranolol or TIPPS.

The recognition of upper gastrointestinal pathology from endoscopic images is part of the syllabus and the examination. Several free endoscopy atlases are available online (see, for example,< www.endoatlas.com> and <http://daveproject.org>). Time is well spent reviewing these images.

Burak K, Lee S and Beck P. Portal hypertensive gastropathy and gastric antral vascular ectasia (GAVE) syndrome. *Gut* 2001; 49: 866–872.

Dulai GS, Jensen DM, Kovacs TO *et al.* Endoscopic treatment outcomes in watermelon stomach patients with and without portal hypertension. *Endoscopy* 2004; 36: 68–72.

Pate GE, Chandavimol M, Naiman SC *et al.* Heyde's syndrome: a review. *Journal of Heart Valve Disease* 2004; 13: 701–712.

6. D. Conscious sedation is defined as the use of medication to depress the central nervous system, thereby enabling treatment, but without the loss of verbal communication. In 2001 the Royal College of Anaesthetists recommended that loss of verbal responsiveness requires the same level of care as for general anaesthesia. In 2004 the National Confidential Enquiry into Patient Outcome and Death (NCEPOD) reported that inappropriate sedation was a factor in 14% of all endoscopy-related deaths. Sedation is the leading factor in endoscopy-related mortality.

Risk factors for complications of sedation include increasing age, obesity, cirrhosis, cardiac disease, respiratory disease, renal disease, prior administration of sedation or opiates, known drug allergies, low resting saturations, and emergency endoscopy. Complications of sedation include over-sedation, paradoxical excitement, respiratory depression and aspiration, cardiac arrhythmias, acute coronary events, hypertension, hypotension, cerebrovascular events, nausea, vomiting, and local or generalized flushing. Risk factors for complications should warrant discussion of unsedated endoscopy, and if sedation is undertaken, adjustment of doses should be considered.

Benzodiazepine: midazolam

- Contraindications: neuromuscular respiratory weakness, severe respiratory depression
- Effects: sedation with amnesia, and no analgesic effect
- Side effects: confusion, paradoxical excitement or agitation, nausea, vomiting, decreased responsiveness and ability to report pain, reduced respiratory effort, hypoxia, hypotension, cardiac or respiratory arrest
- Initial onset time: up to 1 minute
- Time to peak effect: 1–2 minutes
- Adults < 70 years old: initial dose 0–2 mg, increment 0–1 mg, maximum 5 mg
- Adults > 70 years old: initial dose 0–1 mg, increment 0–0.5 mg, maximum 2 mg
- The reversal agent is flumazenil: dosage 0.2–0.5 mg, increment 0.1 mg, peak effect in up to 1 minute, duration of action 1–2 hours
- Flumazenil side effects include flushing, seizures, and late re-sedation.

Opiates: pethidine and fentanyl

- Contraindications: acute respiratory depression, phaeochromocytoma
- Effects: prevention, reduction, and relief of pain
- Side effects: confusion, nausea, vomiting, decreased responsiveness and ability to report pain, reduced respiratory effort, hypoxia, hypotension, cardiac or respiratory arrest
- Synergism: opiates have a synergistic effect with benzodiazepines. It is advised that they are given 3 minutes before benzodiazepines, as doses may need to be reduced by up to fourfold
- Pethidine is metabolized to fentanyl and therefore has less predictable effects, including a higher risk of hypotension, and hallucinations
- Initial onset time: 1–2 minutes
- Time to peak effect: 3 minutes
- Adults < 70 years old:
  - Pethidine: initial dose 25 mg, increment 25 mg, maximum 50 mg
  - Fentanyl: initial dose 50 mg, increment 25 mg, maximum 100 mg
- Adults > 70 years old:
  - Pethidine: initial dose 12.5 mg, increment 12.5 mg, maximum 25 mg
  - Fentanyl: initial dose 25 mg, increment 12.5 mg, maximum 50 mg
- The reversal agent is naloxone: dosage 0.1–0.2 mg, maximum 10 mg, peak effect in 1–2 minutes, duration of action 1–3 hours
- Naloxone side effects include pain, agitation, arrhythmias, pulmonary oedema, and late re-sedation.

Adjuncts: buscopan

- Contraindications: myasthenia gravis, acute closed-angle glaucoma
- Effects: relief of smooth muscle spasm
- Side effects: tachycardia, palpitations, arrhythmias, anti-muscarinic side effects
- Time to peak effect: 4 minutes
- Duration of action: 5 hours
- Dose: 20 mg can be repeated every 30 minutes up to a maximum of 100 mg in 24 hours.

Adjuncts: lignocaine throat spray

- Relative contraindications: unsafe swallow
- Effects: analgesia of oropharynx
- Time to peak effect: up to 1 minute
- Duration of action: 15–60 minutes
- Dose: maximum of '20 squirts' recommended
- Although there is a theoretical risk of aspiration with concurrent sedation, this practice is widely adopted, including at national endoscopy training centres.

Safety in endoscopy is paramount; safe sedation is achieved with careful planning and monitoring.

Preparing the patient

- Discussion and informed consent are required
- Risk factors for sedation are assessed
- It is recommended that patients are starved prior to sedation, but there is no consensus on duration.

Preparing for drug delivery

- Secure intravenous access is mandatory
- All drug vials should be checked, and syringes labelled
- Specific antagonist drugs must be checked and available to hand.

Preparing the equipment

- Monitoring and recording by endoscopy nurse
- All sedated patients must have continuous pulse oximetry
- Blood pressure monitoring and ECG monitoring should be considered in older patients and those with comorbidity
- Pre-oxygenation reduces the risks from desaturation during intubation
- Oxygen and appropriate delivery methods must be available; any saturations below 90% requires immediate attention
- The trolley should be able to be tipped head down
- Resuscitation equipment should be available, and staff should be trained in its use.

Post-sedation advice

- The patient must be accompanied home by a responsible adult and have someone at home overnight
- They must not operate machinery or sign documents for 24 hours.

NCEPOD. *Scoping our Practice: the 2004 Report of the National Confidential Enquiry into Patient Outcome and Death.* www.ncepod.org.uk/pdf/2004/04sum.pdf (accessed 20 January 2012).

Quine A, Bell GD, McCloy RF et al. Prospective audit of upper gastrointestinal endoscopy in two regions of England: safety, staffing, and sedation methods. *Gut* 1995; 36: 462–467.

Royal College of Anaesthetists. *Implementing and Ensuring Safe Sedation Practice for Healthcare Procedures in Adults. Report of an Intercollegiate Working Party chaired by the Royal College of Anaesthetists.* www.rcoa.ac.uk/node/2270 (accessed 20 December 2012).

Lord DA, Bell GD, Gray A et al. *Sedation for Gastrointestinal Endoscopic Procedures in the Elderly: getting safer but still not nearly safe enough.* www.bsg.org.uk/clinical-guidelines/endoscopy/guidelines-on-safty-and-sedation-during-endoscopic-procedures.html (accessed 7 January 2012).

Teague R. *Guidelines on Safety and Sedation during Endoscopic Procedures.* www.bsg.org.uk/clinical-guidelines/endoscopy/guidelines-on-safety-and-sedation-during-endoscopic-procedures.html (accessed 7 January 2012).

7. B. In 2009, the British Society of Gastroenterology (BSG) published updated guidelines on the role of antibiotic prophylaxis in gastrointestinal endoscopy. For the prevention of infective endocarditis in patients with cardiac risk factors, antibiotic prophylaxis is no longer routinely recommended during diagnostic or therapeutic endoscopy. In this question, antibiotic prophylaxis is indicated for the endoscopic retrograde cholangiopancreatography (ERCP) for jaundice secondary to a hilar cholangiocarcinoma, as complete biliary drainage is unlikely to be achieved, and antibiotics are required for the prevention of cholangitis. There are specific situations in endoscopy where antibiotics are indicated. These are summarized in the following table:

Summary of prophylactic antibiotic regimens recommended for gastrointestinal endoscopy

Scenario	Rationale	Antibiotics	Dose/route
1. Patients with valvular heart disease, valve replacement, and/or surgically constructed systemic–pulmonary shunt or conduit or vascular graft	Prevention of infective endocarditis or conduit/graft infection	Not indicated	
2. ERCP in the following:			
a. Ongoing cholangitis or sepsis elsewhere	Prevention of procedure-related bacteraemia	Guide by culture results. Patients should already be established on antibiotics	Microbiology advice
b. Biliary obstruction and/or CBD stones	Prevention of cholangitis	Not indicated unless biliary decompression is not achieved. If biliary decompression is not achieved during the procedure, a full course of antibiotics is indicated	
c. When complete biliary drainage is unlikely to be achieved (e.g. PSC, hilar cholangiocarcinoma) (may need to consider alternative antibiotic prophylaxis if repeated procedures are needed)	Prevention of cholangitis	Ciprofloxacin or Gentamycin	750 mg PO 60–90 mins before procedure 1.5 mg/kg IV over 2–3 mins
d. Communicating pancreatic cyst or pseudocyst	Reducing risk of introducing infection into cavity	As (c)	As (c)
e. Biliary complications following liver transplant	Prevention of cholangitis	As (c) + amoxicillin or vancomycin	1 g IV single dose 20 mg/kg IV infused over at least 1 hour

Scenario	Rationale	Antibiotics	Dose/route
3. EUS in the following:			
a. FNA solid lesions	Prevention of local infections	Not indicated	
b. FNA cystic lesions in or near the pancreas or drainage of a cystic cavity	Prevention of cyst infections	Co-amoxiclav _or_ Ciprofloxacin	1.2 g IV single dose 750 mg PO single dose
4. PEG	Prevention of peristomal infection Possible reduction in risk of other infections, such as aspiration pneumonia	Co-amoxiclav _or_ Cefuroxime Teicoplanin can be used if there is a past history of anaphylaxis or angioedema with penicillin/ cephalosporin	1.2 g IV injection or infusion just before procedure 750 mg IV injection or infusion just before procedure 400 mg IV for adults
5. Variceal bleeding (not strictly prophylaxis)	Prevention of infections such as spontaneous bacterial peritonitis	Piperacillin/ tazobactam _or_ Third-generation cephalosporin Seek microbiology or regional liver unit advice in cases of penicillin allergy	4.5 g IV 3 times a day e.g. cefotaxime 2 g IV 3 times a day
6. Profound immunocompromise (e.g. neutropenia < 0.5 x 10⁹/L or advanced haematological malignancy)	Prevention of procedure-related bacteraemia	Only indicated in procedures with a high rate of bacteraemia (e.g. sclerotherapy, dilatation, ERCP with obstructed system)	Discuss with haematologist and/or clinical microbiologist

CBD, common bile duct; PO, by mouth; IV, intravenous; PSC, primary sclerosing cholangitis; EUS, endoscopic ultrasound; FNA, fine-needle aspiration; PEG, percutaneous endoscopic gastrostomy.

Reproduced from _Gut_, Allison MC _et al._, 'Antibiotic prophylaxis in gastrointestinal endoscopy', 58, 6, pp. 869–880. Copyright 2009, with permission from BMJ Publishing Group Ltd.

Allison MC, Sandoe JAT, Tighe R _et al._ prepared on behalf of the Endoscopy Committee of the British Society of Gastroenterology. Antibiotic prophylaxis in gastrointestinal endoscopy. _Gut_ 2009; 58: 869–880.

8. C. Diabetes is the most common metabolic disorder and it leads to increased morbidities, increased mortality, poor outcome after surgery, and increased length of hospital stay. In April 2011, NHS Diabetes identified a number of factors that contribute to adverse outcomes, including recurrent hyper- and hypoglycaemia, multiple associated comorbidities (including complications), complex polypharmacy, inappropriate use of intravenous insulin, errors made in converting intravenous insulin infusions to usual medication, and peri-operative infections. They published an extensive guideline on the management of patients with diabetes, including operative procedures and endoscopy.

Suggested guidelines for patients are summarized in the tables below. Many units will have their own local policies.

Management of oral medications for endoscopy

Tablets	On the day before the procedure	On the day of a morning-list procedure	On the day of an afternoon-list procedure
Acarbose	For gastroscopy, take your medications as normal For colonoscopy or flexible sigmoidoscopy, *do not* take any oral medications	Omit your morning dose if you have been told to fast from midnight	Take your morning dose if eating breakfast. Do not take your lunchtime dose
Meglitinides (repaglinide or nateglinide)	For gastroscopy, take your medications as normal For colonoscopy or flexible sigmoidoscopy, *do not* take any oral medications	Omit morning dose if you have been told to fast from midnight	Take your morning dose if eating breakfast. Do not take your lunchtime dose
Metformin (once twice, or three times a day)	For gastroscopy, take your medications as normal For colonoscopy or flexible sigmoidoscopy, *do not* take any oral medications	If taken once or twice a day, do not stop If taken three times a day, stop the lunchtime dose only	If taken once or twice a day, do not stop If taken three times a day, stop the lunchtime dose only
Sulphonylureas Once or twice a day (glibenclamide, glipizide, gliclazide/gliclazide MR, glimepiride, gliquidone)	For gastroscopy, take your medications as normal For colonoscopy or flexible sigmoidoscopy, *do not* take any oral medications	If taken once or twice a day, omit the morning dose	If taken once a day, omit the morning dose If taken twice a day, omit both doses
Thiazolidinediones (pioglitazone)	For gastroscopy, take your medications as normal For colonoscopy or flexible sigmoidoscopy, *do not* take any oral medications	Take as normal	Take as normal
DPP-IV inhibitors (sitagliptin, saxagliptin, vildagliptin)	For gastroscopy, take your medications as normal For colonoscopy or flexible sigmoidoscopy, *do not* take any oral medications	Omit your morning dose	Omit your morning dose

Reproduced from 'Management of adults with diabetes undergoing surgery and elective procedures: improving standards', April 2011, NHS Diabetes, with kind permission from Dr Ketan Dhatariya and NHS Diabetes.

Management of diabetic injected medications for endoscopy

Injections	On the day before the procedure	On the day of a morning-list procedure	On the day of an afternoon-list procedure
Once daily evening or morning insulin (Lantus, Levemir, Insulatard, Humulin 1, Insuman)	For gastroscopy, continue your normal regime For colonoscopy, take increased clear fluids and sugary drinks to maintain blood glucose levels Monitor blood levels before administering insulin Take usual dose of insulin	For gastroscopy and colonoscopy: Continue your normal regime.* Check blood glucose levels on admission	For gastroscopy, continue your normal regime* For colonoscopy, halve your normal morning regime. Check blood glucose levels on admission
Twice daily insulin (Novomix 30, Humulin M3, Humalog Mix 25 or 50)	For gastroscopy, continue your normal regime For colonoscopy, take increased clear fluids and sugary drinks to maintain blood glucose levels Monitor blood levels before administering insulin Take half the normal dose of short-acting or mixed insulin	For gastroscopy and colonoscopy: Halve the usual morning dose. Check blood glucose levels on admission. Continue the normal dose of insulin with your evening meal	For gastroscopy and colonoscopy: Halve the usual morning dose. Check blood glucose levels on admission. Continue the normal dose of insulin with your evening meal
Three, four, or five injections daily:	For gastroscopy, continue your normal regime For colonoscopy, follow dietary advice and monitor blood levels before administering insulin Take half the normal doses of short-acting insulin and mixed insulin Take the normal dose of long-acting insulin	For gastroscopy and colonoscopy: Omit the morning insulin if no breakfast is eaten, and the lunchtime short-acting insulin Keep the basal unchanged* If you take premixed insulin, the dose should be halved Check blood sugar levels on admission Resume the normal insulin dose with evening meal	For gastroscopy, continue your normal morning regime For colonoscopy, halve your normal morning regime, and omit the lunchtime dose. Check blood glucose levels on admission Resume the normal insulin dose with evening meal

*Some units may recommend reducing the normal dose of long-acting insulin by one third, especially in patients who require regular snacks.

Table adapted and reproduced from 'Management of adults with diabetes undergoing surgery and elective procedures: improving standards', April 2011 'NHS Diabetes' with kind permission from Dr Ketan Dhatariya and NHS Diabetes.

Frisch A, Chandra P, Smiley D *et al.* Prevalence and clinical outcome of hyperglycemia in the perioperative period in noncardiac surgery. *Diabetes Care* 2010; 33: 1783–1788.

Moghissi ES, Korytkowski MT, Dinardo MM *et al.* American Association of Clinical Endocrinologists and American Diabetes Association consensus statement on inpatient glycemic control. *Diabetes Care* 2009; 32: 1119–1131.

NHS Diabetes. *Management of adults with diabetes undergoing surgery and elective procedures: improving standards.* www.diabetes.nhs.uk/areas_of_care/emergency_and_inpatient/perioperative_management (accessed 23 February 2012).

9. B. Angiodysplasia refers to small vascular malformations that can affect the gastrointestinal tract, particularly the caecum or ascending colon. They consist of dilated, tortuous, thin-walled vessels lined with endothelium and sometimes smooth muscle. They are often multiple, and can present with acute bleeding, giving rise to melaena, or a more chronic occult pattern of bleeding causing symptoms of iron-deficiency anaemia.

Angiodysplasia is found more commonly in patients over the age of 60 years, and is associated with other conditions, such as von Willebrand disease, end-stage renal failure, and possibly aortic stenosis (known as Heyde's syndrome). It can be found at colonoscopy, wireless capsule endoscopy, deep small bowel enteroscopy, CT angiography, and red cell scintigraphy.

There are a number of treatment options available. Endoscopic options using cautery are the most widely used. Argon plasma coagulation involves transmitting high-frequency energy to tissues by means of ionized argon gas. It is widely used, and has been shown to be safe and effective. Bipolar diathermy and heater probe coagulation have also been used effectively, but heater probe coagulation has been associated with a higher rate of colonic and small bowel (beyond the duodenum) perforation. Other endoscopic techniques that have been described include endoscopic clips, injection sclerotherapy, and Nd-YAG lasers. There are case reports of the use of band ligation to treat lesions in the stomach and small intestine; the caecum is too thin-walled for this to be a safe method of managing angiodysplastic lesions.

Systemic medication, which is often used, with varying results, includes antifibrinolytic agents such as tranexamic acid. Oestrogens have been used to control bleeding in conditions such as hereditary haemorrhagic telangiectasia, but their role in sporadic angiodysplastic lesions is not proven. There have been some promising reports on the use of octreotide and thalidomide.

Angiography can be helpful in the localization of the actively bleeding lesions (particularly if they are not visualized at colonoscopy), and allows for embolization. This can be useful in the management of high-risk patients in whom colonoscopy or surgery may not be appropriate. Surgical resection should be considered for those patients with recurrent uncontrolled or life-threatening bleeding.

Vargo JJ. Clinical applications of the argon plasma coagulator. *Gastrointestinal Endoscopy* 2004; 59: 81–88.

Askin NP and Lewis BS. Push enteroscopic cauterization: long-term follow-up of 83 patients with bleeding small intestinal angiodysplasia. *Gastrointestinal Endoscopy* 1996; 43: 580–583.

Moparty B and Raju GS. Role of hemoclips in a patient with cecal angiodysplasia at high risk of recurrent bleeding from antithrombotic therapy to maintain coronary stent patency: a case report. *Gastrointestinal Endoscopy* 2005; 62: 468–469.

Bemvenuti GA and Julich MM. Ethanolamine injection for sclerotherapy of angiodysplasia of the colon. *Endoscopy* 1998; 30: 564–569.

Rutgeerts P, Van Gompel F, Geboes K *et al.* Long term results of treatment of vascular malformations of the gastrointestinal tract by neodymium Yag laser photocoagulation. *Gut* 1985; 26: 586–593.

10. C. The most likely diagnosis in this case is post-polypectomy syndrome (also known as post-polypectomy electrocoagulation syndrome). This is caused by the electrical current used during polypectomy, which extends beyond the mucosa and muscularis propria into the serosal surface of the colon, causing thermal injury without evidence of colonic perforation. This results in a localized inflammatory reaction, and patients often present with fever, tachycardia, abdominal tenderness at the site of polypectomy, rigidity, and leucocytosis. The main differential diagnosis is colonic perforation; the clinical presentation is similar, and the definitive investigation for differentiate between these is a CT scan.

The reported rates of occurrence of post-polypectomy syndrome are between 0.5% and 1% of polypectomies. Patients often present within 12 hours, but can present with symptoms up to 5 days after the procedure. The syndrome occurs after large amounts of thermal energy have been applied over a long period of time, so it is more commonly seen after the removal of larger polyps (> 2 cm in diameter), or when normal mucosa is inadvertently caught within the snare alongside the polyp. It is possible that the injection of fluid submucosally at the polyp site prior to polypectomy may reduce the risk of developing post-polypectomy syndrome, but there are no large studies confirming this.

Investigations invariably consist of plain radiographs and CT scanning. In contrast to perforation, there will be no evidence of free air, but CT scans may show focal thickening of the colon, and periluminal fat stranding. Treatment is conservative, in contrast to perforation, which often requires operative intervention. Management includes nil by mouth, and intravenous fluids and antibiotics, ideally overseen by both gastroenterology and surgical teams. If symptoms and signs are mild, some patients may even be managed as outpatients, with clear fluids and oral antibiotics, such as ciprofloxacin and metronidazole.

There is a very low risk of evolution to frank perforation, and the prognosis is generally excellent. Treatment by conservative measures should be maintained until the symptoms and inflammatory markers have settled.

Waye JD. The postpolypectomy coagulation syndrome. *Gastrointestinal Endoscopy* 1981; 27: 184.

Christie JP and Marrazzo J 3rd. "Mini-perforation" of the colon—not all postpolypectomy perforations require laparotomy. *Diseases of the Colon and Rectum* 1991; 34: 132–135.

Waye JD, Lewis BS and Yessayan S. Colonoscopy: a prospective report of complications. *Journal of Clinical Gastroenterology* 1992; 15: 347–351.

Waye JD, Kahn O and Auerbach ME. Complications of colonoscopy and flexible sigmoidoscopy. *Gastrointestinal Endoscopy Clinics of North America* 1996; 6: 343–377.

11. C. The blood supply of the colon is derived from the superior mesenteric artery (SMA) and the inferior mesenteric artery (IMA). The two systems communicate via a marginal artery that runs alongside the length of the colon and parallel with it. The ascending colon is supplied by the ileocolic and right colic arteries (branches of the SMA), the proximal two-thirds of the transverse colon derives its blood supply from the middle colic artery (a branch of the SMA), and the distal third is supplied by branches of the IMA. This area, between two arterial supplies, is known as the 'watershed area', and it is highly susceptible to ischaemic damage.

The left colic artery (a branch of the IMA) supplies the descending colon, and the sigmoid colon receives blood from multiple branches ('sigmoid arteries') of the IMA. The first two-thirds of the rectum are supplied by the IMA (via the superior rectal artery), while the last third of the rectum receives blood from the internal iliac artery (via the middle rectal artery). As a result of this dual blood supply, ischaemia affecting the rectum is rare.

The main differential diagnoses in this case are ischaemic colitis and Crohn's disease. Ulcerative colitis tends to present as continuous inflammation extending from the rectum, although skip lesions have been reported, and relative rectal sparing can be seen when 5-aminosalicylic acid enemas are used. Acute infection may be clinically difficult to distinguish from acute inflammatory bowel disease, but rectal sparing would be unusual.

NSAIDs can affect the colon and distal small bowel, either by causing a non-specific colitis or by exacerbating a pre-existing disorder such as inflammatory bowel disease or diverticular disease. Colonoscopy may be normal, but abnormalities include inflammation, ulceration, strictures, and the formation of diaphragms. Treatment includes withdrawal or reduction of the offending drug.

12. B. This patient has ischaemic heart disease with recently placed bare metal stents. However, the stent was placed over 1 month ago, and theoretically should no longer require clopidogrel. He has atrial fibrillation, which is a low-risk condition. The polypectomy is a high-risk procedure for bleeding, and therefore the safest approach would be to discuss his case with his cardiologist. Therapeutic procedures can be safely performed in patients on aspirin. However, if the patient required a polypectomy, the clopidogrel would need to be stopped 7 days prior to the polypectomy.

Veitch AM, Baglin TP, Gershlick AH *et al*. Guidelines for the management of anticoagulant and antiplatelet therapy in patients undergoing endoscopic procedures. *Gut* 2008; 57: 1322–1329.

13. E. Endoscopic ultrasound views of the stomach wall appear as five distinct layers. These alternate between hyperechoic (bright) and hypoechoic (dark) layers. From the layer closest to the lumen and therefore the probe they are as follows:

- Interface: bright layer between the probe and the mucosa
- Mucosa (superficial and deep): dark
- Submucosa: bright
- Muscularis propria: dark
- Serosa: bright.

This man had an area of ectopic pancreas or pancreatic rest. These are rare submucosal tumours that consist of endocrine and/or exocrine cells. Pancreatic rest is most often seen in the distal stomach, duodenum, or proximal jejunum. Complications of ectopic pancreas are rare, but can lead to ulceration, gastric outflow obstruction, and (rarely) malignancy. It appears endosonographically as hypoechoic or intermediate echogenic (as in this case) heterogeneous lesions with indistinct borders. The diagnosis is made histologically, and management is guided by symptoms. Asymptomatic lesions can be followed expectantly. Symptomatic lesions can be removed by snare or surgically.

Matsushita M, Hajiro K, Okazaki K *et al*. Gastric aberrant pancreas: EUS analysis in comparison with the histology. *Gastrointestinal Endoscopy* 1999; 49 (4 Pt 1): 493–497.

14. A. This woman has severe acute gallstone pancreatitis. In those patients who have jaundice, cholangitis, or (predicted) severe disease of biliary aetiology, biliary sphincterotomy plus endoscopic stone extraction within 72 hours of presentation is recommended. Percutaneous transhepatic cholangiogram is not indicated, as there is no dilatation of the biliary tree. An elective cholecystectomy should occur 6 weeks after presentation. However, this is not required in the short term. Magnetic resonance cholangiopancreatogram would add little benefit to this woman's management, as a stone has already been seen on the initial imaging.

UK Working Party on Acute Pancreatitis. UK guidelines for the management of acute pancreatitis. *Gut* 2005; 54: 1–9.

15. C. All factors other than raised body mass index (BMI) are known risk factors for post-ERCP pancreatitis.

Complications of endoscopic retrograde cholangiopancreatography (ERCP)

Pancreatitis

- This is generally defined as abdominal pain with an amylase level of three times normal at > 24 hours; it occurs in approximately 5% of cases
- Increased risk is associated with suspected sphincter of Oddi dysfunction (SOD), young age, normal bilirubin, a past history of post-ERCP pancreatitis, difficult or failed cannulation, pancreatic duct injection, pancreatic sphincterotomy, balloon dilation of intact biliary sphincter, and precut sphincterotomy
- Pancreatic stents reduce the risk of post-ERCP pancreatitis, especially if the patient has biliary or pancreatic sphincterotomy for SOD, precut biliary sphincterotomy, difficult cannulation, or endoscopic ampullectomy.

Haemorrhage

- Bleeding is seen at the time of sphincterotomy in 10–30% of cases, but clinically relevant haemorrhage occurs in only 0.5–2%
- Clinical presentation is generally delayed from 1 to 10 days post procedure
- Patients are at increased risk of bleeding if they have a coagulopathy, restart anticoagulation less than 3 days after endoscopic sphincterotomy, have cholangitis prior to ERCP, or have bleeding during sphincterotomy. The risk is also increased in operators with a lower ERCP case volume, precut sphincterotomy, and periampullary diverticulum.

Perforation

- Perforation occurs in less than 1% of cases, and is more common in patients with Billroth II anatomy, sphincterotomy, and suspected SOD.

Cholangitis and cholecystitis

- The occurrence of these conditions is related to failed or incomplete biliary drainage, malignancy, and operator inexperience.

Long-term complications

- Occur in approximately 6–24% of cases
- Recurrent stone formation from sphincterotomy stenosis
- Bacterobilia due to duodenal–biliary reflux
- Recurrent pancreatitis from thermal injury to the pancreatic sphincter after biliary sphincterotomy.

Chapman RW. *Complications of ERCP. BSG Guidelines in gastroenterology.* www.bsg.org.uk/pdf_word_docs/complications.pdf (accessed 6 March 2012).

16. B. The image shows a visible vessel that is oozing blood in the duodenum. The Forrest classification is a grading system that is used to describe bleeding lesions in the upper gastrointestinal tract. It is a useful method of predicting the risk of rebleeding.

The Forrest classification

Forrest classification	Bleeding	Lesion description	Risk of rebleeding (%)	Treatment
Ia	Acute haemorrhage	Spurting haemorrhage	23.6	Dual endoscopic therapy
Ib		Oozing haemorrhage	19.0	Dual endoscopic therapy
IIa	Signs of recent haemorrhage	Visible vessel	19.5	Dual endoscopic therapy
IIb		Adherent clot	17.0	Dual endoscopic therapy
IIc		Haematin on ulcer base	9.7	Medical therapy alone
III	Lesions without active bleeding	Lesions without signs of recent haemorrhage	1.1	Medical therapy alone

Reproduced from Heldwein W et al., 'Is the Forrest classification a useful tool for planning endoscopic therapy of bleeding peptic ulcers?', Endoscopy, 21, 6, pp. 258–262, with permission. doi: 10.1055/s-2007-1010729.

Guglielmi A, Ruzzenente A, Sandri M et al. Risk assessment and prediction of rebleeding in bleeding gastroduodenal ulcer. Endoscopy 2002; 34: 778–786.

Heldwein W, Schreiner J, Pedrazzoli J et al. Is the Forrest classification a useful tool for planning endoscopic therapy of bleeding peptic ulcers? Endoscopy 1989; 21: 258–262.

INDEX

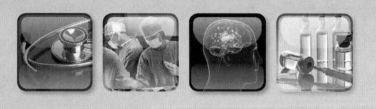
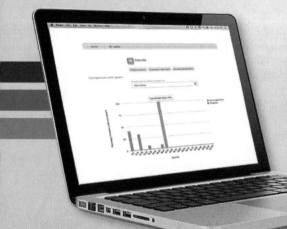